Atherosclerosis and Cardiovascular Diseases

Atherosclerosis and Cardiovascular Diseases

Edited by
S. Lenzi and G.C. Descovich
Istituto di Clinica Medica Generale e Terapia Medica I
dell'Università degli Studi di Bologna

Proceedings of the Sixth International Meeting on
Atherosclerosis and Cardiovascular Diseases held in
Bologna, Italy, October 27-29, 1986

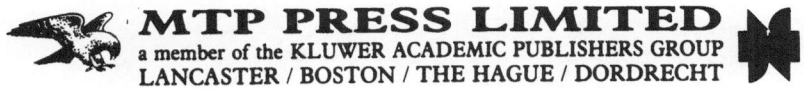

MTP PRESS LIMITED
a member of the KLUWER ACADEMIC PUBLISHERS GROUP
LANCASTER / BOSTON / THE HAGUE / DORDRECHT

Published in the UK and Europe by
MTP Press Limited
Falcon House
Lancaster, England

British Library Cataloguing in Publication Data

International Meeting on Atherosclerosis and
    Cardiovascular Diseases *(6th : 1986 : Bologna)*
    Atherosclerosis and cardiovascular diseases:
    proceedings of the Sixth International Meeting
    on Atherosclerosis and Cardiovascular Diseases
    held in Bologna, October 27-9, 1986.
    1. Coronary heart disease
    I. Title   II. Lenzi, S.   III. Descovich, G.C.
    616.1'23   RC685.C6

    ISBN   978-94-010-7938-9   ISBN   978-94-009-3205-0   (eBook)
    DOI   10.1007/978-94-009-3205-0
Published in the USA by
MTP Press
A division of Kluwer Academic Publishers
101 Philip Drive
Norwell, MA 02061, USA

Library of Congress Cataloging-in-Publication Data

International Meeting on Atherosclerosis and
    Cardiovascular Diseases (6th : 1986 Bologna, Italy)
Atherosclerosis and cardiovascular diseases.

    Includes bibliographies and index.
    1. Atherosclerosis--Congresses. 2. Atherosclerosis--
Etiology--Congresses. 3. Blood lipoproteins--Metabolism--
Disorders--Congresses. I. Lenzi, S. (Sergio) II. Descovich,
G.C. (Giancarlo) III. Title. [DNLM: Arteriosclerosis--
congresses. 2. Atherosclerosis. 3. Cardiovascular Diseases--
congresses. W3 IN756 6th 1986a / WG 550 I607 1986a]

RC692.I476 1986   616.1'36   87-22794

Contents

ACETYLCARNITINE AND AGEING BRAIN SYNDROMES

Preface

1985 and 1986 were milestones for those who study atherosclerosis. In those years took place the USA Consensus Conference, followed first by the Italian Consensus Conference and then by the European one. They marked the final solution to the "querelle" on cholesterol and ischemic cardiopathy. On the basis of the results obtained from the Coronary Primary Prevention Trial (CPPT), plasmatic cholesterol is now no longer considered "a" risk factor in cardiovascular diseases, but "the cause" of atherosclerosis and its organ damages. This was also the basic statement that came out of the 6th International Congress on "Atherosclerosis and Cardiovascular Diseases". The meeting was attended by specialists from various countries representing different experimental approaches to the cardiovascular diseases, from basic research (receptor pathology, apoproteins physiopathology); to epidemiology (both observational study and prevention); to pure cardiology in its aspects of physiopathology, diagnosis and therapy; to the new invasive and non-invasive diagnostic methods; and to the presentation of studies which correlate new variables (serotonin, endogenous opioids) with the atheromasic disease. The final outcome of this research is therapy, be it a pharmacological, nutritional and/or surgical one. Illustrious names from five continents dealt with a wide a range of topics, and their presentations produced a wealth of data. The presentations contained in this volume are the "corpus" of the congress and will serve as a precise updating for all specialists, physicians and students.

Furthermore we wish to underline the expectancy of further progress from the results of primary and secondary prevention programs now in progress both in the USA and in Italy.

It is a great pleasure for us to present this volume containing the result of the co-operation of specialists engaging in further decreasing heart disease observed in some countries and in reversing the dangerously increasing trend to atherosclerosis and its complications still present in most industrialized countries.

Future meetings among experts representing different experimental approaches and operating in different environments, will continue the search for the answer to the still open questions.

Our sincere thanks go the authors for their precious contributions and the publishers MTP Press for their unfailing assistance and expertise in bringing this volume to print.

Sergio Lenzi
Giancarlo Descovich

List of Contributors

G Abate
Istituto Gerontologia e
Geriatria
Università degli Studi
66100 Chieti
Italy

P Avogaro
Divisione Medica II
Ospedali Riuniti
30100 Venezia VE
Italy

ME de Bakey
Department of Surgery
Baylor College of Medicine
Texas Medical Center
Houston, TX 77030
USA

L Barbara
Gastroent. Clinica Med. III
Policlinico S. Orsola
Via Massarenti, 9
40138 Bologna
Italy

P Bernardi
Clinica Medica Generale e
Terapia Medica I
Policlinico S. Orsola
Via Massarenti, 9
40138 Bologna
Italy

S Bertolini
Servizio Prevenzione
Aterosclerosi
ISMI, Ospedale S. Martino
Viale Benedetto XV
16132 Genova GE
Italy

A Beynen
Department of Laboratory
Animal Science
Veterinary Faculty
University of Utrecht
Yalellan 1
3508TD Utrecht
The Netherlands

T Bombardini
Clinica Medica I
Policlinico S. Orsola
Via Massarenti, 9
40138 Bologna
Italy

A Bucci
Istituto Terapia Medica
Systematica
Policlinico Umberto 1°
Viale del Policlinico
00161 Roma
Italy

S Calandra
Istituto di Patologia
Generale
Università di Modena
Via Campi, 287
41100 Modena MO
Italy

A Capurso
Centro di Geriatria e
Prevenzione Aterosclerosi
Clinica Medica II
Piazza Giulio Cesare
70124 Bari
Italy

P Cavallo Perin
Cattedra Patologia Medica B
Ospedale Le Molinette
Corso Polonia, 14
10100 Torino TO
Italy

L Chan
Department of Cell Biology
Baylor College of Medicine
Methodist Hospital
6535 Fannin Street
Houston, TX 77030
USA

G Crepaldi
Cattedra Patologia Med.
Istituto Medicina Clinica
Via Giustiniani, 2
35128 Padova PD
Italy

F Cuccurullo
Patologia Speciale Medica
Ospedale SS. Annunziata
66100 Chieti
Italy

S Coccheri
Servizio di Angiologia
Policlinico S. Orsola
Via Massarenti, 9
40138 Bologna
Italy

M D'Addato
Cattedra Chirurgia
Vascolare
Policlinico S. Orsola
Via Massarenti, 9
40138 Bologna
Italy

GC Descovich
Clinica Medica Generale e
Terapia Medica I
Policlinico S. Orsola
Via Massarenti, 9
40138 Bologna
Italy

JA Dormandy
St James' Hospital
Sarsfeld Road
London SW12 8HW
UK

J Dyerberg
Department of Clinical
Chemistry
Aalborg Hospital
Section North
DK-9000 Aalborg
Denmark

S Eisenberg
Department of Medicine
Hadassah University
Hospital Kyriat Hadassah
PO Box 12000
Jerusalem
Israel

FH Epstein
Lindenstrasse 37
CH-8008 Zürich
Switzerland

C Fieschi
III Cattedra di Clinica
Neurologica
Università degli Studi
Viale dell' Università, 30
00185 Roma
Italy

A Gaddi
Clinical Medica Generale e
Terapia Medica I
Policlinico S. Orsola
Via Massarenti, 9
40138 Bologna
Italy
D Gambi
Clinica Neurologica
Università di Chieti
Via Martiri Lancianesi
66100 Chieti CH
Italy

G Ghiselli
Baylor College of Medicine
Methodist Hospital
6535 Fannin Street
Houston, TX 77030
USA

S Giaquinto
Ospedale San Giovanni
Battista
S.M.O.M.
Via Luigi Dasti, 7
00100 Roma RM
Italy

AM Gotto
Department of Medicine
Baylor College of Medicine
Methodist Hospital
6535 Fannin Street
Houston, TX 77030
USA

SM Grundy
Center for Human Nutrition
5323 Harry Hines Blvd.
The University of Texas
Health Center at Dallas
Dallas, TX 75235
USA

GM Kostner
Institute of Medical
Biochemistry
Department of Protein
Research
University of Graz
Harrachgasse, 21
A 8010 Graz
Austria

PK Kovanen
Wilhuri Research Institute
Kalliolinnantie 4
SF-00140 Helsinki
Finland

D Kritchevsky
The Wistar Institute
36th Street at Spruce
Philadelphia, PA 19104
USA

W Krone
Universitäts-Krankenhaus
Eppendorf
Martinistrasse, 52
D-2000 Hamburg 20
West Germany

L Lalloni
Terapia Medica
Policlinico Umberto 1°
Viale del Policlinico
00161
Roma
Italy

G Lamm
Klinikum der Universität
Heidelberg
Abteilung Klinische
Sozialmedizin
Bergheimer Strasse 58
D-6900 Heidelberg
West Germany

R Laschi
Istituto Microscopia Elettr.
Policlinico S. Orsola
Via Massarenti, 9
40138 Bologna
Italy

GL Lenzi
Clinica Neurologica III
Viale dell' Università 30
00185 Roma
Italy

S Lenzi
Cattedra di Clinica Medica
Generale e Terapia Medica I
Policlinico S. Orsola
Via Massarenti, 9
40138 Bologna
Italy

EF Lüscher
Universitaet Bern
Theodor-Kocher Institut
Postfach 99, Freiestape 1
CH 3000 Bern
Switzerland

M Mancini
Istituto Medicina Interna e
Malattie Dismetaboliche
II Facoltà di Medicina e
Chirurgia
Via Pansini, 5
80131 Napoli
Italy

A Maseri
Cardiovascular Unit
Royal Postgraduate Medical
School
Hammersmith Hospital
Ducane Road
London W12 OHS
UK

A Menotti
Istituto Superiore Sanità
Laboratorio di
Epidemiologia e Biostatistica
Viale Regina Elena, 299
00100 Roma
Italy

U Montaguti
Policlinico S. Orsola
Via Massarenti, 9
40138 Bologna
Italy

M Muggeo
Cattedra Malattie
Metaboliche
Policlinico Borgo Roma
37134 Verona
Italy

G Nappi
Centro Cefalee
Clinica Neurologica
Università
Via Palestro, 3
27100 Pavia
Italy

A Notarbartolo
Cattedra Patologia
Speciale Medica Università
Via Feliciuzza
90127 Palermo
Italy

MF Oliver
Cardiovascular Research
Unit
Hugh Robson Building
George Square
Edinburgh, EH8 9XF
UK

M Onofrj
Clinica Neurologica
Università di Chieti
Via Martiri Lancianesi
66100 Chieti
Italy

P Oriente
Istituto Medicina Interna e
Malattie Dismetaboliche
Nuovo Policlinico
Via Pansini, 5
80131 Napoli
Italy

G Pagano
Cattedra Patologia
Medica C
Ospedale Le Molinette
Corso Polonia, 14
10100 Torino
Italy

A Pagnan
Clinica Medica I
Policlinico Universitario
Via Giustiniani, 2
35100 Padova
Italy

A Palermo
Clinica Medica Generale e
Terapia Medica
Ospedale L Sacco
Via Grassi, 74
20146 Milano
Italy

FM Picchio
Istituto Malattie Apparato
Cardiovascolare
Policlinico S. Orsola
Via Massarenti, 9
40138 Bologna
Italy

A Pierangeli
Clinica Cardiochirurgia
Policlinico S. Orsola
Via Massarenti, 9
40138 Bologna
Italy

P Puddu
Istituto Clinica Medica
Generale e Terapia Medica
Policlinico S. Orsola
Via Massarenti, 9
40138 Bologna
Italy

MT Ramacci
Sigma Tau s.p.a.
Via Pontina Km. 30,400
00040 Pomezia RM
Italy

G Ricci
Istituto Terapia Medica
Sistematica
Policlinico Umberto 1°
00161 Roma RM
Italy

BM Rifkind
National Heart, Lung and
Blood Institute
National Institute of Health
9000 Rockville Pike
Federal 401 Bethesda
USA

WC Roberts
Department of Health and
Human Services
National Institute of Health
Bethesda, MD 20892
USA

F Rovelli
Centro A De Gasperi
Div. Cardiologia
Ospedale Niguarda
Piazza Ospedale Maggiore
20162 Milano
Italy

P Rubba
Clinica Medica
Istituto Medicina Interna e
Malattie Dismetaboliche
II Facoltà di Medicina e
Chirurgia
Via Pansini, 5
80131 Napoli
Italy

GP Salvioli
Istituto Clinico di
Puericultura
Via Massarenti, 11
40138 Bologna
Italy

U Senin
Istituto Gerontologia e
Geriatria
Policlinico Monteluce
06100 Perugia
Italy

C Sirtori
Cattedra di Chemioterapia
Istituto Farmacologia e
Farmacognosia
Via A Del Sarto, 21
20129 Milano
Italy

EB Smith
Department of Chemical
Pathology
University Medical Buildings
Foresterhill
Aberdeen AB9 2ZD
UK

D Sommariva
Institute of Medical
Pathology
University of Milan
Via del Sarto, 21
20100 Milano
Italy

S Spampinato
Istituto Farmacologia
Via Irnerio, 48
40126 Bologna
Italy

G Steiner
Division of Endocrinology
and Metabolism
Toronto General Hospital
Toronto, Ontario
Canada

A Stella
Istituto di Chirurgia
Vascolare
Policlinico S. Orsola
Via Massarenti, 9
40138 Bologna
Italy

J Van Neuten
Janssen Pharmaceutica
Turnhoutseweg, 30
B-2340 Beerse
Belgium

S Ventura
Istituto Clinica Medica
Generale e Terapia Medica
Policlinico Monteluce
06100 Perugia
Italy

G Weber
Istituto Anatomia e Istologia
Patologica
Università degli Studi
Via delle Scotte
53100 Siena
Italy

F Zacà
Clinica Medica Generale e
Terapia Medica I
Policlinico S. Orsola
Via Massarenti, 9
40138 Bologna
Italy

M Zanetti
Servizio Ospedaliero
S. Orsola-Malpighi
Via Massarenti, 9
40138 Bologna
Italy

1
Evaluation of the clinical significance of the discovery of the LDL receptor
S.M. Grundy

Over a decade ago, Goldstein and Brown [1] discovered the cell-surface receptor for low density lipoprotein (LDL). Since this discovery, these investigators and their co-workers have defined the structure, origins, and functions of the LDL receptor in great detail. For this work, Goldstein and Brown were awarded the Nobel Prize in Medicine in 1985. This prize was awarded both for the high quality of their work and for the potential significance of their findings for the control of high blood cholesterol and hence for the prevention of coronary heart disease. This paper will attempt to evaluate the potential clinical significance of the discovery of the LDL receptor.

NORMAL REGULATION OF LDL LEVELS:ROLE OF LDL RECEPTORS

LDL receptors are located on the surface of cells in many tissues, and thus these tissues have the potential for removal of LDL. However, it is further apparent that LDL can be removed from the circulation by other mechanisms which have been collectively called the non-receptor pathway [1]. The cellular events responsible for this non-receptor pathway have not been fully determined, but nonspecific or bulk phase pinocytosis probably is involved. One view of the significance of the LDL receptor is that its activity is the major factor controlling the level of LDL. However, over opinions have been expressed. For example, some have suggested that the non-receptor pathway is the major mechanism for removal of LDL in humans, and the receptor pathway is relatively minor. Another view is that the production of LDL is the major factor controlling concentrations of LDL, and the LDL receptors "passively" accept the LDL that has entered the circulation. Both of the alternative hypotheses for the control of LDL levels will be considered in this discussion.
Perhaps the strongest evidence that the activity of LDL receptors is the major factor regulating LDL levels is found in the disorder called familial hypercholesterolemia (FH). In this condition, the gene encoding for LDL receptors is defective. Normally, one gene for the LDL receptor is inherited from each parent. However, one in 500 people inherit one defective gene for

1

the LDL receptor, and consequently, the affected person has half the normal number of functioning receptors. Further, the LDL cholesterol level is essentially twice normal. Much more rarely, about one in a million, a person will inherit two abnormal genes for the LDL receptor, and the LDL-cholesterol concentration is at least four times normal. The fact that individuals of this kind, called FH homozygotes, achieve a steady state in LDL levels indicate that there are alternative routes of removal of circulating LDL, but their extremely high levels of LDL-cholesterol also attest to the importance of LDL receptors for keeping LDL levels in the normal range. If LDL receptors are lesser importance for regulating LDL levels in the circulation, patients with homozygous FH should not have such high concentrations of LDL. Thus, from the marked hypercholesterolemia noted in patients with FH, it would appear that LDL receptors are potentially very important in controlling concentrations of LDL in humans.

What then led to the concept that non-receptor pathways are more important than the receptor pathway in controlling levels of LDL? It arose in part from the concept that under physiological conditions the LDL receptors normally should be saturated with ambient concentrations of plasma LDL and thus most LDL would have to be removed by non-receptor pathways. Further, a technique was introduced to determine the relative rates of removal of LDL via receptor and non-receptor pathway in humans. This technique involved forming a derivative of the LDL apoprotein (apolipoprotein B or apo B) that would block receptor-binding by LDL. One derivative was formed with cyclohexandione [2]; this agent blocks the arginine groups of apo B which interfere with receptor binding in tissue culture. This technique allows for the simultaneous injection of radiolabeled LDL and cyclohexandione-LDL, radiolabeled differentially, and the difference in their rates of decay should reflect uptake by non-receptors pathways (by the latter) and non-receptor + receptor pathways (by the former). Initial studies in normal humans suggested that about two-thirds of circulation LDL is removed by non-receptor pathways, while only a third is cleared by non-receptor pathways. This finding might suggest that LDL receptors provide the lesser pathway for clearance of LDL. However, further studies using this general approach have provided a different result. When LDL is extensively glucosylated, to block lysine residues, the fraction of LDL removed by the non-receptor pathway appears to be less, usually about one-third or one-fourth of the total clearance [3]. Seemingly, the cyclohexandione method did not completely obliterate receptor-mediated uptake of LDL, while extensive glycosylation does. In summary, therefore, by completely blocking receptor mediated clearance of LDL, it now appears that the non-receptor pathway is the lesser of the two pathways.

Another concept that might lessen the importance of the LDL receptor is that production rates of LDL are the dominate factor regulating LDL levels. For example, Kesaniemi and Grundy [4] reported that production rates of LDL were more important in determining concentrations of LDL over a broad range of LDL levels than fractional catabolic rates FCRs of LDL. Subsequently, other investigators have affirmed the importance of production rates for regulating LDL-cholesterol concentrations [5]. An early view regarding the significance of these two parameters of LDL metabolism was that fractional catabolic rates (FCRs) of LDL are a reflection of removal processes, notably LDL receptor activity, while production rates of LDL reflect rates of synthesis (or input) of lipoproteins into plasma. If this concept is valid, then the finding that production rates of LDL are the major determinant of LDL levels would mean that the de novo synthesis of lipoproteins is the major factor controlling LDL concentrations.

Actually, isotope kinetic studies have suggested that there were two sources of LDL, namely, the catabolism of very low density lipoproteins (VLDL) and "direct" synthesis of LDL by the liver. The possibility of direct synthesis of LDL was suggested by the observation that in isotope kinetic studies the quantities of LDL formed from VLDL cannot account for the total production of LDL [6]. For instance, in patients with homozygous FH, production rates for LDL are extremely high, and most of this excess production of LDL appears to be derived from "direct" synthesis. If so, an abnormality in activity of LDL receptors in FH patients might stimulate the synthesis of excess apo B, which could cause an abnormally high secretion of LDL by the liver.

The importance of production of LDL in regulating the input of LDL is further suggested by the analysis of LDL kinetics by Meddings and Dietschy [7]. These investigators suggest that rates of production of LDL determine FCRs of LDL by the process of saturation of LDL receptors. In other words, high input rates of LDL should "saturate" LDL receptors and thereby reduce FCRs for LDL. Thus, not only is the production of LDL the determining factor for regulating LDL concentrations, but FCRs of LDL may not be a good reflection of activity of LDL receptors, as originally thought.

In spite of these interpretations, questions can be raised about their validity, and consequently, the activity of LDL receptors may be much more important in regulating concentrations of LDL than they would suggest. For example, there is growing evidence that LDL receptor activity affects production rates of LDL. This is because LDL receptors can remove the precursors of LDL as well as LDL itself. The major precursors of LDL are remnants of VLDL. The liver secretes triglyceride-rich VLDL, and the triglycerides of these lipoproteins are hydrolyzed in the peripheral circulation by lipoprotein lipase. The particles remaining after lipolysis of triglycerides is almost complete are called VLDL remnants. These remnants can have two fates. They can be removed directly by the liver, or they can be converted to LDL [8]. Hepatic uptake of VLDL remnants by the liver appears to be mediated mainly by LDL receptors. Not only can these receptors recognize the apo B contained on remnants, but LDL receptors also bind to the apolipoprotein E (apo E) present on VLDL remnants. Thus, VLDL remnants actually are better ligands for LDL receptor than LDL itself.

If the activity of LDL receptors is reduced, then uptake of VLDL remnants will be retarded as well as that of LDL. The result will be an increased conversion of VLDL to LDL, or overproduction of LDL. Thus, the overproduction of LDL in patients with FH probably can be explained by a reduced number of LDL receptors, decreased uptake of VLDL remnants, and enhanced conversion of VLDL remnants to LDL. This mechanism complicates the analysis of Meddings and Dietschy [7] who have viewed the production and clearance of LDL as independent processes. In other words, not only can LDL particles compete among themselves for LDL receptors but the same can occur for VLDL remnants. Consequently, increased removal of VLDL remnants should reduce the production of LDL and at the same time reduce FCRs of LDL; this is because of competition between LDL and VLDL remnants for receptors. In other words, production rates for LDL and FCRs for LDL can no longer be considered to be reflections of hepatic secretion rates of apo B-containing lipoproteins and LDL receptor activity, respectively, but the two parameters both are intimately connected to receptor activity in a complicated fashion.

Another concept that has come under question is the liver secretes LDL directly. In normal laboratory animals, hepatic secretion of LDL-sized lipoprotein has not been identified, even though cholesterol-fed animals may produce such particles. We recently suggested that isotope kinetic studies in humans suggesting direct secretion of LDL may be an artifact of the methodology [9]. We postulated the existence of a pool of LDL in plasma that has a very rapid turnover rate, and while most of the lipoprotein in this pool is rapidly cleared by the liver, a small fraction of it may be converted to LDL. The presence of such a pool in humans is suggested by investigations on turnover rates of subfractions of VLDL carried out by two groups [10,11]. A very rapid pool of VLDL would not be traced by conventional isotope kinetic methods, and these latter methods could erroneously suggest that the liver directly secretes lipoproteins into plasma. If a portion of VLDL passes through this very rapid pathway and the major fraction of it is cleared by the liver, the activity of LDL receptors could significantly affect the metabolic fate of VLDL in this compartment. In other words, a reduced activity of LDL receptor would enhance the quantity of LDL that apparently is synthetized directly.

In summary, several lines of evidence suggest that LDL receptors are crucially important in the regulation of LDL concentrations. The strongest evidence comes from patients with FH who have a specific defect in the gene encoding for LDL receptors. However, improved methodology has indicated that the non-receptor pathway is quantitatively of lesser significance than suggested by early studies. Further, while the production of LDL undoubtedly is a major determinant of LDL concentrations, recent investigations suggest that the activity of LDL receptors can have a major influence on the rate of input of LDL by affecting catabolism of VLDL remnants, the precursors of LDL. Finally, the concept of direct synthesis of LDL has been brought into doubt, which lessens the potential importance of de novo production of lipoproteins in regulating LDL concentrations.

RISE OF LDL LEVELS WITH AGE: ROLE OF LDL RECEPTORS

A well-documented phenomenon in many societies is a rise of LDL concentrations with age. The mechanisms responsible for this rise have not been elucidated. In a recent report, Miller [12] pooled all existing data from many different turnover studies and concluded that the FCRs for LDL decline with age; he interpreted this finding to mean that the activity of LDL likewise declined with age. We subsequently examined LDL kinetics in a group of young men and middle-aged men to examine the same question [13]. The younger men had significantly lower concentrations of LDL on the average than the older men, clearly indicating a rise of LDL levels with age. Our isotope kinetic data indicated that the older men had both higher production rates of LDL and lower FCRs for LDL. This finding could mean that the activity of LDL receptors had declined with age. The higher production rates might be explained by decreased uptake of VLDL remnants with a greater conversion of VLDL to LDL, while the reduced FCRs for LDL could be the result of a lesser number of LDL receptors available for uptake of LDL.

Although this interpretation may be correct, it is possible that a true overproduction of lipoproteins containing apo B may have contributed to the higher LDL levels in the older group. The older men were somewhat more obese, and it has been shown that obesity raises the production of VLDL as well as LDL [14]. Thus, the role of synthetic rates of lipoproteins in the rise of LDL concentrations with age has not been determined with certainty, and production rates of VLDL, and not inherent activity of LDL receptors, could be the major determinant of the rise of LDL levels with age. Increasing body weight is a well documented factor with aging, while no mechanisms responsible for a natural decline in activity of LDL receptors with age have been discovered.

INFLUENCE OF DIET ON LDL CONCENTRATIONS: ROLE OF LDL RECEPTORS

One of the dietary factors that raises the LDL level is dietary cholesterol. This effect is seen most dramatically in experimental animals, but it also is evident in humans in carefully-controlled studies carried out in the metabolic ward. The mechanism of increase in LDL-cholesterol associated with high intakes of cholesterol probably is mediated by a decrease in activity of LDL receptors. Goldstein and Brown [15] have shown that the synthesis of LDL receptors is under feedback control by amounts of cholesterol in cells. When the concentration of cholesterol within cells increase, this excess cholesterol suppresses the promoter for the gene for the LDL receptor, and the activity of the gene is reduced. Therefore, the number of receptors synthesized is decreased. In converse, when concentrations of cholesterol in cells fall, the number of receptors synthesized by cells increases. When the intake of cholesterol in the diet is high, the quantity of cholesterol reaching the liver is enhanced, and this excess cholesterol apparently inhibits the synthesis of LDL receptors; consequently, the level of plasma LDL increases.

One study by Packard et al [16] showed that feeding cholesterol causes an increase in the production of LDL and a decrease in FCRs for LDL. However, as discussed earlier, this dual effect could be mediated entirely by a decrease in number of LDL receptors on liver cells. First, the increased production of LDL could be due to an inhibition of clearance of VLDL remnants, the precursors of LDL, and the reduced FCRs for LDL could be the result of reduced clearance of LDL by receptors. The extent to which dietary cholesterol contributes to a rise in plasma cholesterol levels thus is largely a function of the degree of suppression of the synthesis of LDL receptors by this excess cholesterol. Certainly, there are compensatory mechanisms (e.g. suppression of cholesterol synthesis, reexcretion of cholesterol into bile, and enhanced conversion of cholesterol into bile acids) to minimize the effects of dietary cholesterol on LDL receptor activity, but nonetheless, there usually is a finite increase in LDL levels as a result of increasing the quantity of cholesterol in the diet [17].

Another dietary factor that raises the plasma cholesterol is saturated fatty acids. The saturated acids are of several carbon chain lengths, and of these, palmitic, myristic, and palmitic acids appear to be the most hypercholesterolemic [18]. The major effect of dietary saturated fatty acids is to raise the plasma level of LDL-cholesterol. Although the precise mechanisms by which saturated fatty acids raise the cholesterol levels are not known, available evidence from studies in laboratory animals suggest that they decrease the removal of LDL though receptor-mediated pathways [19]. Studies of LDL kinetics in humans are compatible with this mechanism. Thus, it appears that both dietary cholesterol and saturated fatty acids increase the plasma LDL level by suppressing the activity of LDL receptors.

Another category of fatty acids, the polyunsaturated fatty acids, have been reported to lower plasma total cholesterol and LDL-cholesterol levels. The exact mechanism for this cholesterol lowering effect has not been determined, and a variety of theories have been set forth. However, recent evidence suggests that polyunsaturated fatty acids, of which linoleic acid is the major form, do not have an inherent LDL-lowering action, but instead, reduce LDL levels by replacing saturated fatty acids. In other words, when polyunsaturated fatty acids are substituted for saturated fatty acids, they allow for a return of the natural activity of LDL receptors that had been suppressed by saturated fatty acids.

This concept can be extended to other fatty acids. For example, we recently showed that substitution of monounsaturated fatty acids (oleic acid) for saturated fatty acids will produce the same degree of lowering of LDL-cholesterol as substituting linoleic acid [20]. The action of oleic acid to lower the LDL level likewise appears to be to remove the LDL-receptor suppressing activity of saturated fatty acids. As a result of these studies we have suggested that monounsaturated fatty acids are just as effective as substitutes for saturated fatty acids in the diet as polyunsaturates [20]. Indeed, the monounsaturates may have certain advantages. For instance, they do not reduce the HDL concentration as do polyunsaturates. Further, in laboratory animals, polyunsaturates tend to suppress the immune system and predispose animals to development of chemically-induced cancer [21]. Finally, no large population has ever consumed large quantities of polyunsaturates for long periods with proven safety. In contrast, monounsaturates have been consumed in large amounts in the form of olive oil in the Mediterranean region for centuries without evidence of adverse effects; further, in this region, levels of plasma cholesterol are relatively low as are rates of coronary heart disease [22]. Therefore, in our opinion, monounsaturates have previously been underrated as a potential replacement for saturated fatty acids in the diet.

Yet another way to remove saturated fatty acids from the diet is to eat a low-fat diet. In this way, saturated fatty acids can be replaced by carbohydrates. Our studies have revealed that low-fat, high-carbohydrate diets are just as effective as those high in monounsaturated fatty acids for lowering LDL levels [23]. These diets have the advantage of having been proven to be associated with low rates of coronary heart disease in many societies throughout the world, especially in Asia. A further advantage of low-fat diets is that they may help to prevent the development of obesity. Finally, epidemiology studies raise the possibility that low-fat diets may reduce the risk for certain cancers, i.e., colon cancer and breast cancer, which are common in populations that consume high fat diets.

In summary, diets high in cholesterol and saturated fatty acids seemingly suppress the activity of LDL receptors and thereby raise the plasma cholesterol. Such diets may contribute significantly to development of coronary heart disease in several societies, particularly those of the Western culture. Thus, a decreased activity of LDL cholesterol, secondary to diet may be one of the major causes of coronary heart disease. Decreasing intakes of cholesterol and replacement of saturated fatty acids with polyunsaturates, monounsaturates, and carbohydrates should reverse the "mass" hypercholesterolemia that is such an important factor in causation of coronary heart disease.

DRUG TREATMENT OF HYPERCHOLESTEROLEMIA BY MODIFICATION OF LDL RECEPTOR ACTIVITY

Since the hepatic synthesis of LDL receptors is under feedback regulation by amounts of cholesterol in liver cells, it should be possible to increase the synthesis of LDL receptors by reducing the cholesterol content of the liver. This in fact can be accomplished in several ways using drugs. Three major pathways can be altered to reduce hepatic content of cholesterol. These are (a) the conversion of cholesterol into bile acids, (b) the absorption of cholesterol, and (c) the synthesis of cholesterol. Drugs that affect these three major pathways will be discussed.

First, the bile acid sequestrants (cholestyramine and colestipol) enhance the conversion of cholesterol into bile acids. This is accomplished by binding of bile acids in the intestine, which reduces return of bile acids to the liver and thereby releases the inhibition of bile acids on their own synthesis. The resultant increase in synthesis of bile acids lowers hepatic contents of cholesterol and stimulates the synthesis of LDL receptors. This causes a fall in LDL levels, although the degree of fall is mitigated by a compensatory increase in synthesis of cholesterol. The potential for bile acid sequestrants for treatment of hypercholesterolemia is illustrated in the Lipid Research Clinic's Coronary Primary Prevention Trial [24,25]. This trial demonstrated that the lowering of LDL by cholestyramine will reduce rates of coronary heart disease.

Second, absorption of cholesterol can be inhibited by either neomycin or plant sterols. Both agents will reduce concentrations of LDL. The mechanism of action presumably is by inhibiting return of intestinal cholesterol to the liver and thus reducing hepatic content of cholesterol; this should increase the synthesis of LDL receptors and in this way lower plasma LDL levels. At present, none of agents available for inhibiting absorption of cholesterol have proven to be practical therapeutic drugs, but this approach to lowering LDL levels should hold considerable promise if effective and safe drugs can be identified that will inhibit the absorption of cholesterol.

Third, hepatic cholesterol concentrations can be reduced by inhibiting the synthesis of cholesterol. A new class of drugs have been identified that have this action. The drugs competitively inhibit the activity of 3-hydroxy-3-methylglutaryl coenzyme A (MHG Co A) reductase, the rate limiting enzyme in the synthesis of cholesterol [26]. One drug of this class, lovastatin (mevinolin) has proven to be highly effective in lowering LDL concentrations [27,28]. Studies from our laboratory [27] provide strong evidence that lovastatin promotes LDL-receptor mediated clearance of LDL and VLDL remnants. This drug, which is effective in relatively small doses and apparently is safe, can produce reductions in LDL concentrations ranging from 30 to 40%. Many investigators believe that HMG Co A reductase inhibitors will eventually replace other agents for lowering LDL levels for the majority of patients with hypercholesterolemia. They demonstrate the power of reducing LDL levels by enhancing the activity of LDL receptors.

Finally, it has been shown that the combination of HMG CoA reductase inhibitors and bile acid sequestrants can induce a very marked reduction of LDL levels [29,30]. This combination should doubly lower hepatic concentrations of cholesterol, because the former will reduce the formation of cholesterol while the latter will promote the transformation of cholesterol into bile acids. We have demonstrated that this combination will induce a 50 to 60% reduction in LDL-cholesterol concentrations in patients with hypercholesterolemia.

8

SUMMARY

This review attempts to demonstrate the great clinical importance of the discovery of the LDL receptor. It points out that the activity of LDL receptors is critical in regulation of LDL levels for most people. Further, it indicates that dietary factors affect LDL-receptor activity, and high intakes of cholesterol and saturated fatty acids, which suppress the activity of LDL receptors, probably account for most of the "mass hypercholesterolemia" that afflicts high-risk societies. It points out that replacement of saturated fatty acids in the diet with other nutrients--polyunsaturated fatty acids, monounsaturated fatty acids, and carbohydrates--will allow for a return of activity of LDL receptors to normal. Consequently, there is great potential for prevention of coronary heart disease through dietary enhancement of activity of LDL receptors. Finally, for individuals who are hypercholesterolemic for genetic reasons, the activity of LDL receptors can be enhanced by drugs that promote the conversion of cholesterol into bile acids, that inhibit the reabsorption of cholesterol, or interfere with the formation of cholesterol. Of these mechanisms, drugs that retard the synthesis of cholesterol appear to hold the greatest promise for dramatic lowering of LDL-cholesterol and thus for greatly reducing the risk for coronary heart disease in patients with genetic forms of hypercholesterolemia.

REFERENCES

1.   Goldstein, JL and Brown, MS (1982). The LDL receptor defect in familial hypercholesterolemia: Implications for pathogenesis and therapy. Med Clin North Amer, 66, 335.
2.   Shepherd, J, Bicker, S, Lorimer, AR, and Packard, CJ (1979). Receptor-mediated low density lipoprotein catabolism in man. J Lipid Res, 20, 999.
3.   Kesaniemi, YA, Witztum, JL and Steinbrecher, UP (1983). Receptor-mediated catabolism of low density lipoprotein in man: Quantitation using glucosylated low density lipoproteins. J Clin Invest, 71, 950.
4.   Kesaniemi, YA and Grundy, SM (1982). Significance of low density lipoprotein production in the regulation of plasma cholesterol level in man. J Clin Invest, 70, 13.
5.   Turner, PR, Revil, J, Ville, AL, Cortese, C, Konarska R, Masana, L, Jackson, P, Swan, AV and Lewis, B (1984). Metabolic study of variation in plasma cholesterol level in normal men. Lancet, 2, 663.
6.   Soutar, AK, Myant and NB, Thompson, GR (1977). Simultaneous measurement of apolipoprotein B turnover in very-low and low-density lipoproteins in familial hypercholesterolemia. Atherosclerosis, 28, 247.
7.   Meddings, JB and Dietschy, JM (1986). Regulation of plasma levels of low-density lipoprotein cholesterol: Interpretation of data on low-density lipoprotein turnover in man. Circulation, 74, 805.
8.   Brown, MS and Goldstein, JL (1983). Lipoprotein receptors in the liver: Control signals for plasma cholesterol traffic. J Clin Invest, 72, 743.
9.   Beltz, WF, Kesaniemi, YA, Howard, BV and Grundy, SM (1985). Development of an integrated model for analysis of kinetics of apolipoprotein B in plasma very low density lipoproteins, intermediate density, lipoproteins, and low density lipoprotein. J Clin Invest, 76, 575.
10. Packard, CJ, Munro, A, Lorimer, AR, Gotto, AM and Shepherd J (1984). Metabolism of apolipoprotein B in large triglyceride-rich very low density lipoproteins of normal and hypertriglyceridemic subjects. J Clin Invest, 74, 2178.
11. Stalenhof, AFH, Malloy, MJ, Kane, JP and Havel, RJ (1984). Metabolism of apolipoproteins B-48 and B-100 of triglyceride-rich lipoproteins in normal and lipoprotein lipase-deficient humans. Proc Natl Acad Sci, 81, 1839.
12. Miller, NE (1984). Why does plasma low density lipoprotein concentrations in adults increase with age? Lancet, 1, 263.
13. Grundy SM, Vega, GL and Bilheimer DW (1985). Kinetic mechanisms determining variability in low density lipoprotein levels and their rise with age. Arteriosclerosis, 5, 623.
14. Egusa, G, Beltz, WF, Grundy, SM and Howard, BV (1985). The influence of obesity on the metabolism of apolipoprotein B in man. J Clin Invest, 76, 596.

15. Goldstein JL and Brown MS (1977). The low density lipoprotein pathway and its relation to atherosclerosis. Annu Rev Biochem, 46, 897.
16. Packard, CJ, McKinney, L, Carr, K and Shepherd, J (1983). Cholesterol feeding increases low density lipoprotein synthesis. J Clin Invest, 72, 45.
17. Hegsted, PM (1986). Serum-cholesterol response to dietary cholesterol: a re-evaluation. Am J Clin Nutr, 44, 299.
18. Keys, A, Anderson, JT and Grande, F (1965). Serum cholesterol responses to changes in diet. IV. Particular saturated fatty acids in the diet. Metabolism, 14, 776.
19. Spady, DK and Dietschy, J (1985). Dietary saturated triglycerides suppress hepatic low density lipoprotein receptors in the hamster. Proc Natl Acad Sci, 82, 4526.
20. Mattson, FH and Grundy SM (1985). Comparison of dietary saturated, monounsaturated, and polyunsaturated fatty acids on plasma lipids and lipoproteins in man. J Lipid Res, 26, 194.
21. Bennett, M, Uauy, R and Grundy, SM (1987). Dietary fatty acid effects on T cell-mediated immunity in mice infected with Mycoplasma pulmonis or injected with carcinogens. Am J Pathol 126, 103.
22. Keys, A (ed) Coronary heart disease in seven countries (1970). Circulation, 41, I-1.
23. Grundy, SM (1986). Comparison of monounsaturated fatty acids and carbohydrates for plasma cholesterol lowering. N Engl J Med, 314, 745.
24. Lipid Research Clinics Program (1984). The Lipid Research Clinics Coronary Primary Prevention Trial Results. I. Reduction in incidence of coronary heart disease. JAMA, 251, 351.
25. Lipid Research Clinics Program (1984). The Lipid Research Clinics Primary Prevention Trial Results. II. The relationship of reduction in incidence of coronary heart disease to cholesterol lowering. JAMA, 251, 365.
26. Endo, A, Kurodo, M and Tsujita, G (1976). ML-236A, ML-236B, and ML-236C, new inhibitors of cholesterol-genesis produced by Penicillum citrinum. J Antibiot, 29, 1346.
27. Bilheimer, DW, Grundy, SM, Brown, MS and Goldstein, JL (1983). Mevinolin and colestipol stimulate receptor-mediated clearance of low density lipoprotein from plasma in familial hypercholesterolemia heterozygotes.
28. Illingworth, DR and Sexton, GJ (1984). Hypocholesterolemic effects of mevinolin in patients with heterozygous familial hypercholesterolemia. J Clin Invest, 74, 1972.
29. Grundy, SM, Vega, GL and Bilheimer, DW (1985). Influence of combined therapy with mevinolin and interruption of bile-acid reabsorption in low density lipoproteins in heterozygous familial hypercholesterolemia. Ann Int Med, 103, 339.
30. Vega, GL and Grundy, SM (1987). Treatment of primary moderate hypercholesterolemia with mevinolin and colestipol. JAMA, 257, 33.

2
Social aspects of atherosclerosis
M. Zanetti and U. Montaguti

If one is to follow the evidence produced by authorities
such as Oliver (1) on the one hand and Winkelstein and
Marmot (2) on the other it certainly cannot be argued that
the measures taken so far to prevent atherosclerosis and its
most common complication (coronary heart disease, CHD) have
been truly effective. The scarce results of the Multiple
Risk Factor Intervention Trial have not made it possible to
say whether the decrease in mortality due to CHD is
attributable to reductions in the three classic risk factors
(smoking, hypertension and hypercholesterolemia) or whether
this decrease is due to the general trend towards a
reduction in CHD which is manifest in the USA and many
European countries and which in turn is due to a combination
of social and environmental factors not yet clearly defined
(2).
In the "North Karelia Project" (3), for example, there was
no significant decrease in CHD morbidity despite a
substantial reduction in the target risk factors.

Similar results have been reported from other major projects
to control atherosclerosis biological risk factors (4).

This does not mean of course that we should abandon attempts
to control smoking, hypertension and hypercholesterolemia.
The evidence regarding their role in CHD is far too
consistent to warrant any doubts in this connection.
Rather we should ask ourselves whether the inability of
preventive measures to meet expectations is not in fact a
direct result of a limited conception of the problem which
has led to there being few attempts at integrated control of
the biological and social risk factors. All or nearly all of
the resources in this field have been tied up with the three

classic risk factors which are however strongly conditioned by two things:

- the presence of risk factors can "only" explain 50 - 60% of CHD cases (5),
- these factors correspond to a "biomedical" model of illness (6, 7), that is, a model which excludes any defect in the formula "organic morbose state/organic cause/cure by medical intervention".

Or in other words an approach to the problem of atherosclerosis which treats the biological risk factors at the level of the individual without taking into account social causes influencing behaviour and the probability of exposition to these factors in society; an approach which does not see the illness holistically and thus makes it difficult to treat the condition satisfactorily especially from the point of view of preventive medicine.

The behaviour of the organism and the social situation (understood as a system of relationships between the organisms present and interacting in a particular environment) cannot be excluded as variables in the equation regarding the probable contact between organisms and pathogenic factors.

Stallones expressed this concept succinctly when he stated that the distribution of a morbose process in a community is a social phenomena and one should therefore expect it to reflect social factors (9).

If we are to shift the emphasis from the biological causes of atherosclerosis to its social causes then it is necessary to examine the pathogenetic link between illness and society.

Stress is widely indicated as the pathogenetic link between atherosclerosis and society.

There are still broad, undefined areas and the passage from the "social situation" (varied and difficult to define in terms of its single components) to the "stressing element" often requires oversimplification. Despite this however it is possible, on the basis of the results of experiments conducted mainly with animals (10 - 12), to hypothesise the following process (13):

1) Some of the important precursors (anatomic and physiological) of clinical atherosclerosis (essential hypertension, coronary spasms, ventricular extrasistole, the formation of atheroma) have a (functional) relationship with substantial neurohormonal imbalances.

2) Neurohormonal imbalances can be produced by, among other things, a sinergic activation of the sympatho-adrenergic (with augmented incretion of cathecolamyne) and the hypophysis-cortico-adrenergic system (with an increase in serum corticosteroids).

3) Obviously situations which the nervous system identifies as a threat to the organism and which have defence or preservatory reflexes are those which require a homeostatic mechanism (14, 15). In fact in Cannon's opinion (16) good health is not the absence of illness but rather the ability of the human organism to function in a given environment; that is, to maintain homeostasis. Climate, micro-organisms, chemical pollutants, the psychological pressures of everyday life arising from relationships with other human beings all modify the environment in which the human organism lives. It cannot be argued however that every homeostatic act is a source of stress since the capacity of a situation to induce the hormonal imbalances

previously referred to, depends on the individual's perception of the stressor and his/her perception of its significance rather than on objective indicators of the situation's capacity to cause stress.

4) Defensive and preservatory responses are triggered by experiences or fears threatening emotive and social bonds and relationships on the one hand and threats to physical and social preservation on the other.

The threatening element is the "stressor", the situation in which it occurs is "stressful" and the psycho-physiological state induced is "stress".

For Schwab and Pritchard (17) the duration and the type of stimulus are important.

Looked at from the point of view of duration there are three classes of stressful situation:

- short term (from a few seconds to several hours)
- moderate (days or weeks)
- severe (weeks, months and years).

Examples of stressors causing short term stress are an annoying insect, a slamming door, a public appearance in front of an audience, in other words those light and habitual daily commitments that probably do not trigger pathological processes.

Stressors which cause moderate stress are, for example, overwork, the temporary absence of a loved one and those minor psychological disturbances generated during social interaction.

Examples of severe stress are the death of a loved one, serious economic problems, the protraction of a socially intolerable situation, illness.

To remain within the subject matter chosen for this paper we may mention the scale drawn up by Holmes and Rahe (18) which has often been used to identify the correlations between cardio-vascular pathologies and unpleasant events during life (Table 1).

It should however be emphasised that the link betweeen stress and atherosclerosis seems to be more complex than that mediated by a simple neurohormonal response. In fact, Friedman et al (19) have shown that the cholesterolemia of bank workers with a moderate work load increased significantly during periods when the work load increased because the annual returns were being prepared. There are also studies (20 - 22) showing considerable increases in the cholesterolemia of medical students at exam time this period also being accompanied by small changes in eating habits.

What then is the evidence currently available firmly supporting the hypothesis of a correlation between social factors and atherosclerosis?

In replying to this question it should first be pointed out that there have been various attempts to draw up classifications of social factors in order to identify those characteristics useful at the operational level. Among these attempts there are three which in our opinion warrant attention; the study by Graham and Reeder, that by Badura and that by Lisa Berkman.

TABLE   1.   Life   Events   and   Weighted   Values   (adapted   from
                T. H. Holmes and R.H. Rahe,"The Social Readjustment
                Rating Scale",   1967).

Life Event	Value	Life Event	Value
Death of spouse	100	Son or daughter leaving home	29
Divorce	73	Trouble with in-laws	29
Marital separation	65	Outstanding personal	
Jail Term	63	achievement	28
Death of close family member	63	Wife beginning or topping	
Personal injury or illness	53	work	26
Marriage	50	Beginning or ending school	26
Fired at work	47	Revision of habits	24
Marital reconciliation	45	Trouble with boss	23
Retirement	45	Change in works hours	20
Change in healt of family	44	Change in residence	20
Pregancy	40	Change in schools	20
Sex difficulties	39	Change in recreation	19
Gain of new family member	39	Change in social activity	18
Change in financial state	38	Change in sleeping habits	16
Death of close friend	37	Change in number of family	
Change of work	36	get-togethers	15
Change in number of		Change in eating habits	15
arguments with spouse	35	Vacation	13
Foreclusure of mortgage	30	Minor violations of law	11
Change of responsability			
at work	29		

Graham and Reeder (8), viewing social relations in terms of the individual, identified four general categories as follows:

- family characteristics
- socio-economic status
- ethnic and religious group membership
- socio-cultural and psycho-social processes such as:
  . cultural changes
  . mobility and migration
  . personal status incongruence
  . events and changes during life

Badura (23), taking into account only that which is expressed dynamically in the social environment, argued that there are three types of stress factor:

a) unpleasant events during life and experiences involving the loss of relationships:
   . serious illness
   . unemployment
   . loss of a loved one

b) chronic tensions involved in various social roles:
   . excessive work load
   . interpersonal conflicts (with colleagues or superiours)
   . chronic problems with spouse or family
   . frustrated career expectations

c) psycho-social transitions during life:
   . from infancy to school
   . from school to work
   . from work to retirement

Lisa Berkman (24), in emphasising the pre-eminence of personal relationships, maintained that the correlation between social environment and disease could be explained on the basis of three categories:

- factors apertaining to social class
- factors relating to socio-cultural change
- factors relating to the network of social relations.

Each of the above authors has applied, to a greater or lesser degree, their classification scheme to the problem of CHD. In this paper we will limit ourselves to the classification put forward by Berkman.

Social Class

Some authors have maintained that the most striking weakness in the traditional epidemiological studies of the role of social factors in the aetiology of an illness has been the oversimplification of the social variables (25, 26). This seems to be particularly true when examining membership of a particular social class which presupposes certain levels of education and wealth, type of work, life-style etc., all characteristics which it might otherwise be convenient to describe separately.

Social class is however an important indicator of risk despite the approximate nature of the information which it circumscribes. In the cases of both general mortality and CHD mortality (27) the finding is: the lower the social class, the higher the probability of death.

The classic study of British civil servants by Marmot et al (28) found a strong inverse correlation between employment grade and CHD mortality rate not influenced by classic risk factors (Figure 1).

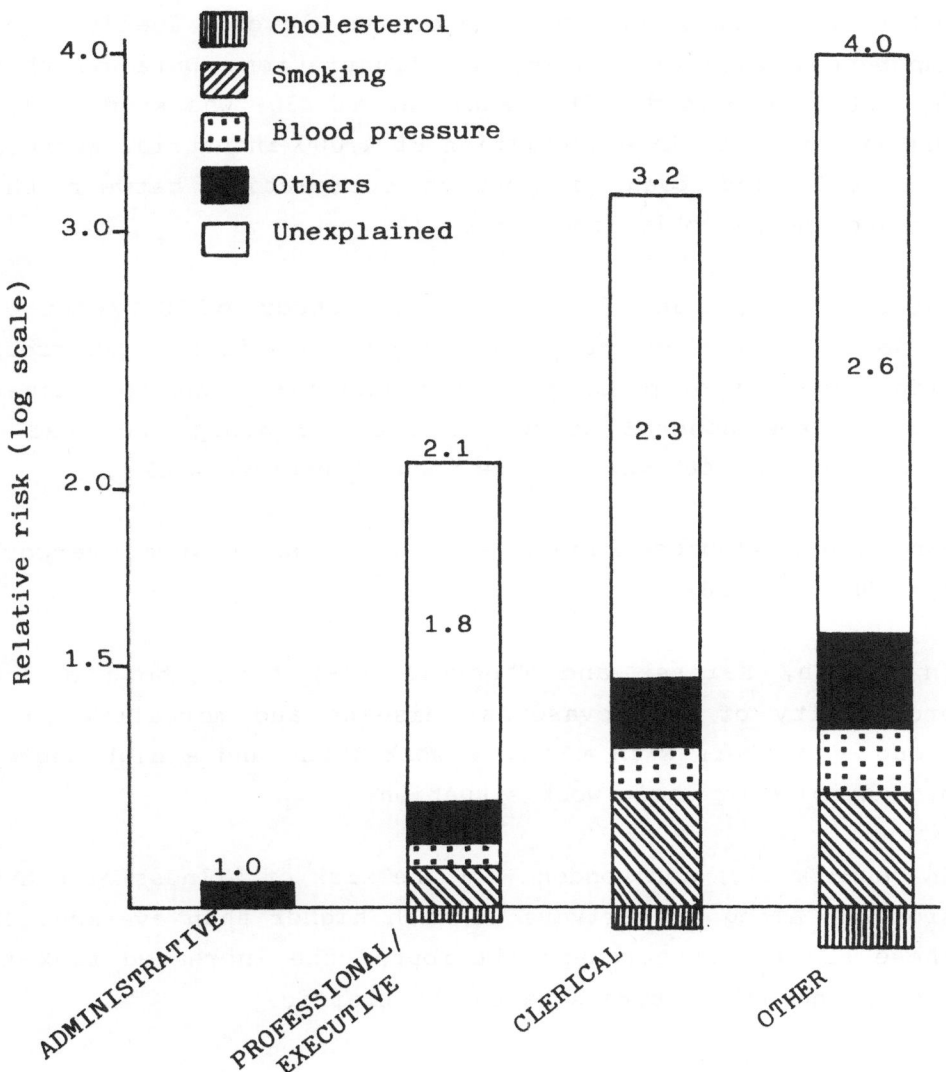

FIGURA 1: RELATIVE RISK OF DEATH FROM CORONARY HEART
DISEASE ACCORDING TO EMPLOYMENT GRADE, AND
PROPORTIONS OF DIFFERENCES THAT CAN   BE
EXPLAINED STATISTICALLY BY VARIOUS   RISK
FACTORS.

21

This result is difficult to explain if we consider the results of the analyses conducted on this subject (Table 2). The most common finding however concerns alienation at work where lack of control over the productive process, uneven distribution of incomes and fragmentary and competitive work relations cause, at the subjective level, feelings of impotence, dissatisfaction and frustration. Data on this subject is provided by Kritsikis et al (30) who studied 150 angina sufferers in a population of 4,000 industrial workers in Berlin and found a postive correlation between the disease and assembly line work.

Russek and Zohman (31) in a case study of CHD/control subjects found that the number of subjects in the CHD group with a history of prolonged emotional stress was four times that of the control group. In the CHD group, 20% had a second job and 46% worked more than 60 hours a week.

Many other studies confirm a correlation between overwork and CHD (32 - 38).

In Sweden, Karasek and Theorell (39) have shown a low probability of cardiovascular disease and mortality in a group of workers with moderate work loads and a high degree of control over their work situation.

In Denmark (40) and London (41) the risk of illness or death from CHD among bus drivers is much higher than average. In these studies researchers attributed the increased risk to the psychological stress caused by traffic.

These are all problem arising from the "external" environment; those caused by the "internal" psychological environment also seem to be important.

TABLE 2. Technostress: A working model (adapted from D.H.J., Caro and A.S. Sethi, 1985).

STRESSORS

environmental stressors

. light
· noise
· temperature
· humidity
· pollution

technostressors

· technological innovations
· technological policies/procedures
· rate of technological diffusion

individual stressors

· role conflict
· role ambiguity
· workload
· lack of career mobility
· job management

social group stressors

· peer group conflict
· lack of supportive relationships
· lack of good congruence
· conflict in values and norms
· group think

organizational stressors

· lack of participation
· weak organizational structure
· occupational level
· lack of clear policies
· lack of procedures

Since the beginning of the 1970's there have been many studies concerning the behavioural pattern, described by Friedman and Rosenman (42 - 53), known as Type A. The Type A person is engaged in a chronic struggle aimed at obtaining an unlimited number of vaguely defined things in the shortest possible time in competition, if necessary, with other persons or things present in the same environment. The Type A person tends to be found in work situations where competition is intense. Studies in this field have so far provided conflicting results. For example, in the study of British civil servant already quoted above (28) the Type A person is more common in the higher employment grades where however the incidence of CHD mortality is lower.

As regards educational background it can be said that the lower the educational level, the higher the CHD risk (54). Weinblatt et al. (55) in an investigation conducted under the Health Insurance Plan of Greater New York, found that a low level of education (less than 8 years of schooling) doubled CHD risk irrespective by classic risk factors.

Mortality statistics by socio-economic class also tend to show that low incomes are accompanied by increased risk.

Socio-cultural changes

A substantial part of the epidemiological literature on CHD is dedicated to the impact of the processes of industrialisation and urbanisation and the phenomenon of migration and geographical and occupational mobility.

Just as cardiovascular diseases of atherosclerosis origin are the prerogative of industrialised and urbanised countries so it seems that these diseases increase among people from "underdeveloped" regions when they adopt an urban or "modern" life style (24). This has been

demonstrated in studies of Zulus in South Africa (56),
Polynesians on the Cook Islands (57) and on the island of
Palau (58) and among the inhabitants of Tonga (59).

Successive studies based on these findings followed three
main hypotheses (24):

1 - In modern industrial countries stressful situations
    are created which can cause CHD;

2 - the process of cultural and social change can in
    itself be stressful and create a predisposition
    towards CHD;

3 - there is a type of selective bias whereby people with
    a predisposition to CHD migrate towards certain social
    environments.

The first two hypotheses concentrate on the fact that if an
individual finds him/herself in a situation for which s/he
has not been prepared for reasons of social discontinuity or
some breakdown in cultural or traditional links then the
situation itself becomes stressful and increases
vulnerablity to the disease (60, 61).

In a series of studies conducted at the beginning of the
1960's, Cassel and Tyroler (62) showed that persons employed
in industry for a short time had CHD rates much higher than
those of second generation industrial workers; they also
found that persons with a stable domicile but whose
community had undergone urbanisation had a similarly
increased CHD risk.

Syme (63 -, 65) was able to demonstrate the same phenomena
in a comparison between stable groups and groups
experiencing occupational and geographical mobility. More
recent studies have both confirmed (66, 67) and conflicted

(68, 69) with the hypothesis of a correlation between mobility and CHD; a fact which ought to make us think about the methodological problems in defining social factors of this type. Studies on immigrants, however, provide further proof of the influence of social mobility on mortality and CHD morbidity. Marmot (70) has shown that immigrants to the U.S.A have a higher incidence of CHD than their compatriots irrespective of country of origin.

Other authors (71, 72) found that the CHD rates of immigrants where midway between those of their compatriots and those of native Americans.

We should not forget the long-term study (73) of the inhabitants of the Tokelau islands whose arterial pressure was higher after immigration to New Zealand. It is interesting to note in this study that immigrants whose social and work relations were mainly with New Zealand institutions and New Zealanders of European origin had higher arterial pressure than those immigrants who had more contact with other immigrants from the Tokelau islands.

We ought also to mention those studies conducted among Japanese immigrants to the U.S.A. Many researchers (74, 75) have found high CHD mortality rates among Japanese immigrants when compared to those of Japan. Japan being an industrialised country with a high standard of living but an exception among advanced industrial nations in that it has very low mortality rates for coronary heart disease.

Marmot and Syme (76) found that Japanese-Americans who were more attached to the traditions of their country of origin had an incidence of CHD which was between three and five times less than that of those Japanese-Americans who had adopted the culture of the U.S.A. and that this difference was not influenced by any of the main risk factors (arterial pressure, smoking, cholesterol, diet).

In 1970 Matsumoto (77) argued that the considerable differences between the Japanese culture and the American culture is linked to the fact that traditional group values in Japan have continued to prevail despite great social change; in America, on the other hand, individualist tendencies predominate which although they increase the level of personal autonomy they also decrease the possibilities for giving and receiving support at home and at work.

These considerations provide a suitable introduction to a discussion of the last group of factors, that is, those factors which can be traced back to the network of social relations.

The network of social relations

Situations such as social mobility and emigration are stressful in the sense that they cause breaks in the fabric of social contacts which surround an individual and which according to psychologists, sociologists and anthropologists provide great support in facing to problems generated by daily life (78).

For the sake of clarity it should be emphasised that the social network provides the individual with support both in the form of help with emotional, material, economic and cognitive problems and also in the form of a system of values which the individual uses for reference in self-evaluation (79).

The social network, just like all the other social factors, is a synthesis of many elements and characteristics; from the moment in which the individual enters into relations with other persons in his/her surroundings we may identify the following elements (24):

1 - **density and complexity** (the extent to which members of a network know and interact with each other)

2 - **size** (number of persons in the network)

3 - **symmetry and reciprocity** (extent to which the support and obligations between network members is reciprocated)

4 - **geographical closeness** (extent to which network members live close to focus individual)

5 - **homogeneity** (extent to which network members are similar in terms of age, social class, religion)

6 - **accessibility** (ease with which the focus person can make contact with other network members)

7 - **quality, frequency, intensity, duration and strength** of the interaction process (80 - 84).

Studies (85 - 88) to test the importance of the social network in general have been limited to analysis of general mortality. For coronary heart disease the literature uses the customary simplifications. Much of the research concerns widowhood (89 - 94), a typical example of irreparable breakdown in social relations. Widowhood is not only accompanied, in the short term at least (94), by an increased mortality risk but also provokes, according to Koskenvuo (95) in a Finnish study, an increase in the incidence of CHD which can only in part be explained by a varied distribution of the conventional risk factors.

Retirement and losing your job are other examples of breaks in social relations. Some authors (96) have shown increased CHD risk in these cases.

Widowhood, dismissal but also celibacy, a state which implies a lack of "important" relationships, increases CHD risk. Weiss (97) found an excess of deaths due to CHD in unmarried persons over the age of 25 which could not be explained on the basis of biological risk factors.

The discussion so far has, to a greater or lesser extent, implied something that should now be stated clearly. The most obvious weakness of traditional epidemiological research into the role of social factors in the aetiology of heart disease is the oversimplification of social variables (25, 26).

Karasek (98) demonstrates this point using the example of "job decision latitude"; this is something which contains the concept of "decision taking responsibility" together with that of "latitude of decision taking responsibility", two concepts which are antithetical in that "responsibility" is stressful while "autonomy" is gratifying. Panico (99) analysed the methodological problems involved in defining social class in relation to this factor in the context of epidemiological studies and came to the conclusion that substantial modifications in the interpretation of the results were possible depending on the standpoint chosen (education, cultural background, income level, job).

The situation is complicated further if we take into accont the fact that the response to stress factors is mediated by individual behavioural characteristics which are difficult to check but which should always be taken into account because they might explain variations in the intensity and expression of social factors. These behavioural characteristics, known as "coping capacities" presuppose a reflex or creative ability to adapt in difficult conditions (100) and are recognisable in all the processes for handling stress situations (101 - 103).

The special terms used such as "problem solving", "adaption", "defence" and "mastery" have never been clearly defined even though they identify various ways of coping with stress (104).

Operational solutions to these problems are not available: we cannot however overlook their importance either in research design or in the evaluation of results. Some authors (7, 8) have put foward the hypothesis that a possible solution would be to incorporate the instruments of social epidemiology into medical epidemiology.

We believe that this means constantly bearing in mind the social factors and studying them with the same scientific determination and meticulousness as that used for studying biological risk factors.
This also involves the integration of biological and social factors.

The question now presents itself of whether we can exclude a priori that the distribution of biological factors is not significantly determined by other factors present at the social level; in other words, are things such as smoking and eating habits risk factors on the basis of which it is possible to identify groups with a predisposition towards certain types of disease?

Factors such as these can only be studied through the social environment which influences motives, and values and through values behaviour and life style.

Today in the United States smoking and poor eating are becoming more and more the exclusive habits of the lower social classes. Membership of such classes is in itself a risk factor since it entails the assumption of a life-style which in turn increases the risk of CHD and other degenerative patholologies.

This approach to the problem, which is nothing more than considering life style from the broader medical/social viewpoint rather than from the restricted medical viewpoint, is in our opinion of great importance in the planning of effective preventive measures in the future.

The same conclusion emerges from an analysis of the social aspects of atherosclerosis by Antonovsky (105); an analysis which provides, in our opinion, a further confirmation of the author's intuition but also a confirmation that an integrated approach to the biological and social problems of disease is the key element in the changeover from the field of pathogenesis, useful but not exhaustive, to that exhaustive and gratifying field of salutogensis.

BIBLÍOGRAFIA

1 - M.F.Oliver: "Does Control of Risk Factors Prevent Coronary Heart Disease?", Brit. Med. J., vol. 285, 16 oct. 1982, 1065.

2 - W. Wilkenstein Jr., M.Marmot: "Primary Prevention of Ischemic Heart Disease: Evaluation of Community Interventions", Ann. Rev. Publ. Hlth, 1981, 2: 253.

3 - P.Puska: "The Community Based Strategy to Prevent Coronary Heart Disease: Conclusions from Ten Years of the North Karelia Project", Ann. Rev. Publ. Hlth, 1985, 6: 147.

4 - G.Rose, H.D.Tunstall-Pedoe, R.F.Heller: "U.K. Heart Disease Prevention Project: Incidence and Mortality Results", Lancet may 14, 1983, 1062.

5 - A.Menotti: "Cardiopatia ischemica in prevenzione", Corriere Medico, 6 giugno 1986, p. 17.

6 - P.I.Ahmed, A.Kolker: "The Role of Indigenous Medicine in Who's Definition of Health", in "Toward a New Definition of Health Psychosocial Dimension", ed by P.I.Ahmed e G.V.Coelho, Plenum Press, 1979, p. 113.

7 - H.Fabrega Jr.: "Disease and Illness from a Biocultural Standpoint" in "Toward a new Definition of health Psychosocial Dimensions", ed. by P.I.Ahmed e G.V.Coelho, Plenum Press, 1979, p. 236.

8 - S.Graham, L.G.Reeder: "Social Epidemiology of Chronic Diseases" in "Handbook of Medical Sociology", ed. by H.E.Freeman, S.Levine, L.G.Reeder, Prentice-Hall, 3° edition, 1979.

9 - R.A.Stallones: "To Advance Epidemiology", Ann. Rev. Public Hlth, 1980. 1: 69.

10 - J.B.Calhoun: "Population Density and Social Pathology", Scientific American, 206 (2): 139, 1962.

11 - R.Ader, A.Kreutner, H.L.Jacobs: "Social Environment Emotionality and Alloxandiabetes in the Rat", Psycosom.Med., 25: 60, 1963.

12 - H.L.Ratcliffe,   M.I.T.Cronin: "Changing Frequency of
      Arteriosclerosis in Mammals and Birds at the Philadelphia
      Zoological Garden", Circulation, 18: 41, 1958.

13 - J.Siegrist, K.Siegrist, I.Weber: "Sociological Concepts in
      the Etiology of Chronic Disease: the Case of Ischemic Heart
      Disease", Soc.Sci.Med., vol. 22, N. 2, p. 249, 1986.

14 - J.P.Henry, P.Stephens: "Stress, Health and the Social
      Environment", Springer, New York, 1977.

15 - W.C.Cockerham: "Medical Sociology", 2° edition, Prentice-
      hall, 1982.

16 - W.B.Cannon: "The Wisdom of the Body", Norton, New York,
      1932.

17 - R.S.Schwab, J.S.Pritchard: "Situational Stresses and Extra
      Pyramidal Disease in Different Personalities", in "Life
      Stress and Disease", Proceedings of the Association for
      Research in Nervous and Menal Disease, Williams & Wilkins,
      Baltimora, 1950 (Quoted by W.C.Cockerham in 16).

18 - T.H.Holmes, R.H.Rahe: "The Social Readjustment Rating
      Scale", J.Psychosom. Res., 11: 213, 1967.

19 - M.Friedman, R.H.Rosenman, V.Carol: "Changes in the Serum
      Cholesterol and Blood Clotting Time in Men Subjected to
      Cyclic Variation of Occupational Stress", Circulation, 17
      (may): 152, 1958.

20 - F.Dreyfus: "Blood Cholesterol and Uric Acid of Healthy
      Medical Students under the Stress of an Exam", Arch.
      Intern. Med., 103: 708, 1959.

21 - S.M.Grundy: "Relationship of Periodic Mental Stress to
      Serum Lipoprotein and Cholesterol Levels", JAMA, 171: 1794,
      1959.

22 - C.Thomas, E.Murphy: "Cholesterol in Medical Students with
      Exam Stress", J.Chron.Dis., 8: 861, 1958.

23 - B.Badura: "Life-style and health: Some Remarks on Different
      Viewpoints", Soc.Sci.Med., vol. 19, 4: 341, 1984.

24 - L.F.Berkman: "Physical Health and the Social Environment: a Social Epidemiological Perspective", in "The Relevance of Social Science for Medicine", ed. by L.Einsenberg & A.Kleinman, D.Reidel, Publishing Co. 1980, p. 51.

25 - D.V.McQueen, J.Siegrist: "Social Factors in the Etiology of Chronic Disease: an Overview", Soc.Sci.Med., 16: 353, 1982.

26 - P.A.Thoits:" Conceptual, Methodological, and Theoretical Problems in Studying Social Support as a Buffer Against Life Stress", J. Hlth Soc.Behav., 23: 146, 1982.

27 - A. Antonovsky: "Social class and the Major Cardiovascular Diseases", J. Chron.Dis., vol. 21, 65, 1968.

28 - M. G.Marmot, G.Rose, M. Shipley, P.J.Hamilton: "Employment Grade and Coronary Heart Disease in British Civil Servants", J. Epid. Comm. Hlth, vol. 32, 4: 244, 1978.

29 - D.H.J.Card, A.S.Sethi:"Strategic Management of Technostress - the Chaining of Prometheus", J.Med.Syst., vol. 9, nos. 5/6: 291, 1985.

30 - S.Kritsikis, A.Heinemann, S.Eitner: "Die Angina Pectoris im Aspect Ihrer Korrelation mit Biologischer Disposition, Psychologishen und Soziologischen Einfluss Faktoren", Deutsch Gesundh., 23: 1878, 1968. Quoted in S.Kiritz, R.H.Moos "Psychological Effects of Social Environment", Psychosom. Med., 36 (2): 96, 1974.

31 - H.I.Russek, B.L.Zohman: "Relative Significance of Heredity, Diet, and Occupational Stress in Coronary Heart Disease in Young Adults", Am.J.Sciences, 235: 266, 1958.

32 - S.Sales: "Organization Role as a Risk Factor in Coronary Disease", Admin.Sci.Quart., 14: 325, 1969.

33 - E.Biorck, G.Blomquist, J.Sievers: "Studies in Myocardial infarction in Malm_ 1935-54: II.Infarction Rate by Occupational Group", Acta Med.Scand., 161: 21, 1958.

34 - P.Buell, L.Breslow: "Mortality from Coronary Heart Disease in California Men Who Work Long Hours", J.Chron.Dis., 11: 615, 1958.

35 - R.Theorell, R.H.Rahe: "Behaviour and Life Satisfaction Characteristics of Swedish Subjects with Myocardial Infarction", J.Chron.Dis., 25: 139, 1972.

36 - H.E.S.Pearson, J.Joseph: "Stress and Occlusive Coronary-Artery Disease", Lancet, 1: 415, 1963.

37 - H.G.Thiel, D.Parker, T.Bruce: "Stress Factors and the Risk of Myocardial Infarction", J.Psychosom.Res., 17: 43, 1973.

38 - J.Garfield: "Alienated Labor, Stress, and Coronary Disease", Int.J.Hlth Serv., vol. 10, 4: 551, 1980.

39 - R.Karasek, D.Baker, F.Marxer, A.Ahlbom, T.Theorell: "Job Decision Latitude, Job Demands, and Cardiovascular Disease: a Prospective Study of Swedish Men", Am.J.Publ.Hlth, vol. 71, 7: 694, july 1981.

40 - P.Laursen: "Work Environment for Busdrivers 1", Institute for Social Medicine, Copenhagen University, N. 11, 1980, Quoted in B.Gardell "Scandinavian Research on Stress in Working Life", Int.J.Hlth Serv., vol. 12, 1: 31, 1982.

41 - J.N.Morris: "Coronary Heart Disease and Physical Activity at Work", Lancet, 2: 1111, 1953.

42 - R.H.Rosenman, M.Friedman, R.Straus: "A Predictive Study of Coronary Heart Disease", JAMA, 189: 103, 1964.

43 - C.D.Jenkins, S.J.Zizanski, R.H.Rosenman: "Progress Toward Validation of a Computer Scored Test for the Type A Coronary Prone Behaviour Pattern", Psychosom.Med., 33: 193, 1971.

44 - C.D.Jenkins: "Psychologic and Social Precursors of Coronary Disease" (First of Two Parts), N.Engl.J.Med., vol. 284, 5: 244, feb. 4, 1971.

45 - M.Friedman, R.H.Rosenman: "Type A Behaviour and Your Heart", Knopf, New York, 1974.

46 - C.D.Jenkins: "Recent Evidence Supporting Psychologic and Social Risck Factors for Coronary Disease", (Two Parts), N.Engl.J.Med., vol. 294, 18: 987, 19: 1033, 1976.

47 - S.G.Haynes, M.Feinleib, W.B.Kannel: "The Relationship of Psychosocial Factors to Coronary Heart Disease in the Framingham Study. III. Eight Year Incidence of Coronary Heart Disease", Am.J.Epid., 111: 37, 1980.

48 - R.J.Brand, R.H.Rosenman, C.D.Jenkins: "Comparison of Coronary Heart Disease Prediction in the Western Collaborative Group Study Using the Structured Interview and the Jenkins Activity Survey Assessment of the Coronary Prone Type A Behaviour Pattern", (Abstract), Am.Heart Ass. CVD Epid. Newsletter, 24, 1978.

49 - J.B.Cohen, D.Reed: "Type A Behaviour and Coronary Heart Disease Among Japanese Men in Hawaii", J.Behav.Med., 8: 343, 1985.

50 - R.B.Shekelle, S.B.Hulley, J.D.Neaton: "The MRFIT Behaviour Pattern Study. II. Type A Behaviour and Incidence of Coronary Heart Disease", Am.J.Epid., 122: 559, 1985.

51 - G.De Backer, M.Kornitzer, F.Kittel: "Behaviour, Stress, and Psychosocial Traits as Risk Factors", Prev.Med., 12: 32, 1983.

52 - J.M.Siegel: "Type A Behaviour: Epidemiologic Foundations and Public Health Implications", Ann.Rev.Publ.Hlth, 5: 343, 1984.

53 - K.A.Matthews, S.G.Haynes: "Type A Behaviour Pattern and Coronary Heart Disease Risk - Update and Critical Evaluation", Am.J.Epid., vol. 123, 6: 923, 1986.

54 - D.C.Jenkins: "Low Education: a Risk Factors for Death", New Engl.J.Med., 299, 2: 95, 1978.

55 - E.Weinblatt, W.Ruberman, J.D.Golberg, et Al.: "Sudden Death After Myocardial Infarction in Relation to Education", New Engl.J.Med., 299, 2: 111, 1978.

56 - N.A.Scotch: "Sociocultural Factors in the Epidemiology of Zulu Hypertension", Am.J.Publ.Hlth, 53 (8): 1205, 1963.

57 - I.A.Prior: "Cardiovascular Epidemiology in New Zealand and the Pacific", New Zealand Med.J., 80: 245, 1974.

58 - D.Labarthe, D.Reed, J.Brody, R.Stallones: "Health Effects of Modernization in Palau", Am.J.Epid., 98: 161, 1973.

59 - World Health Organization for the Western Pacific: "The Prevention and Control of Cardiovascular Disease", 1975.

60 - J.Cassel, R.Patrick, D.Jenkins: "Epidemiological Analysis of Culture Change: a Conceptual Model",Ann.N.Y.Acad.Sci.,84: 938.

61 - J.Henry, J.Cassel: "Psycosocial Factors in Essential Hypertension", Am.J.Epid., 40: 171.

62 - J.Cassel, H.Tyroler: "Epidemiological Studies of Cultural Change. I. Health Status and Recency of Industrialization", Arch.Env.Hlth, 3: 31, 1961.

63 - S.L.Syme, M.M.Hyman, P.E. Enterline: "Some Social and Cultural Factors Associated With the Occurrence of Coronary Artery Disease", J.Chron.Dis., 17: 272, 1964.

64 - S.L.Syme, M.M.Hyman, P.E. Enterline: "Cultural Mobility and the Occurence of Coronary Artery Disease", J.Hlth Behav., 6 (Winter): 178, 1965.

65 - S.L.Syme, N.D.Borhani, R.W.Buechley: "Cultural Mobility and Coronary Heart Disease in an Urban Area", Am.J.Epid., 82: 334, 1966.

66 - B.H. Kaplan, J. Cassel, H.Tyroler, et Al.: "Occupational Mortality and Coronary Artery Disease", Arch.Intern.Med., 128: 398, 1971.

67 - I. Lehr, H.B.Messinger, R. Rosenman: "A Sociobiological Approach to the Study of Coronary Heart Disease", J.Chron.Dis., 2: 13, 1973.

68 - W.Wardwell, C.Bahnson: "Behavioral Variables and Myocardial Infarction in the Southeastern Connecticut Heart Study", J. Chron.Dis., 26: 447, 1973.

69 - C.Bengtsson, T.Hallstrom, G.Tibblin: "Social Factors, Stress Experience and Personality Traits in Women With Ischaemic Heart Disease", ACTA MED. SLAND., SUPPL. 589:82, 1973

70 - M. Marmot: "Migrants, Acculturation and Coronary Heart Disease", MIMED, Dept. of Epidemiology, Univ. California, Berkeley, 1975.

71 - J. Stamler, Hykjelsberg, Y. Hall, N. Scotch, "Epidemiologic Studies on Cardiovascular-Renal Disease. III. Analyses of Mortality by Age-Sex-Nationality", J. Chron. Dis., 12:464, 1960.

72 - D. Krueger, I. Moryama, "Mortality of the Foreign Born", Am. J. Publ, Hlth, 57:496, 1967.

73 - I.A. Prior, "Migration and Physical Illness", in "Epidemiologic Studies in Psychosomatic Medicine", S. Kasl Ed., S. Karger, Basel, Switzerland, 105, 1977.

74 - T. Gordon, "Mortality Experience among the Japanese in the United States, Hawaii, Japan", Publ. Hlth Rep., 72:543, 1957.

75 - R. Worth, A. Kagan, "Ascertainment of Men of Japanese Ancestry in Hawaii through WWII Selective Service Registration", J. Chron. Dis., 23:389, 1970.

76 - M. Marmot, S.L. Syme, "Acculturation and Coronary Heart Disease in Japanese-Americans", Am. J. Epid., 104 (3):225, 1976.

77 - Y. Matsumoto, "Social Stress and Coronary Heart Disease in Japan: a Hypothesis", Milb. Mem. Fund Quart., 48-9, 1970.

78 - L.F. Berkman, "Assessing the Physical Health Effects of Social Networks and Social Support", Ann.Rev.Publ.Hlth, 5-413, 1984.

79 - J. House, "Work, Stress and Social Support", Addison-Wesley Reading, Mass., 1981.

80 - A. Fisher, R. Jackson, C. Steve, et Al., "Networks and Places: Social Relations in the Urban Setting", Free Press, New York, 1977.

81 - E. Laumann, "Bonds of Ruralism: the Form and Substance of Urban Social Networks, Wiley, New York, 1973.

82 - J.C. Mitchell, "The Concept and Use of Social Networks", in "Social Networks in Urban Situations", J.C. Mitchell Ed., Manchester Univ. Press, Manchester, U.K., 1969.

83 - B. Kellman, "The Community Question", Am. J. Sociol., 84, 1201, 1979.

84 - M. Granovetter, "The Strength of Weak Ties", Am. J. Sociol., 78, 1360, 1973.

85 - L.F. Berkman, L. Breslow, "Health and Ways of Living: Findings from the Alameda County Study", Oxford Univ. Press, New York, 1983.

86 - L.F. Berkman, S.L. Syme, "Social Networks, Host Resistance, and Mortality: a Nine Year Follow-up Study of Alameda County Residents", Am. J. Epid., 115:684, 1979.

87 - J. House, C. Robbins, H. Metzner, "The Association of Social Relationships and Activities with Mortality: Prospective Evidence from Tecumseh Community Health Study", Am. J. Epid., 116:123, 1982.

88 - D. Blazer, "Social Support and Mortality in an Elderly Community Population", Am. J. Epid., 115:684, 1982.

89 - H.S. Kraus, A.M. Lilienfeld, "Some Epidemiologic Aspects of the High Mortality Rates in the Young Widowed Group", J. Chron. Dis., 10:207, 1959.

90 - M. Young, B. Benjamin, C. Wallis, "The Mortality of Widows", Lancet, 2:454, 1963.

91 - P.R. Cox, J.R. Ford, "The Mortality of Widows Shortly after Widowhood", Lancet, 1:163, 1964.

92 - W.P. Rees, S.G. Lutkin, "Mortality of Bereavement", Brit. Med. J., 4:13, 1967.

93 - A.N. Ward, "Mortality of Bereavement", Brit. Med. J., 1:700, 1972.

94 - K.J. Helsing, M. Szklo, "Mortality after Bereavement", Am. J. Epid., 114 (1):41, 1981.

95 - M. Koskenvuo, J. Kaprio, M. Romo, H. Langinvainio, "Incidence and Prognosis of Ischaemic Heart Disease with Respect to Marital Status and Social Class - A National Record Linkage Study", J. Epid. Comm. Hlth, 35:192, 1981.

96 - C. D'Arcy, C.M. Siddique, "Unemployment and Health: an Analysis of Canada Health Survey Data", Int. J. Hlth Serv., 15 (4):609, 1985.

97 - N.S. Weiss, "Marital Status and Risk Factors for Coronary Heart Disease: the United States Health Examination Survey of Adults", Brit. J. Prev. Soc. Med., 27:41, 1973.

98 - K.A. Karasek, "Job Demands, Job Decision Latitude and Mental Strain: Implication for Job Redesign", Admin. Sci. Quart., 24:268, 1979.

99 - S. Panico, "Social Class and Coronary Heart Disease", Term Paper, Dept. Epidemiology, London School of Hygiene and Tropical Medicine, 1980.

100- W. Karmaus, "Working Conditions and Health: Social Epidemiology, Pattern of Stress and Change", Soc. Sci. Med., 19, 4:359, 1984.

101- R.S. Lazarus, "Psychological Stress and the Coping Process", London, 1966

102- L.J. Pearlin, C. Schooler, "The Structure of Coping", J. Hlth Soc. Behav., 19:2, 1978.

103- L.J. Pearlin, E.C. Menagham, M.A. Lieberman, J.J. Mullan, "The Stress Process", J. Hlth Soc. Behav., 22:337, 1981.

104- G.U. Coelho, D.A. Hamburg, J.E. Adams, "Coping and Adaptation", Basic, New York, 1974.

105- A. Antonowsky, "Health Stress and Coping", London, 1979.

3
Primary and secondary prevention of atherosclerosis and coronary heart disease
A.M. Gotto

The focus of my presentation will be plasma cholesterol and lipoproteins and their relationship to prevention of coronary heart disease (CHD). Data from the Framingham Study shows that cardiovascular risk increases linearly with the level of cholesterol. [1] Hypercholesterolemia is the only one of three risk factors for CHD; the other two are cigarette smoking and hypertension. Other factors include a low level of HDL cholesterol, an elevation of serum plasma triglycerides, lack of exercise, diabetes mellitus, obesity, a high saturated fat diet, excessive stress, personality type A, and other psychosocial factors, and factors related to coagulation and platelet aggregation which have not been precisely defined. Figure 2 illustrates the increasing risk of CHD when multiple risk factors are involved. The most preventable cause of CHD is cigarette smoking. The risk from cigarette smoking and from hypertension tends to remain relatively constant between ages 30 and 60. By contrast, the risk of an elevated serum cholesterol is much greater at age 30 than at age 60, although HDL cholesterol, and to a lesser extent, LDL cholesterol are still important even after age 60. HDL is as strong a

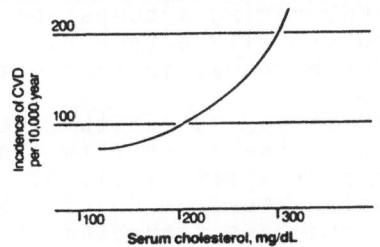

Figure 1. Cardiovascular risk and cholesterol. From the Framingham Study [1].

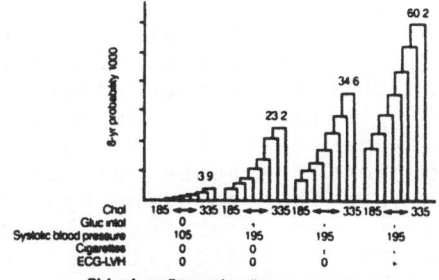

Figure 2.

risk factor as is known, the risk of CHD being inversely related to the concnetration of this lipoprotein fraction.

The recent European Cholesterol Consensus Conference emphasized the importance in detecting and intervening on all risk factors, including hypertriglyceridemia. Hypertriglyceridemia was an independent risk factor for CHD in females in the Framinhgam Study, and in studies reported from Sweden. Hypertension, cigarette smoking, obesity, and diabetes are also given importance in the European consensus report.

New studies recently reported at the 10th World Congress of Cardiology, in Washington D.C., September, 1986, support the concept that reducing risk factors and changing lifestyles of populations will reduce CHD. A study carried out in the United States [2] with 356,000 males between ages 35 and 57 reported that during a 6 year period, 7948 non-smokers with low levels of cholesterol and low levels of blood pressure had a death rate of only 0.8 per thousand; this amounted to only 6 deaths over 6 years for this group of individuals. In the overall group, 6.3 per thousand died of CHD during a comparable period of time. The rate for smokers with either hypertension or hypercholesteorlemia or both was increased to 21.4 per thousand.

Another study from China [3] accounted for the fact that the Chinese have about one half the death rate from CHD as Americans. This study of approximately 11,000 subjects attributed the lower death rate from CHD to the fact that the Chinese diet contained less saturated fat, cholesterol, and in this group of Chinese individuals, a lower intake of salt. Blood pressure levels were also lower than in the U.S. Finally, a Russian [4] study was performed over a period of 5 years and involved approximately 6,000 subjects between ages 40-59. Of 3000 individuals that enrolled in a CHD prevention program, the overall mortality was decreased by 21% and CHD death was decreased by 41%. These studies all reinforced the view that primary prevention can and will reduce CHD morbidity and mortality.

The death rate from CHD in the United States has declined by almost 40% over the past 20 years and the death rate from cerebrovascular disease by about 50%. No single factor can account for these changes, but it is assumed that changes in lifestyle represent major contributions. A number of intervention trials have established that reducing hypertension decreases overall mortality and cerebrovascular death. A disappointing aspect of these studies is that coronary heart disease morbidity and mortality is not greatly corrected by normalization of blood pressure. For example, based on analysis of risk from the Framingham data, the reduction in blood pressure has produced only about 25% of the decrease in

CHD one might have predicted.

In the United States, the National Institutes of Health, the American Heart Association, and the Citizen's for Public Action on Cholesterol have called for a national cholesterol education program. The message of this program is aimed at the physician and at the public, and is relatively simple. High blood cholesterol increases the risk of CHD, hypercholesterolemia produces no symptoms for many years, and when symptoms occur, the disease may be far advanced. Hypercholesterolemia may be detected by a simple blood test, and effective measures are available for lowering cholesterol through diet and/ or medication. Evidence now extsts that lowering cholesterol and specifically LDL cholesterol, reduces CHD.

Several recent primary and secondary trials have established the benefits of cholesterol lowering. The Coronary Primary Prevention Trial [5] has provided the firmest evidence to date in support of the cholesterol or LDL hypothesis. Reducing cholesterol by approximately 8.5%, and LDL cholesterol by approximately 11%, CHD, measured as CHD death, or non-fatal myocardial infarction, were reduced by 19%. (Figure 3.) There were also significant reductions in the number of coronary bypasses performed, in the appearance of new positive exercise electrocardiograms, and in the occurrence of angina pectoris. Overall, a reduction of 1% in cholesterol reduced CHD by 2%. This finding is similar to what would be predicted by the Framingham Study.

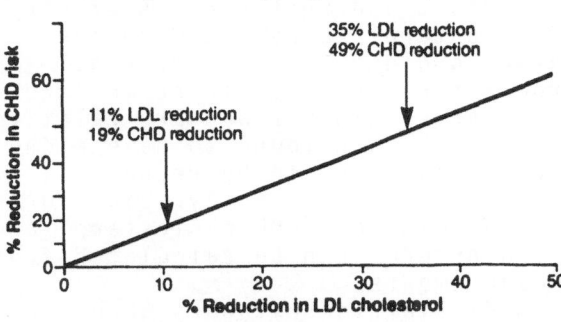

Figure 3. Relation of reduction in LDL to reduction of CHD. The Coronary Primary Prevention Trial [5].

Several secondary studies have also been reported. A small controlled study on peripheral atherosclerosis was performed by Duffield [6] in London, a Type II intervention study [7] was carried out at the NIH using cholestyramine, and a diet study without a control group was performed in the Netherlands [8]. These studies showed that reducing cholesterol and LDL decreased the rate of progression of atherosclerosis confirmed by femoral and/ or coronary arteriography. The ratios which correlated best with rate of progression were the total cholesterol to HDL cholesterol, or the LDL to HDL cholesterol. Raising HDL per se has not yet been proven to prevent or reduce coronary disease; the Helsinki heart trial with gemfibrozil may provide valuable information concerning the HDL hypothesis.

Based on an extensive review of existing evidence, the NIH Cholesterol Consensus Conference, [9] and more recently the European Cholesterol Consensus Conference recommended a new set of guidelines for defining hyper-cholesterolemia. (Table 1) Moderate risk was defined as cholesterol levels between the 75th and 90th percentiles, and high risk as cholesterol above the 90th percentile. For adults age 40 and over, these translate respectively into cholesterols of 240 mg/dl and 260 mg/dl. These are not ideal levels of cholesterol;

Blood Cholesterol Values for Selecting Men and Women Who Require Treatment

Age	Moderate Risk (75th percentile)	High Risk (90th percentile)
20–29	200–220 mg/dl	220–240 mg/dl
30–39	220–240 mg/dl	240–260 mg/dl
≥40	240–260 mg/dl	>260 mg/dl

Table 1. From the Cholesterol Consensus Conference. [9]

it was further advised that a desriable objective would be that the entire population have cholesterol levels under 200 mg/dl above age 30, and under 180 mg/dl below age 30.

A two-pronged strategy was recommended to achieve these goals-- a high risk strategy and a mass approach strategy. It was recommended that cholesterols be measured at every physician contact and that every American should know his or her cholesterol value. New devices are available for measuring cholesterol by a drop of blood or serum taken from a fingerprick. These measurements can be done in a matter of minutes and are relatively inexpensive. Individuals who are found to have a cholesterol above the 75th percentile should be rechecked, and if confirmed, should be referred to a physician for a fasting sample of plasma cholesterol, HDL cholesterol and triglyceride. The LDL cholesterol can be calculated from a formula using these measurements.

Individuals in the moderate risk catagory should be treated with diet, beginning with the Phase I diet of the American Heart Association [10]. In this diet, total fat intake is reduced to 30% of the total calories, and is equally divided between polyunsaturated, saturated and monounsaturated fats. Total cholesterol is reduced to 250-300 mg/day depending upon the caloric intake. It is also advised that ideal body weight be achieved and maintained, and that sodium

Dietary Goals of Phases 1, 2 and 3 of the American Heart Association Diet

Phase	1	2	3
Fat (% calories)	30	25	20
Carbohydrate (% calories)	55	60	65
Protein (% calories)	15	15	15
Cholesterol (mg)	300	200–250	100–150
P/S (ratio polyunsaturated fat to saturated fat)	1	1	1–2

Adapted from AHA Special Report. Recommendations for treatment of hyperlipidemia in adults. Circulation 1984;69:1065A-1090A.

Table 2.

intake be limited to no more than 3 gm daily. For those whose cholesterol levels are not normalized by diet, a drug may be needed. For those with cholesterol values above the 90th percentile, diet and often drugs will be required for treatment. As a mass strategy approach, these recommendations are also made to the general population. Thus, the cholesterol level for the entire population would be shifted downward.

Several first-line drugs are available for treating hypercholesterolemia and hyperlipidemia. [11] The bile acid sequestrants reduce mainly cholesterol and LDL. Cholestryramine is the only drug to date which has been allowed by the FDA to make the claim that lowering cholesterol and LDL with this drug has been shown to reduce CHD. Nicotinic acid reduces cholesterol, triglyceride, LDL and VLDL, and at the same time, raises HDL cholesterol. Probucol reduces total cholesterol and LDL cholesterol, and lowers HDL. Gemfibrozil decreases primarily trilgyceride and raises HDL in individuals with hypercholesterolemia and with elevated LDL, but without hypertriglyceridemia. LDL and cholesterol are also reduced by 10-15%. Clofibrate, the prototype of the fibric acid derivative is a primary drug used only in Type III hyperlipidemia, since the World Health Organization reported an increase in overall mortality in patients treated with this drug.

Removal of LDL through an extracorporeal procedure has been introduced, and various adaptations of this technique have been used. In one procedure, antibodies to LDL are used; in another, heparin and separose are used to remove LDL and VLDL. Initially, plasmapheresis per se was employed. More recently, filters to remove particles of the LDL size have been employed. In a few patients who are homozygotes for familial hypercholesterolemia, liver transplantation has been done. This procedure will provide LDL receptors in a patient who has no functioning receptors; in other words, who is receptor negative and a homozygote for familial hypercholesterolmeia. Finally, an ileal bypass procedure is being tested in a secondary prevention trial in the United States. In this trial, ileal bypass surgery is being undertaken in men with above average levels of cholesterol and LDL and who have had myocardial infarction. The procedure reduces cholesterol by about 30% and LDL by about 40%. It remains to be determined if CHD mortality and overall mortality will be reduced by this intervention.

New drugs are currently being tested, and include inhibitors of cholesterol synthesis, particularly a competitive inhibitor of HMG CoA reductase called mevinolin, which is based on the Japanese drug compactin, originally isolated from a fungal agent. As a pill in the dosage of 20 mg b.i.d., mevinolin will reduce cholesterolby about 20-25% in heterozygotes for familial hypercholesterolemia. Taken in conjunction with a bile acid sequestrant in heterozygotes, LDL has been reduced by over 50%.

Based on the work of Brown and Goldstein [12], it is possible to explain the action of drugs such as the bile acid sequestrants and mevinolin, and on a hypothetical basis, at least, of diet on plamsa cholesterol and LDL based on the LDL receptor. Approximately 2/3 to 3/4 of

LDL is removed from the circulation via the LDL or B/E receptor. This recpetor is heavily concentrated in the liver and recognizes apoB-100 or apoE. ApoB-100 appears to be the primary ligand recognized. The relationship between concentrations of LDL receptors in the liver is a primary determinant of LDL cholesterol. (Figure 5)

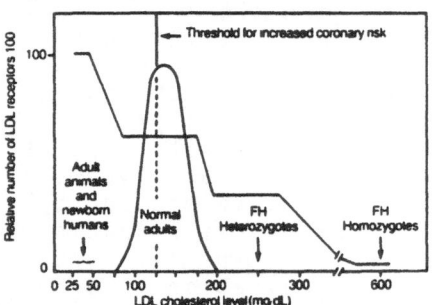

Figure 5.

This approach assumes that there is a critical level of LDL which is necessary for atherosclerosis to develop. By reducing the intrahepatic concentration of cholesterol, it has been postulated that bile acide sequestrants and HMG CoA reductase inhibitors will increase the activity of the LDL receptor on the surface of liver cells, and thus increase the rate of LDL removal from the circulation.

In addition to the LDL, or B/E or high affinity receptor, approximately 1/3 of the LDL is removed by another pathway known as the lower affinity pathway. This includes the scavenger pathway, which involves the macrophages, monocytes and cells of the reticulo endothelial system. Uptake of altered LDL by these cells may actually contribute to the accumulation of atherosclerosis in the arterial wall, and thus may be a factor in the development of atherosclerosis. A diet high in cholesterol and saturated fat could chronically suppress the activity of the LDL receptors and lead to an increase in the circulating level of LDL.

A potential cholesterol synthesis inhibitor, a polar sterol called 15-ketosterol, has been shown to increase HDL while decreasing LDL concentraitons in primates. Other potential approaches to the prevention of atherosclerosis include inhibitors of acyl cholesterol acyl transferase, which might prevent conversion of dietary cholesterol to cholesteryl ester, and prevent cholesterol esterification within the arterial wall; substances which increase the level of or mimic the acvitity of HDL; and maneuvers which increase the level of lipoprotein lipase, and/or decrease the level of hepatic lipase.

It is hoped that with these new approaches, it will be possible not only to retard the progression of atherosclerosis, but actually to halt it and effect a reversal of this process.

REFERENCES

1. Dawber, TR. (1980) The Framingham Study: The Epidemiology of Atherosclerotic Disease.(Cambridge: Harvard University Press)

2. Stamler, J, Wentworth DN, Neaton JD, for the MRFIT Research Group. Middle-aged American men at ver low risk of coronary death: 6-year findings on 356,222 screenees of the Multiple Risk Factor Intervention Trial (MRFIT). (abstr.) X World Cong Cardiol Abstract Book, 1986.

3. Tao, SC, Huang, ZD, Tsai, RS, et al. Dietary patterns serum lipids, urinary electrolytes and blood pressure: middle-aged male and female workers and farmers in North and South China. (abstr) X World Cong Cardiol Abstract Book, 1986.

4. Oganov, RG, Chazova, LV, Pavlova, LI, et al. Multifactoral prevention of coronary heart disease in a population. (abstr.) X World Cong Cardiol Abstract Book, 1986.

5. Lipid Research Clinics' Program: (1984) The Lipid Research Clinics' coronary primary prevention trial results. I. Reduction in incidence of coronary heart disease. II. The relationship of reduction in incidence of coronary heart disease to cholesterol lowering. JAMA 261: 351-364.

6. Duffield, RGM, Miller NE, Brunt, JNH, et al. (1983) Treatment of hyperlipidemia retards progression of symptomatic femoral atherosclerosis. A randomized controlled trial. Lancet 2:639-642.

7. Brensike, JF, Levy RI, Kelsey, SF, et al. (1984) Effects of therapy with cholestyramine on progression of coronary arteriosclerosis: results of the NHLBI Type II coronary intervention study. Circ 69:313-324.

8. Artzenius, AC, Kromhout, D, Barth, JD, et al. (1985) Diet, lipoproteins, and progression of coronary atherosclerosis. The Leiden Intervention Trial. N Engl J Med 312:805-811.

9. Consensus Conference. (1985) Lowering blood cholesterol to prevent heart disease. JAMA 253:2080-2086.

10. AHA Special Report. Recommendations for treatment of hyperlipidemia in adults. Circ 1984; 69:1065a-1090a.

11. Gotto, AM Jr, Jones, PH, Scott, LW (1986) The diagnosis and management of hyperlipidemia. DM 32:245-311.

12. Brown, MS, Goldstein, JL (1977) Atherosclerosis: The low density lipoprotein receptor hypothesis. Metabolism 26:1257-1275.

4
The "CNR Progetto Finalizzato Obiettivo 44 Progression e/o regression" an update on studies in Italy

S. Lenzi

The possibility of regression of the atheromatous plaque is a crucial problem of the present atherosclerosis (ATS) investigation (1-6).

Therefore in 1982 in Italy started a Finalized Project, launched by the National Research Council, aimed: a) to detect the age and sex related differences between the ATS lesion prevalence in carotid and ileo-femoral vessels territories; b) to assess if the ATS lesions were correlated to main ATS Risk Factors, namely to the total plasma cholesterol (TC) levels; c) to follow the atheromatous plaques evolution in asymptomatic subjects submitted to a different drug and/or dietetic treatment (9).

Nine Operative Units, from different Italian areas collaborate to the program (Tab.I).

All diagnosis procedures (clinical data records, biochemical determinations, echotomographic and Doppler techniques) were standardized and validated as reported elsewhere (9).
The study was performed by means of non invasive techniques applied on the carotid and ileo-femoral vascular territories (7-8).

TABLE I

CNR Finalized Project on Preventive and Rehabilitative
Medicine
Degenerative Diseases: Arteriosclerosis
OBJECTIVE 44

Town	Operative Unit	Principal Investigator
Bologna	Clinica Medica I	Prof.S.Lenzi (Chairman)
Milano	Farmacologia	Prof.R.Paoletti
Padova	Patologia Medica	Prof.G.Crepaldi
Siena	Anatomia Patologica	Prof.P.Tanganelli
Perugia	Clinica Medica II	Prof.A.Ventura
Roma I	Terapia Medica Sistematica	Prof.A.Bucci
Roma II	Anatomia Patologica	Prof.L.G.Spagnoli
Roma III	Istituto Superiore Sanita'	Prof.A.Menotti
Napoli	Clinica Medica II	Prof.P.Rubba

The second step of the study concerned the evaluation of
the ATS lesion prevalence in different population
samples: geographically randomized free living subjects,
and hyperlipoproteinaemic (HLP) patients.
The enrollment criteria of the free living citizens
comprehended males and females selected from different
Italian geographical areas, aged from 45 to 64 years and
without symptoms of vascular damage.
For the HLP patients the enrollment criteria were to
elect males and females having total plasma cholesterol
concentration more than 239 mg/dl and/or triglyceride
(TG) more than 199 mg/dl (Type IIa, IIb and IV HLP
phenotype), excluding subjects with secondary HLP.
The third step of the Project, regarding to regression or
progression of ATS plaques, consisted in the enrollment
of IIa aand IIb HLP patients which were randomly
allocated in two treatment groups: the first one was
submitted only to prudent diet and the second to diet
plus drugs.
Cholestyramine (8-20 g/day) was the first drug
administered to all the patients of the second group: if,
after 2 months of treatment the TC fall was less than 25%
of the baseline values, fenofibrate (100 mg t.i.d) will
be added, and if the TC values decrease do not reach the
25% decline, acipimox (a nicotinic acid derivative) was
also added.
The study protocol stated a complete check of
biochemical, clinical and instrumental parameters every 2
months for 36 months.

The October 1986 situation is summarized in Tab.II.

TABLE II
Subjects enrolled

	GROUP I (Diet)	GROUP II (Diet + Drugs)
IIa Type	33.3%	33.3%
IIb Type	11.7%	21.5%
Males	45.6%	48.3%
Females	54.3%	51.7%
Age (mean y.)	51.4	51.8
Diet	100.0%	100.0%
DRUGS:		
CHOLESTYRAMINE	----	100.0%
+ FENOFIBRATE	----	46.4%
+ ACIPIMOX	----	23.2%

The maximal time of follow up reached by the patients in October 1986 was 18 months, as illustrated in Tab.III.
At moment it is impossible to drawn definitive conclusions about the regression, progression or steady state of ATS plaques.
However the biochemical data confirm the efficacy of the drug treatment both in IIa and IIb HLP patients: in fact TC mean decrease was 21.7% and TG was in IIb patients of 23.5%.
An evident increase of HDL-Cholesterol mean values was recorded only in drug treated group.
Preliminary data indicate a good compliance in the two groups and a significant reduction of plasma lipids in pharmacological treated subjects.
The next period of follow up will give some answer to the basic problem of the regression of ATS plaques.
At moment it is possible to underline that no one of the subjects admitted to the study underwent to surgery treatment for some vascular complications, nor became symptomatic.
This may confirm, at least, the rationale of the study protocol and the efficacy of both diet and drug treatment.

TABLE III
Follow up

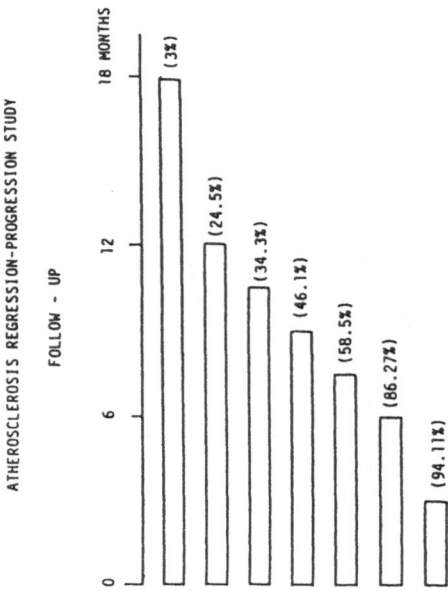

REFERENCES

1) Wissler R.V., Vesselinovitch D.: Regression of atherosclerosis in experimental animals and man.
Mod. Concepts Cardiovasc. Dis. 46, 27, 1977.

2) Malinow M.R.: Atherosclerosis: regression in nonhuman primates (review).
Circulation Res. 46, 311, 1980.

3) Blanckenhorn D.H.: Progression and regression of femoral atherosclerosis in man. In: Paoletti R., Gotto A.M. (Eds.): "Atherosclerosis Reviews". Raven Press, New York, 3, 169, 1978.

4) Olsson A., Erikson U.: Study on femoral artery atheromatous plaque regression by computerized digital angiography.

In: Lenzi S., Descovich G.C. (Eds.): "Atherosclerosis and Cardiovascular Disease". MTP Press, Lancaster, Boston, The Hague, 231, 1984.

5) Mc Gill H.C. Jr.: Characterization of atherosclerotic lesions as they pertain to noninvasive techniques. In: Hegyeli R.J.: "Atherosclerosis Reviews", Raven Press, New York, 10, 1, 1983.

6) Insull W. Jr.: Highlights on regression or progression of the atheromatous plaque. In: Lenzi S., Descovich G.C. (Eds.): "Atherosclerosis and Cardiovascular Disease". MTP Press, Lancaster, Boston The Hague, Dordrecht, 231, 1984.

7) Strandness D.A. Jr.: Invasive and non-invasive techniques in the assessment of the atheromatous plaque. In: Lenzi S., Descovich G.C. (Eds.): "Atheroslcerosis and Cardiovascular Disease". MTP Press, Lancaster, Boston, The Hague, Dordrecht, 237, 1984.

8) Bond M.G., Barnes R.W., Sawyer J.K., Ball M., Riley W.A.: Preliminary data on validation of noninvasive techniques for arterial imaging. In: Hegyeli R.J.: "Atherosclerosis Reviews". Raven Press, New York, 10, 175, 1983.

9) Lenzi S., Bucci A., Crepaldi G., Mancini M., Menotti A., Paoletti R., Spagnoli L.G., Ventura A., Weber G.: The CNR Program of Preventive Medicine - SP4 Objective 44. Non-invasive techniques for the evaluation of atherosclerotic plaque progression or regression. In: Ventura A., Crepaldi G., Senin U.: "Extracoronary atherosclerosis". Karger Verlag, Basel, Munchen, Paris, London, New York, New Delhi, Singapore, Tokyo, Sidney, 83, 1986.

Appendix

This work has been supported by the Italian Consiglio Nazionale delle Ricerche (CNR); Progetto Finalizzato "Medicina Preventiva e Riabilitativa", Sottoprogetto 4 (SP 4), "Arteriosclerosi", Obiettivo 44, "Progressione e Regressione", under contracts 82.02208.56, 83.02612.56, 84.02386.56, 85.00635.56, and 86.01837.56.
The following Operative Units are collaborating:
Bologna (Clinica Medica Generale e Terapia Medica I):

S.Lenzi (Principal Investigator and Chairman), ´ M.S. Benassi, G. Dalmonte, G.C. Descovich, A. Dormi, A. Gaddi, G.L. Magri, G. Mannino, S. Rimondi, Z. Sangiorgi, M. Trianni, F. Zaca´.

Milano (Farmacologia e Farmacognosia): R. Paoletti (Principal Investigator), G. Mora, A. Poli, E. Tremoli.

Padova (Patologia Speciale Medica e Metodologia Clinica): G. Crepaldi (Principal Investigator), A. Calabro´, R. Fellin, L. Lusiani, A. Pagnan, A. Rossi, A. Visona´.

Siena (Anatomia e Istologia Patologica):P. Tanganelli (Principal Investigator), G. Bianciardi, L. Centi, M.T. Novelli, M. Salvi, P. Toti, G. Weber.

Perugia (Clinica Medica Generale e Terapia Medica II): A. Ventura (Principal Investigator), E. Mannarino, L. Moggi, U. Senin, E. Signorini, C. Susta, A. Tazza.

Roma I (Terapia Medica Sistematica): A. Bucci (Principal Investigator), E. Del Monaco, L. Lalloni, G. Ricci, P. Ricci, A.G. Scarno, G.L. Sotis.

Roma II (Anatomia e Istologia Patologica): L.G. Spagnoli (Principal Investigator).

Roma III (Istituto Superiore di Sanita´): A. Menotti (Principal Investigator).

Napoli (Clinica Medica Generale e Terapia Medica II): P.O.F. Rubba (Principal Investigator), A.L. Ferrara, M. Mancini, P. Postiglione, G. Riccardi.

5
Atherosclerosis and the CNR Progetto Finalizzato "Medicina Preventiva e Riabilitativa"
G. Ricci

The Special Project "Preventive Medicine and Rehabilitation" (P.F.-MPR) of the Italian National Research Council (CNR) was started in July 1982 as a second generation Project, as it followed the one which had taken place in the 76-81s under the direction of Prof. L. Bonomo. It articulates in 8 subprojects, with 84 objectives and involves 570 Operational Units, with an average assignement per year of 12.5 billion lire.

Such efforts clearly illustrate how the PF-MPR undoubtedly had the great merit of conveying towards preventive medicine and rehabilitation a large number of researchers as well as a remarkable quota of financial resources.

Since in this volume several data will be presented concerning the PF-MPR, I chose to take into consideration only two sectors: 1) epidemiology of risk factors for atherosclerosis, and 2) intervention and prevention programmes.

At the moment when the PF-MPR Feasibility Study was outlined, we could dispose of the first map of the so-called main risk factors for atherosclerosis in Italy, which had been obtained during the so-called Fase A of the Special Project "Preventive Medicine", Research Line ATS-RF2 (Atherosclerosis, Risk Factors) (1), as well as of the results of the multifactor prevention trial of coronary heart disease, i.e. the Rome Project of Coronary Heart Disease Prevention (PPCC), carried out on a male working population aged 40-59 years (2).

The above Research Line had described for the first time the mean values in Italy of the main risk factors for atherosclerosis (cholesterol and triglycerides, cigarette smoking, physical activity and dietary habits) in nine Italian population samples distributed in Northern, Central and Southern Italy as well as on the Islands. On the whole, we disposed of 6699 subjects of both sexes, aged 20-59 years (populations AB). In such a way it was shown that mean cholesterol levels were largely higher than those deemed desirable,

as well as that in many areas there was a high prevalence of hypercholesterolemic subjects. In addition, such data confirmed the high
frequency of hypertensives, above all of the ones so far ignored,
or,somehow, inadequately treated.Finally,the relevance of smoking was
evidenced, with its high prevalence in women of the younger generation. In practice, thanks to this study, we were able to dispose
for the first time of a useful tool to assess the prevalence of the
main risk factors for atherosclerosis in our country, also important
to the purpose of planning intervention and prevention procedures.

The PPCC data had shown unequivocally that an intervention aiming at modifying the main coronary risk factors, carried out fun-
damentally through programmes of health education, was able to reduce significantly the incidence of coronary heart disease. The
above through the reduction, however modest, of the mean levels of
its risk factors. At that time we did not know yet, as we would
know two years later, that even the prevalence of atherosclerotic
lesions in carotid and femoral beds, assessed through Echo-doppler,
was significantly lower in the group of men treated, as compared
to controls (3).

Such was then the epidemiologic knowledge as well as the intervention and prevention data we could dispose of when the PF-MPR
activity was started.

Table 1 shows the research programmes carried out or under way
within the PF-MPR, concerning the aspects which will be considered
in this report.

Table 1. Programmes of PF-MPR

Epidemiology of risk factors for atherosclerosis:
Project ATS-RF2 -(Ob.43)

Studies on the prevalence of atherosclerotic lesions
assessed by non invasive techniques-(Ob.44)

Intervention programme on populations AB of Project
ATS-RF2 -(Ob.43)

Community control programme: "Distretto Sezze
Controllo Comunitario" - Di.S.Co. Project

Studies on epidemiology of atherosclerosis and its risk factors

One of the aims of Research Line ATS-RF2, Ob.43, which continues
the activity of ATS-RF2 of the previous Special Project, was that
of measuring the levels of known main risk factors, and of adding

Table 2. Age standardized mean differences of risk factors in the pool of men and women belonging to populations AB (1978-79) and populations C (1983-84).
$*p<0.05;$ $**p<0.01;$ $***p<0.001$

	MEN			WOMEN		
	POPULATIONS AB	POPULATIONS C	CHANGE	POPULATIONS AB	POPULATIONS C	CHANGE
	M ± SD	M ± SD	%	M ± SD	M ± SD	%
SERUM CHOLESTEROL (mg/dl)	211.3 ± 46.7	212.0 ± 43.5	+0.3	205.2 ± 43.7	204.6 ± 38.5	-0.3
SYSTOLIC BLOOD PRESSURE (mmHg)	132.4 ± 17.0	131.2 ± 16.4	-0.9**	131.2 ± 18.5	127.3 ± 16.6	-3.0***
DIASTOLIC BLOOD PRESSURE (mmHg)	84.7 ± 10.9	82.9 ± 10.4	-2.1***	83.1 ± 10.9	79.9 ± 10.0	-3.9***
BODY MASS INDEX (kg/m^2)	25.3 ± 3.3	25.4 ± 3.1	+0.5	25.3 ± 4.5	24.6 ± 3.7	-2.8***
PREVALENCE SMOKING (%)	55.0 ± 0.8	50.1 ± 0.7	-8.9***	26.0 ± 0.4	28.2 ± 0.4	+8.5**
N. CIGARETTES/DAY IN ALL SUBJECTS	10.1 ± 11.9	9.4 ± 11.7	-7.1*	2.8 ± 5.8	3.2 ± 6.9	+13.9**

Table 3. Means $\pm$ SD values of total serum cholesterol (mg/dl) in Northern, Central and Southern regions of Italy. Comparison of populations AB (ATS-RF2 project) and C (Ob. 43). *p<0.01; **p<0.001

	POPULATIONS AB (1978-79)	POPULATIONS C (1983-84)	POPULATIONS AB (1978-79)	POPULATIONS C (1983-84)
Northern Italy (Venezia, Padova, Pavia)	215.1 + 44.7 (1201)	217.9 + 42.3 (840)	207.0 + 40.1 (1188)	208.0 + 37.7 (872)
Central Italy (Bologna, Siena, Roma)	202.3 + 53.3 (1057)	218.2 + 43.1** (856)	215.0 + 34.0 (1185)	189.5 + 36.2** (852)
Southern Italy (Napoli, Cagliari, Palermo)	195.8 + 42.0 (921)	201.2 + 38.5* (977)	193.8 + 40.0 (1124)	199.3 + 36.3* (1105)

new ones, such as HDL-cholesterol, apo A-I, apo B, erythrocyte
fatty acid composition, stress, thyroid hormones in nine new samples
of the Italian general population with age ranging from 20 to 59
years. In 1983-84 it was possible to collect information on a sample
of 5548 additional subjects (populations C). Table 2 reports a comparison of the mean values of the main risk factors in populations C
with those of populations AB. Whereas in men it was possible to observe a significant reduction in blood pressure levels as well as
in smoking habits (a datum referring both to prevalence of smokers
and to number of cigarettes smoked per day), in women, beside a significant reduction in blod pressure mean levels and body weight, it
was possible to observe a statistically significant increase of cigarette smoking. Though cholesterol mean values did not turn out to be
significantly different in the two population samples, it was possible to notice a significant worsening in populations C in central and
southern Italy as compared to what had been observed in the same
areas five years before (table 3).

As a whole, the results of the present study show that the unfavorable situation of risk factors in 1978-79, assessed by the Research Line ATS-RF2, still persisted in 1983-84, except for a better
control of hypertension. Thus, the number of coronary heart disease
cases expected in 10 years in populations C is 9.9% and 14.3% lower
in men and women respectively as compared to the one expected in populations AB. Another aspect clearly emerging from the data of Ob.43
is the remarkable worsening of mean cholesterol levels in the Italian areas so far considered "protected" from this risk factor.

As for the new risk factors measured during the screening of
populations C, table 4 reports the first national data of mean HDL-
cholesterol levels in both sexes and in the different age groups.

Table 4. Means $\pm$ SD of HDL-choesterol levels in the pool of men and
women belonging to populations C (1983-84).

AGE CLASSES	M E N	W O M E N
20 - 29	46.9 $\pm$ 10.7 (403)	53.6 $\pm$ 12.1 (421)
30 - 39	46.1 $\pm$ 10.3 (546)	53.4 $\pm$ 12.0 (576)
40 - 49	46.4 $\pm$ 11.9 (665)	53.7 $\pm$ 12.6 (701)
50 - 59	47.8 $\pm$ 12.4 (719)	54.0 $\pm$ 13.3 (780)

Moreover, in a subsample of populations C the erythrocyte fatty acid composition, considered as a tool for the objective evaluation of dietary acids (4) was also determined. Table 5 shows the mean values of polyunsaturated/saturated (P/S) ratio in both sexes in Northern, Central and Southern Italy. Going from South toward North, P/S values show a significantly decreasing trend which confirms the relatively low contents of saturated fatty acids in the diet of southern regions.

Table 5. Means ± SD values of erythrocyte polyunsaturated/saturated fatty acids (P/S) ratios in Northern, Central and Southern Italy. ATS-RF2. Ob. 43
*p<0.05; **p<0.001 vs. Northern Italy
§p<0.05; §§p<0.001 vs. Central Italy

	MEN	WOMEN
Northern Italy (Pavia)	0.80 ± 0.20	0.80 ± 0.20
Central Italy (Bologna, Siena, Roma)	0.90 ± 0.10**	0.85 ± 0.18*
Southern Italy (Napoli, Palermo, Cagliari)	0.94 ± 0.26**§	0.94 ± 0.26**§§

Another PF-MPR Research Line on the epidemiologic aspects of atherosclerosis is worthy being mentioned : the study of the prevalence of atherosclerotic lesions in extracoronary beds through non invasive techniques (Ob.44).

Table 6 shows the data obtained so far and referring to 716 subjects of both sexes with age ranging from 45 to 55 years. It is important to keep in mind that these are the first Italian data systematically obtained in population samples, for which reason Italy holds a leading position in this field.

Table 6. Prevalence of extracoronary atherosclerotic lesions in free living subjects (n=716).

	MEN %	WOMEN %
CAROTID BED	18.9	19.4
ILEO-FEMORAL BED	15.5	--
Age range	45-55 years	

Such is then the situation we intended to modify. To this purpose PF-MPR followed two different approaches:
1) a multifactor intervention trial on coronary heart disease prevention (Fase B of ATS-RF2,Ob.43) which, in practice, applies to the general population the intervention methodologies already tested and validated on working population samples;
2) a comprehensive community-based intervention programme (Di.S.Co. Project).

The aim of the first intervention trial was that of bringing about in populations AB a modification of risk factors for coronary heart disease, both through health education programmes covering all subjects and through a more intensive intervention on subjects at a higher risk (that is with cholesterol levels >240 mg/dl, blood pressure levels >160 and/or 95 mmHg, or smoking more than 10 cigarettes per day). The guidelines of the intervention programme were the following: 1) dietary information aiming at reducing consumption of total fat, saturated fats and cholesterol, and increasing consumption of polyunsaturated ones; 2) intensive pharmacological treatment with the aid of ambulatorial services and recording service for hypertensives; 3) recommendations to stop smoking. To evaluate the intervention effectiveness a comparison was made between the baseline data and the final screening results of populations AB. Such comparison, whose results have been already published (5),was carried out in two ways:
1) comparison of mean levels of all participants at entry screening with the means of all those participating in the final one;
2) comparison of entry vs.final means of those participating in both entry and final screenings.
In short, although the first comparison may suggest that the low participation rates observed at the final screening (between 24% and 72%) can be ascribed to autoselection, it was possible to notice a significant reduction of cigarette smoking in males and of blood pressure in both sexes, and an increase of cholesterol, triglycerides, body weigth and blood glucose in both sexes. The picture changes rather drastically when considering only the subjects who took part in both screenings, who were obviously most motivated. A significant reduction of all risk factors (except for body weight and triglycerides) can be observed.

More over, a comparison of males of populations AB aged 40-59 years (who attended both screenings) with a reference group (randomly selected from the PPCC control population), offers a very favourable picture since in the former a 35% reduction of the estimated coronary risk is observed (table 7), which is in line with what obtained in other intervention trials on coronary heart disease.

Table 7. Estimated coronary risk changes as a consequence of variations in serum cholesterol, blood pressure and cigarette smoking in men aged 49-59 years. Risk estimated by multiple logistic function obtained from the Italian data of the Seven Countries Study.

Area	N	Changes %
Venezia-Marghera	135	- 10.1
Mirano	162	- 4.3
Stradella-Broni	95	- 18.3
Bologna-Murri	163	- 19.1
Sovicille	123	- 21.3
Roma-Tuscolano	97	- 4.9
Mugnano	31	+ 2.9
Sinnai	81	- 5.7
Trabia	73	- 22.8
Pool 9 areas	960	- 12.7
PPCC controls	369	+ 22.6

As a matter of fact, this result shows that the intervention programme was accepted by a sheer two thirds of the population initially enrolled, and a preliminary analysis indicates an unsatisfactory participation rate: there was a higher participation of subjects at high risk, of the less young and of women. More over, interventions on an individual basis - equivalent to the traditional relationship doctor-patient - were liked most. Therefore, this approach proved to be beneficial to a limited number of subjects, and I think that coronary heart disease-oriented intervention programmes could better fit a working population. For such reason particular attention was given to the community medicine project.

The Project "Distretto Sezze Controllo Comunitario" (Di.S.Co.), is a community - based project intending to: 1) modify multipredictable risk factors; 2) identify subjects at high risk; 3) reorient health services towards prevention; and 4) bring about a reproducible intervention model not too expensive. It is based on the theory of "multipredictability" of several risk factors and on an intervention providing:
- systematic collection of epidemiological information;
- screenings to the purpose of measuring risk factors;
- detection of ill people who ignore to be such;
- treatment of some risk conditions or factors in the community and large portions of the population;

- activation of mass health education measures;
- organization of therapeutic and rehabilitation activities.

Our Project has interested other bodies and institutions beside the Institute of Systematic Medical Therapy of the Rome University "La Sapienza", where the Operational Unit of the CNR holds its seat:
- Italian National Health Institute;
- Italian National Cancer Institute "Regina Elena", Rome;
- U.S.L. LT/4 (Local Health Service -Latina);
- Municipalities of Bassiano, Roccagorga and Sezze

In short, it covers an intervention area including the whole population (from 20 years upward) of the above mentioned towns for a total of about 25.000 subjects, and a control area formed by the inhabitants of the Priverno district (totalling about 12.000 subjects). Both these areas are part of the Latina area of the MONICA Project, whose aim is that of monitoring mortality trends in about 700.000 individuals aged 25-74 years, and whose activity is likely to continue till 1990. Before starting the intervention activities, in 1983 the screening of a representative subsample of the intervention as well as of the control populations was carried out. In this examination additional parameters, such as blood glucose, blood cell count, hemoglobin, hematocrit, uric acid, serum creatinine, respiratory function were measured, and information on habits of taking preventive measures against cancer was collected.

The participation rates at baseline screenings were 54.0% and 65.0% in the intervention, and 72.2% and 77.5% in the control population, in men and women respectively.

The mean values of the main risk factors in the population samples of the intervention and control areas, as compared with those obtained by ATS-RF2, both in males and females, are shown in table 8 and 9. Although mean cholesterol levels (in males) and diastolic blood pressure levels as well as the number of cigarettes smoked per day (in females) were respectively higher and lower at Priverno, the two samples turned out to be rather well comparable.

Through the cooperation with local social and health structures it was possible to initiate intervention activities, consisting in:
- preparation and distribution of printed material;
- creation of counselling units;
- organization of conferences and exhibitions;
- theoretical and practical training course for teachers and health operators;
- pilot programme for the informatization of general practitioners and for the adoption of diagnostic as well as therapeutic protocols.

The following are examples of some of the intervention activities carried out or under way:

Table 8. Means + SD and prevalence of major risk factors for atherosclerosis in the intervention (Distretto Sezze) and control (Priverno) areas of Di.S.Co. Comparison with data of ATS-RF2 Project. BMI = body mass index (weight (kg)/height (m)^2; SBP and DBP = systolic and diastolic blood pressure.

*p<0.05; **p<0.01; Sezze vs Priverno

RISK FACTORS	DISTRETTO SEZZE	PRIVERNO	CNR ATS-RF2	
	M ± SD	M ± SD	M ± SD	(RANGE)
BMI	26.4 ± 3.7	26.2 ± 3.5	25.3 ± 3.3	(24.8-26.2)
TOTAL CHOLESTEROL (mg/dl)	216.0 ± 46.5	220.6 ± 47.1*	211.3 ± 46.7	(188.1-231.8)
HDL-CHOLESTEROL (mg/dl)	48.6 ± 13.3	47.5 ± 12.5	------	------
TOTAL SERUM TRIGLYCERIDES (mg/dl)	151.6 ± 126.6	160.9 ± 113.5	132.9 ± 114.9	(119.4-153.5)
SBP (mmHg)	136.7 ± 21.0	135.5 ± 20.8	132.2 ± 17.0	(124.2-138.6)
DBP (mmHg)	87.1 ± 12.3	85.3 ± 11.6**	84.7 ± 10.9	(81.2-88.4)
N. CIGARETTES SMOKED/DAY	10.3 ± 11.6	8.6 ± 10.5**	10.1 ± 12.0	(8.1-14.7)
HYPERCHOLESTEROLEMIA	29.1%	36.2%	27.9%	
HYPERTRIGLYCERIDEMIA	26.8%	36.3%	20.3%	
HYPERTENSION	28.4%	28.1%	22.4%	
SMOKERS	54.5%	53.9%	55.0%	

Table 9. Means + SD prevalence of major risk factors for atherosclerosis in the intervention (Distretto Sezze) and control (Priverno) areas of Di.S.Co.. Comparison with data of ATS-RF2 Project. BMI = body mass index (weight (kg)/height (m)^2); SBP and DBP = systolic and diastolic blood pressure.
**p<0.01; ***p<0.001 Sezze vs Priverno

RISK FACTORS	DISTRETTO SEZZE	PRIVERNO	CNR ATS-RF2	
	M + SD	M + SD	M + SD	(RANGE)
BMI	28.6 + 5.1	27.3 + 5.1***	25.3 + 4.5	(23.9-27.9)
TOTAL CHOLESTEROL (mg/dl)	214.7 + 44.8	214.5 + 46.6	205.3 + 43.7	(181.5-226.2)
HDL-CHOLESTEROL (mg/dl)	53.9 + 12.1	53.0 + 12.0	-----	------
TOTAL SERUM TRIGLYCERIDES (mg/dl)	123.4 + 81.6	122.9 + 92.9	99.0 + 65.4	(87.5-115.3)
SBP (mmHg)	138.2 + 25.8	132.1 + 23.1***	131.2 + 18.2	(121.4-143.5)
DBP (mmHg)	87.0 + 13.2	82.8 + 11.9***	83.1 + 10.9	(79.0-85.8)
N. CIGARETTES/DAY	1.6 + 4.1	1.1 + 3.5**	2.8 + 5.8	(0.75-5.44)
HYPERCHOLESTEROLEMIA	25.9%	32.1%	25.2%	
HYPERTRIGLYCERIDEMIA	17.9%	26.0%	9.4%	
HYPERTENSION	33.4%	26.2%	23.4%	
SMOKERS	17.1%	15.6%	26.0%	

- preparation of diets for children attending kindergarten;
- training of schoolchildren to blood pressure measurement;
- informatization of five doctors operating in the three towns of the district;
- briefing and training of diabetic patients;
- enhancing existing services for the early diagnosis of woman cancer;
- conferences and discussions in elementary and secondary school with the paticipation of teachers, families and social and health workers;
- "smoking bubbles": one TV and two radio broadcasts dealing with smoking (interviews of Sezze schoolchildren);
- booklets of a "Health Series".

The intervention programme undertaken is a complex and comprehensive one, which cannot disregard local living habits and is strictly linked with the existing health service (though oriented towards prevention), with the effect of stimulating the general public to take a more active interest in health. To assess the effectivenes of intervention, a final screening of representative subsamples of the intervention and control areas is being planned at the moment.

A Special Project is a research project, where the Director is not only in charge of following research activities but also of making his presence felt in all fields relating to its specific interests. This was certainly true of PF-MPR and I think it is much to the point to mention here the Italian Consensus Conference - Lowering Blood Cholesterol to Reduce Coronary Hearth Disease - which took place in June 1986 in Rome, with the participation of the Italian Scientific Community, to the purpose of examining the guidelines extablished by the US Consensus Conference, of analysing Italian data to take up a position regarding this matter, and proposing possible intervention strategies. The Italian Consensus Conference produced a document (6), with large circulation, which recommended systematic intervention for cholesterol control, specifying its objectives and levels. In addition, it contains several suggestions regarding health, and stresses the importance of a national health education programme on cholesterol. It is now being examined by Ministry of Health to the purpose of appointing a Committee for a National Cholesterol Project, similar to the NHI one.

REFERENCES

1) Gruppo di Ricerca ATS-RF2 (1980). I fattori di rischio dell'arteriosclerosi in Italia. Giorn.Ital.Cardiol.10,suppl.3,1
2) Gruppo di Ricerca del Progetto Romano di Prevenzione della Cardiopatia Coronarica (1982). Il Progetto Romano di Prevenzione della Cardiopatia Coronarica. Risultati finali. Giorn.Ital.Cardiol.12,541

3) Bucci.A..Conti.R..Lalloni.L..Scarno.A.G.,Stefanutti,C.,Ricci,G.
(1984). The Rome Project of Coronary Heart Disease Prevention(PPCC):
B-scan detection of atherosclerotic lesions. A subsample population
study. CVD Epidemiology Newsletter 36,115.

4) Angelico,F.,Amodeo,P.,Borgogelli,C.,Cantafora,A.,Montali,A.,Ricci
G.(1980). Red blood cell fatty acids composition in a sample of italian middle-age men on free diet. Nutr.Met.24,148.

5) The Research Group for Atherosclerosis Risk Factors (ATS-RF2)
(1986). Three year intervention on risk factors for atherosclerosis
in the Italian Nine Communities Study. Clin.Ter.Cardiovasc.3,151

6) Consensus Conference Italiana - Abbassare la Colesterolemia per
Ridurre la Cardiopatia Coronarica. Roma 11-12 giugno,1986.

6
Cardiac and vascular surgery: results, perspectives and hopes
M.E. DeBakey

Despite the sporadic accumulation of knowledge about cardiovascular diseases beginning with antiquity, few advances were made in the development of effective treatment until several decades ago. As late as 1940, treatment was based primarily on indirect methods of increasing blood flow by vasodilation through drugs or sympathectomy [1]. At the turn of the century, extensive experimental studies demonstrated the feasibility of cardiac and renal transplants, as well as of excision of arterial segments and restoration of continuity by end-to-end anastomosis or by insertion of arterial grafts. To be sure, a few patients with aneurysms or peripheral arterial injuries were successfully treated in this way. In 1923, Leriche [2] described aorto-iliac occlusive atherosclerotic disease (Leriche's syndrome) and predicted that excision of the diseased segment and its replacement with an aortic graft would be the ideal treatment for this condition. It was almost 30 years later, however, before this prediction became a reality when Oudot [3] performed the procedure for the first time (1951).

A number of factors were responsible for this long delay in the successful clinical application of these earlier, well-developed principles of vascular surgery: the development and maturation of certain ancillary measures such as induction of anesthesia, readily available and safe blood transfusions, effective chemotherapy to control infection, and most important, safe and readily available arteriography. Haschek and Lindenthal [4] first demonstrated the feasibility of arteriography in 1896, shortly after Roentgen's discovery of roentgen-ray, by injecting a radiopaque substance into the arteries of an amputated hand, but a safe and effective radiopaque solution was developed only after almost fifty years of extensive research. Perhaps the most important event in the development of vascular surgery was the advent of arteriography, which provides accurate and precise visualization of the atherosclerotic process.

Certain clinically successful surgical procedures performed shortly after World War II stimulated more widespread interest in experimental and clinical studies of aneurysmal and occlusive arterial disease: successful surgical treatment of aortic coarctation [5], successful repair with aortic homografts after excision of coarctation [6,7], first successful application of this method in a patient with atherosclerotic occlusive disease of the aorto-iliac segment (Leriche's syndrome) [3], and first successful surgical procedure for aneurysm of the abdominal aorta [8]. During the next few years, we successfully performed this procedure for all types of aneurysms of the thoracic aorta, including dissecting aneurysms [9-13].

The early aortic and arterial homografts that were used to replace excised segments of aneurysmal and occlusive disease had several disadvantages: their limited availability, inconvenience of procurement and preservation, and subsequent deterioration. Intensive investigations with various fabrics made of Dacron, Orlon, Teflon, and Nylon were therefore undertaken by a number of researchers. From our studies [14] we concluded that Dacron was the most desirable fabric for this purpose. Since we first used it in a patient in 1954, several decades of experience have confirmed this original observation [15].

Other significant technical contributions made during this early period included thromboendarterectomy devised by dos Santos [16] in 1947. When he tried to perform thrombectomy in the femoral artery of some patients, he noted that the superimposed thrombus along with the atheroma could be peeled away easily from the remaining wall of the artery by finding the proper cleavage plane. In certain types of well-localized atheromatous occlusive disease, this procedure has proved to be highly successful.

Perhaps a more important development, because it is more widely applicable, is the bypass principle devised originally by Kunlin [17] of France. He observed that the atherosclerotic occlusive process in the superficial femoral artery was well-localized with a fairly normal popliteal artery distal to the occlusion. He reasoned that he should be able to restore circulation around the obstructed segment by attaching a vein-graft to an opening in the artery above and below the occlusion and thus shunt blood around the obstructed segment. His successful performance of this procedure in a patient with such an occlusive process in the superficial femoral artery established the bypass principle and its application for a wide variety of occlusive arterial diseases. A final useful technical contribution to vascular surgery was patch-graft angioplasty [18].

The availability of these surgical techniques to restore normal circulation and arteriography to visualize precisely the arterial bed and the location of the occlusive atheroma resulted in accumulation of considerable clinical experience that provided important concepts about atherosclerosis. It has now been established that the disease tends to assume characteristic anatomic, pathologic, and clinical patterns. Of particular therapeutic significance is the fact that it often tends to be segmental with relatively normal proximal and distal arterial beds.

These patterns have been classified into four major categories according to the anatomic site and distribution of the disease in the major arterial beds as follows [19]: the coronary arterial bed, the major branches of the aortic arch, the major branches of the abdominal aorta, and the terminal abdominal aorta and its major branches. In each category the occlusion may be incomplete or complete, and in most patients the disease is segmental and well localized. The proximal, mid-proximal, or distal parts of the arterial bed may be affected. Occlusions of the proximal and mid-proximal arterial beds, which are the more common forms, are amenable to surgical correction.

Analysis of our long-term follow-up studies after surgical treatment, including angiography, over a period of three decades indicates that the rates of progression may be classified into three groups: rapid rate of progression, usually within 1 to 4 years from insignificant stenosis (less than 50%) to significant stenosis (more than 50%); moderate rate of progression, usually within 5 to 8 years; and slow rate of progression, usually more than 8 years.

The urgent need for an effective mechanical assistor to support the failing human heart has been well recognized, and the feasibility of temporary mechanical cardiac assistance has been firmly established. An effective method of prolonged cardiac assistance, however, remains to be found.

Concerted efforts must be directed toward improving current techniques of circulatory assistance to enhance their clinical applicability. In the future, attention should be focussed on development of biocompatible materials and a pulsatile output that is controlled by biosensors such as the bioreceptor system.

In the broader aspect of treatment of heart disease, the artificial heart must be considered a temporary expedient. The ideal solution to the control of this disabling disease is, of course, prevention. Until a complete understanding of the cause of heart disease is achieved, and effective prophylactic measures are established, development of partial and total mechanical cardiac assistance remains an appropriate approach to atherosclerotic coronary arterial disease.

During the past three decades, considerable progress has been made in the surgical treatment of cardiovascular disease. Assessment of many of these disorders by noninvasive techniques (radionuclide scanning, ultrasound, and computerized tomography) should result in earlier diagnosis of cardiovascular disease and improved results of surgical treatment as well as provide more accurate follow-up evaluation of the patient's cardiovascular condition. Continuing research should eventuate in the development of an artificial prosthesis suitable for replacement of small vessels. Intensifying our research to find the causes of atherosclerosis and to devise methods to prevent or control it should enhance the late surgical results in patients with atherosclerosis. The next decade thus holds promise of further improvements in the results of surgical treatment for cardiovascular disease.

REFERENCES

1. Ochsner A and DeBakey M (1940). Peripheral vascular disease: a critical survey of its conservative and radical treatment. Surg Gynec & Obstet, 70, 1058-1072

2. Leriche R (1923). Des oblitérations artérielles hautes (oblitération de la terminaison de l'aorte) comme causes des insuffisances circulatoires des membres inférieurs. Bull Mem Soc Chir (Paris), 49, 1404-1406

3. Oudot J (1951). La greffe vasculaire dans les thromboses du carrefour aortique. Presse med, 59, 234-236

4. Haschek VE & Lindenthal OT (1896). Ein Beitrag zur praktischen Verwerthung der Photographie nach Röntgen. Wien Klin Wochenschr, 9, 63-64

5. Craafoord C & Nylin G (1945). Congenital coarctation of the aorta and its surgical treatment. J Thorac Surg, 14, 347-361

6. Gross RE (1945). Surgical correction for coarctation of the aorta. Surgery, 18, 673-678

7. Hufnagel CA (1947). Preserved homologous arterial transplants. Bull Am Coll Surg, 32, 231

8. Dubost C, Allary M & Oeconomos N (1952). Resection of an aneurysm of the abdominal aorta. Arch Surg, 64, 405-408

9. DeBakey ME & Cooley DA (1953). Successful resection of aneurysm of thoracic aorta and replacement by graft. JAMA, 152, 673-676

10. DeBakey ME, Cooley DA & Creech O Jr (1955). Surgical considerations of dissecting aneurysm of the aorta. Ann Surg, 142, 586-612

11. DeBakey ME, Creech O Jr & Morris GC Jr (1956). Aneurysm of thoraco-abdominal aorta involving the celiac, superior mesenteric, and renal arteries. Report of four cases treated by resection and homograft replacement. Ann Surg, 144, 549-573

12. DeBakey ME et al. (1957). Successful resection of fusiform aneurysm of aortic arch with replacement by homograft. Surg Gynec & Obstet, 105, 657-664

13. DeBakey et al. (1982). Dissection and dissecting aneurysms of the aorta: twenty-year follow-up of five hundred twenty-seven patients treated surgically. Surgery, 92, 1118-1134

14. DeBakey ME et al. (1958). Clinical application of a new flexible knitted Dacron arterial substitute. Am Surg, 24, 862-869

15. DeBakey ME (1979). The development of vascular surgery, Am J Surg, 137, 697-738

16. dos Santos JC (1947). Sur la désobstruction des thromboses artérielles anciennes, Mém Acad de chir, 73, 409-411

17. Kunlin J (1951). Le traitement de l'ischémie artéritique par la greffe veineuse longue. Rev chir, 70, 206-235

18. DeBakey ME et al. (1962). Patch graft angioplasty in vascular surgery. J Cardiovasc Surg, 3, 106-141

19. DeBakey ME, Lawrie GM & Glaeser DH (1985). Patterns of atherosclerosis and their surgical significance. Ann Surg, 201, 115-131

APOPROTEINS -
CLINICAL ASPECTS

7
Genetic basis of apolipoprotein disorders
L. Chan, S. Datta, Chi-Cheng Luo and
Wen-Hsiun Li

INTRODUCTION

The protein components of plasma lipoproteins are known as apolipoproteins. The major function of apolipoproteins is lipid transport in the intravascular and extravascular compartments. Many apolipoproteins have, in addition, acquired highly specialized functions. For example, apolipoprotein B (apoB) is an important determinant in the binding of LDL to the LDL receptor [1]. ApoE also appears to confer receptor binding capability to lipoprotein particles to both the LDL receptor [2] and a specific apoE receptor [3]. ApoC-II activates lipoprotein lipase and is important in chylomicron and VLDL metabolism [4,5]. Conversely, apoC-III seems to inhibit the apoC-II activation of lipoprotein lipase [6]. It also modulates the uptake of apoE-containing lipoproteins by liver cells. ApoA-I [7] and possibly apoC-I [8], apoE [9] and apoA-IV [10] are thought to activate lecithin-cholesterol acyltransferase.
     Our laboratory has been interested in the molecular biology of apolipoprotein synthesis for many years. We have studied the structural organization and chromosomal localization of a number of apolipoprotein genes. In this communication, we have further analyzed the structures of some recently cloned cDNAs for some canine and rat apolipoproteins. Our analysis provide interesting information on the evolution of apolipoprotein genes and the possible structural constraints on apolipoprotein structure.

MATERIALS AND METHODS

Molecular Cloning of Dog Apolipoprotein cDNAs

Two dog liver cDNA libraries were constructed in pUC18 and in λgt11. Canine apoC-II and apoC-III cDNA clones were identified by cross hybridization of these clones to 32 P-labelled cloned human apoC-II and apoC-III cDNAs. DNAs from these clones were isolated by standard procedures. They were sequenced by the dideoxynucleotide chain termination technique of Sanger et al. [11], following subcloning into the M13 vectors mp18 and mp19.

Genomic and cDNA Structures of Human Apolipoproteins

Our laboratory has reported the structures of th following cDNAs: Human apoB, apoA-I, apoA-II and apoC-II, and rat apoA-II; we also isolated and characterized the genomic sequences for human apoA-II and apoC-II [12, 13]. In our analysis, we have used information from our laboratory as well as published information from other laboratories on the cDNA and genomic structures of other apolipoprotein genes [for additional references, see 14].

Statistical Analysis of Nucleotide Substitution Rates

In estimating the number of substitutions between two genes, we have used the method of Li et al [15].

RESULTS

Isolation and Sequence Analysis of Cloned Dog ApoC-II and ApoC-III cDNAs

The pUC-18 library was initially screened. Three positive clones for apoC-II and four positive clones for apoC-III were isolated after 40,000 colonies were screened using duplicated filters. The clones were purified by secondary screening. Confirmation of the clones was obtained initially by isolating the inserts, fractionating them on an agarose gel and hybridizing them with the respective human probes on the dried gel. The largest of the positive clones, designated pC-II and pC-III, corresponding to the canine apolipoproteins C-II and C-III, respectively, were then sequenced by the dideoxynucleotide chain termination technique of Sanger et al. [11] following subcloning in the M13 vectors mp18 and mp19.

Both of the plasmid clones turned out to be incomplete. They were thus used for screening the dog liver cDNA library cloned in λgt11. Since this screening was with homologous DNA, the conditions of hybridization were maintained at the standard temperature of 68°C under standard salt concentrations. The largest of the positive clones from the λgt11 library were full-length clones. They were named λC-II and λC-III respectively for the two apolipoproteins. There were completely sequenced.

Genomic Structures of ApoA-II and ApoC-II

In our laboratory, we have determined the structural organization and nucleotide sequence of the chromosomal genes for apoA-II and apoC-II. These 2 genes both have 3 introns and 4 exons. The structural organization of these genes has also been studied by electron microscopic analysis of RNA-DNA hybrids. Both biochemical and morphological studies indicate that the locations of the introns are quite similar to those in other apolipoprotein genes.

Sequence of Human apoB-100

Our laboratory has recently reported the complete sequence of human apoB-100 [16, 17]. The cDNA codes for a protein of 4563 amino acid residues, including a 27-amino acid signal peptide. The sequence is characterized by high hydrophobicity, being 0.916 kcal per residue. Secondary structure analysis indicates that apoB-100 contains 43%, 21% and 20% α-helical, β-sheet, and random structures, and 16% β-turns, respectively.

DISCUSSION

Genomic Structure of Human Apolipoproteins

The genomic structures of a number of human apolipoprotein have been determined [for references, see 14]. The availability of the structural organization of six human apolipoprotein genes (apoA-I, apoC-III, apoA-II, apoC-II, apoA-IV and apoE) has allowed us to formulate some generalizations on apolipoprotein genomic structure which may be of functional, structural, and evolutionary significance.

All apolipoprotein genes have a general structural organization of 4 exon-3 intron. The locations of the individual introns are remarkably similar. Intron 1 is always in the 5' untranslated region of the gene, intron 2 is located close to the signal peptidase cleavage site, and intron 3 interrupts the mature peptide coding region within 200 nucleotides from the second intron. The sizes of exons 1, 2, and 3 are quite similar from one gene to the next. The difference in length in the individual mRNAs involves mainly exon 4. ApoA-IV differs from the other apolipoproteins in that it has only 2 introns which correspond to introns 2 and 3 of the other genes. Analysis of DNA and amino acid sequence data have indicated that all apolipoproteins contain multiple repeats of 22 amino acids, each of which is a tandem array of two 11-mers [14, 19-21]. Based on this observation, we have concluded that the apolipoprotein genes have evolved from a primordial gene through multiple partial (internal) and complete gene duplications [14].

Internal Repeats and Rates of Evolution of Apolipoproteins

Our laboratory has defined the internal repeats found in all mammalian apolipoproteins [14]. We could also align the sequences of apolipoproteins from various species. Thus the availability of sequences of apoA-I, apoA-II, apoA-IV, apoE, and apoC-II in two species, and of apoC-III in three species, has allowed us to examine the rate of nucleotide substitution in the individual genes, to speculate on the rate of evolution of these genes in humans, rat, and dog, and to infer the stringency of the structural constraints on apolipoprotein functional domains. It appears that the apolipoprotein genes have all evolved rapidly, at a rate considerably faster than that of β-globin [15]. Certain domains, such as the receptor-binding region of apoE, seem to be much better conserved than others [14]. Finally, the rate of evolution of rat apoC-III seems to be several times faster in rat than in humans or dog.

Structure and Evolution of ApoB-100

Analysis of apoB-100 sequence also reveals that the protein is almost entirely made up of internal repeats [17]. Compared to other apolipoproteins these repeats are generally much larger, many spanning over 100 residues. The relationship of these repeats to the 11-residue repeats found in other apolipoproteins is currently under study. Finally, using synthetic peptides of a specific region of apoB-100, we have identified a potential LDL receptor-binding domain (residues 3345-3381) which is capable of binding to the LDL receptor and suppressing 3-hydroxy-3-methyl-glutanyl coenzyme A reductase activities in cultured human fibroblasts. When additional apoB-100 sequences from other species become available, it will be interesting to study the rate of nucleotide substitution in the various subdomains of apoB-100 and to infer the structure-function relationships and the structural constraints of individual subdomains in this important protein.

ACKNOWLEDGEMENT

This work was supported by grants GM-30998 and HL-27341 for a Specialized Center of Research in Arterioscleroses from the U.S. National Institutes of Health, and a grant from the National Foundation March of Dimes.

REFERENCES

1. Brown, MS and Goldstein, JL (1986). A Receptor-Mediated Pathway for Cholesterol Homeostasis. Science 232, 34-47.
2. Innerarity, TL and Mahley, RW (1978). Enhanced Binding by Cultured Human Fibroblasts of Apo-E-Containing Lipoproteins as Compared with Low Density Lipoproteins. Biochemistry 17, 1440-1447.
3. Sherrill, BC, Innerarity, TL and Mahley, RW (1980). Rapid Hepatic Clearance of the Canine Lipoproteins Containing Only the E apoprotein by a High Affinity Receptor. J. Biol. Chem. 255, 1804-1807.
4. LaRosa, JC, Levy, RI, Herbert, P, Lux, SE and Frederickson, DS (1970). A Specific Apoprotein Activator for Lipoprotein Lipase. Biochem. Biophys. Res. Commun. 41, 57-62.
5. Breckenridge, WC, Little, JA, Steiner, G, Chow, A and Poapot, M (1978). Hypertriglyceridemia Associated with Deficiency of Apolipoprotein c-II. N. Engl. J. Med. 298, 1265-1273.
6. Brown, WV and Baginsky, ML (1972). Inhibition of Lipoprotein Lipase by an Apoprotein of Human Very Low Density Lipoprotein. Biochem. Biophys. Res. Commun. 46, 375-382.

7. Fielding, CJ, Shore, VG and Fielding, PE (1972). A Protein Cofactor of Lecithin: Cholesterol Acyltransferase. Biochem. Biophys. Res. Commun. 46, 1493-1498.

8. Soutar, AK, Garner, CW, Baker, HN, Sparrow, JT, Jackson, RL, Gotto, AM, Jr and Smith, LC (1975). Effect of the Human Plasma Apolipoproteins and Phosphatidylcholine Acyl Donor on the Activity of Lecithin: Cholesterol Acyltransferase. Biochemistry 14, 3057-3064.

9. Zorich, N, Jones, A and Pownall, HJ (1985). Activation of Lecithin Cholesterol Acyltransferase by Human Apolipoprotein E in Discoidal Complexes with Lipids. J. Biol. Chem. 260, 8831-8837.

10. Steinmetz, A and Uterman, G (1985). Activation of Lecithin: Cholesterol Acyltransferase by Human Apolipoprotein A-IV. J. Biol. Chem. 200, 2258-2264.

11. Sanger, F, Coulson, A, Barrell, B, Smith, A and Roe, B (1980). Cloning in Single-stranded Bacteriophage as an Aid to Rapid DNA Sequencing. J. Mol. Biol. 143, 161-178.

12. Tsao, YK, Wei, CF, Robberson, DL, Gotto, AM, Jr and Chan, L (1985). Isolation and Characterization of the Human Apolipoprotein A-II Gene. J. Biol. Chem. 260, 15222-15231.

13. Wei, CF, Tsao, YK, Robberson, DL, Gotto, AM, Jr, Brown, K and Chan, L (1985). The Structure of the Human Apolipoprotein C-II Gene. J. Biol. Chem. 260, 15211-15221.

14. Luo, C-C, Li, W-H, Moore, MN and Chan, L (1986). Structure and Evolution of the Apolipoprotein Multigene Family. J. Mol. Biol. 187, 325-340.

15. Li, W-H, Wu, C-I and Luo, C-C (1985). A New Method for Estimating Synonymous and Non Synonymous Rates of Nucleotide Substitution Considering the Relative Likelihood of Nucleotide and Codon Changes. Mol. Biol. Evol. 2, 150-174.

16. Chen, SH, Yang, CY, Chen, PF, Setzer, D, Tanimura, M, Li, W-H, Gotto, AM, Jr and Chan, L (1986). The Complete cDNA and Amino Acid Sequence of Human Apolipoprotein B-100. J. Biol. Chem. 261, 12918-12921.

17. Yang, CY, Chen, SH, Gianturco, SH, Bradley, WA, Spanow, JT, Tanimura, M, Li, WH, Sparrow, DA, DeLoof, H, Rosseneu, M, Lee, FS, Gu, ZW, Gotto, AM and Chan, L (1986). Sequence, Structure, Receptor-binding Domains, and Internal Repeats of Human Apolipoprotein B-100. Nature 323, 738-742.

18. McLachlan, AD (1977). Repeated Helical Pattern in Apolipoprotein A-I. Nature 267, 465-466.

19. Fitch, WM (1977). Phylogenies Constrained by the Crossover Process as Illustrated by Human Hemoglobins and a Thirteen-cycle, Eleven-Amino Acid Repeat in Human Apolipoprotein A-I. Genetics 86, 623-644.

20. Karathanasis, SK, Zannis, VI and Breslow, JL (1983). Isolation and Characterization of the Human Apolipoprotein A-I Gene. Proc. Natl. Acad. Sci. USA 80, 6147-6151.

21. Boguski, MS, Elshourbagy, N, Taylor, JM and Gordon, JI (1984). Rat Apolipoprotein A-IV Contains 13 Tandem Repetitions of a 22-Amino Acid Segment with Amphipathic Helical Potential. Proc. Natl. Acad. Sci. USA 81, 5021-5025.

8
Apolipoproteins in differential diagnosis of patients at high risk for atherosclerosis

G.M. Kostner, E. Marth and K.H. Pfeiffer

INTRODUCTION

The multifactorial ethiology of atherogenesis has been documented in many studies and review articles. Recently, 246 risk factors for atherosclerosis have been compiled (1) and it was of interest to note that many of them were directly or indirectly connected with abnormalities of the lipid metabolism. To mention only few of the pathophysiological events leading to deposition of lipids or other atheromatous material, the monocyte macrophage system seems to play a key role with that respect. In addion, derangements of the platelet reactivity, unfavorable prostacyclin/ thromboxan ratios, excess catabolism of lipoproteins via the scavenger- or low affinity receptor pathway among others are causally linked with atherosclerosis, causing myocardial infarction (MI) peripheral vascular diseases (PVD) cerebrovascular diseases (CVD) and stroke.

The Normal Lipoprotein Metabolism

The human plasma lipoproteins comprise a complex system of macromolecules designated to solubilize, transport and metabolize neutral lipids (triglycerides and cholesteryl esters :TG,CE) as well as the surface lipids free cholesterol (FC) and phospholipids (PL). This complicated task is managed by apolipoproteins, enzymes and transfer/exchange proteins. Today, there are more than 20 different apolipoproteins known (2) with partly different and partly similar function. With that respect it is of interest to note that evolutionary, most if not all of the apo-Lp have emerged from an ancestren gene by gene duplication, crossing over and partial mutation. Thus it is not much of surprise that the lack or a low concentration of one apo-Lp does not necessarily lead to lethal or fatal pathophysiological events. In a simplificated view, the Lp metabolism can be summarized as follows (Fig.1):

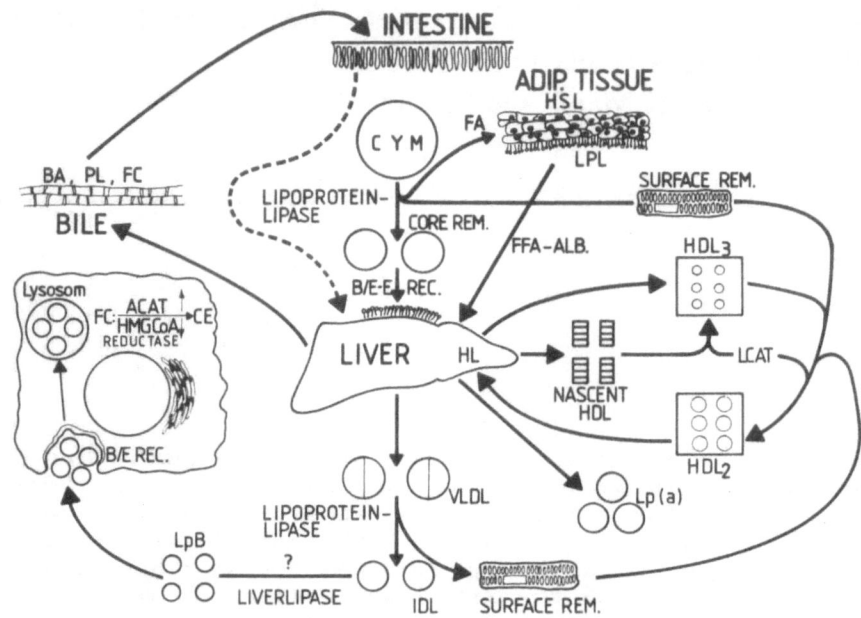

FIGURE 1   The physiological lipoprotein metabolism.

TG, CE and other nutritional lipids wich are taken up
by the intestine after hydrolysis, are resynthesized in
the mucosal cells, envelopped into chylomicrons (CYM)
and reach the blood stream via the intestinal lymph.
During circulation, TG and CE as well as other lipids
and some apo-Lp are transferred to other Lp-fractions,
or exchange one with aonther. The lipoprotein lipase
(LPL) from adipose tissue and muscle, responsible for
TG hydrolysis not only rapidly degrades the core lipids
but also directs the deliberated fatty acids into target organs. CYM as well as CYM-remnants have a very
short half life in circulation, the latter beeing bound
by the CYM-remnant receptor (E-receptor) on the liver
and internalized as well as degraded. The liver as a
consequence produces endogenous Lp, VLDL, which are
hydrolyzed in a similar way by LPL yielding IDL and
finally LDL. In the latter step, the hepatic lipase
(HL) most probably is involved. LDL (LpB) the final
degradation product of VLDL catabolism have a relatively long half life of several days. They are taken up
mainly by the B/E receptor of various tissues followed
by intracellular processing in the Brown & Goldstein
pathway (3). Derangements of this later catabolism not
only leads to increased plasma LDL levels but also to
prolonged half lives and susceptibility to chemical

alterations. This latter process favours the uptake by scavenger cells and possibly starts the atherogenic process. In addition to LDL, IDL and also Lp(a), a Lp which seems to be metabolized independently from other TG-rich Lp (4), play a key role in development of atherosclerosis.

HDL on the other hand which are partly secreted in a nascent form from the liver and the intestine, partly originate from catabolism of TG-rich Lp inthe form of surface lipids, are attacked by the enzyme lecithin:-cholesterol acyl transferase (LCAT), the key enzyme for CE production in circulation. All the HDL-lipids are in active exchange and transfer with or to VLDL, LDL, Lp(a) and other fractions. HDL-lipids, notably CE are also taken up by the liver and catabolized to bile acids and excreted. In all these metabolic pathways, apo-Lp play a key role as transport proteins, cofactors or activators of enzymes, agonists for specifc receptor binding and substances which mediate the export of lipids from cells.

From all these metabolic processes, which are known today in much more detail as discussed here, it follows that lipids by themselves hardly represent the athero-genic agents but rather the Lp or better apo-Lp do. Whenever lipids or Lp-lipids are measured, one necessa-rily obtains only limited information on the metabolic status of a given individual. The optimum probably would be to analyze enzyme activities of LPL, HL, LCAT and exchange proteins in combination with turnover rates of various Lp classes. Since this seems rather utopic at present time, we conceptualized the idea, that absolute concentrations of as many apo-Lp as pos-sible in combination with lipids and Lp-lipids probably reflect as close as rationally can be achieved, the metabolic situation of single individuals. With that in mind we analyzed these parameters in healthy subjects as well as in patients with different forms of atheros-clerosis, aimed at the selection of optimal risk indi-cators.

Evaluation of Risk Indicators by Discriminant Analysis

We are fully aware, that this task should optimally be approached by long term prospective epidemiological studies, including a great number of individuals of both sexes and several socio-economic groups. Not only that such studies are extremely expensive and time consuming as it is true e.g. for the LRC-CCPT study (5), they proved in the past to provide not much more information as already anticipated from well designed case control studies. In any case, case control studies can be considered as a basis for further prospective evaluations. With that in mind, we designed three

independent studies for risk factor evaluations in MI,
CVD and PVD (6-8). Here we will give only a summary of
our results:
In the peripheral vascular disease (PVD) study, approx.
90 male individuals have been examined by doppler
ulrasound and partly also by angiography. The following
laboratory parameters were measured from fasting plasma: TC,TG, PL, LDL-C, HDL-C, HDL-PL, FC, apo-AI, AII,
and B. In addition ratios of these parameters were
calculated. Furthermore, BP, the number of cigarettes,
uric acid and glucose tolerance were recorded. The date
were evaluated in terms of univariate and multivariate
discriminant analysis. The results are shown in Tab.1:

Table 1. Risk indicators in PVD.

Parameters	Cut-Off Points	Error Rate(E.R.)
TG	>154 mg/dl	34%
TC	>192 mg/dl	31%
ApoB	>116 mg/dl	29%
ApoAI/AII	<108/40 mg/dl	40%
LDL/HDL-C	>3.0	34%
ApoAI/apoB	<0.9	25%

Multivariate Analysis:

Independent Variables	Sensitivity	Specificity	E.R.
ApoB + apoAII	0.78	0.79	21%
TC + LDL-C + HDL-C + Apo-AI + AII +B	0.84	0.89	13%

In another study on MI- survivors a similar analysis of
plasma lipids and lipoproteins was performed. Approx.
90 MI-survivors were tested and compared with a control
group matched for age , sex and soci-economic status.
The results are shown in Tab.2.

Table 2. Risk indicators for myocardial infarction

Parameters	Cut-Off Points	Error Rate
TG	>184 mg/dl	41%
TC	>284 mg/dl	35%
HDL-C	< 33 mg/dl	38%
LDL/HDL-C	>3.5	31%
Lp(a)	> 35 mg/dl	36%
ApoAI/apoB	<0.8	23%

By multivariate analysis, similar results were obtained
as shown in Tab.1. In MI, however, Lp(a) was an important indepentent risk factor. In a model with the variables LDL-C, HDL-C, Lp(a), apoAI, -AII and -B a sensi-

tivity of approx. 0.92 and an error rate of 7% was found.
Finally we also studied 72 patients suffering from cerebrovascular arteriopathy as evidenced by electro-encephalography, cerebral arteriograms, brain scan and CFS examinations. The blood lipid and Lp parameters of these patients were compared with those of a healthy control group matched for age, sex an living habits. The following results were obtained:

Table 3. Risk indicators for cerebral atherosclerosis

Parameters	Median Values(mg/dl) patients	controls	Cut-Off Values	E.R.
TC	185	201	>202	41%
LDL-C	129	134	>138	43%
HDL-C	29	48	<38	27%
HDL-PL	62	95	<77	14%
Apo-AI	81	122	<98	9%
Apo-AII	29	45	<33	16%
Apo-B	86	91	>91	44%
ApoAI/apoB	0.96	1.34	<1.09	34%
LDL/HDL-C	4.2	3.1	>3.4	37%

Multivariate Analysis:

Independent Variables	Sensitivity	Specificity	E.R.
FC+TG+HDL-2C + HDL-3C	0.95	0.93	5.6%
TG + HDL-C + apo-AI + + apoAII + sys.BP	0.98	0.97	3.1%

It is worth noting that in CVD-patients, TC and LDL-C were lower than in controls. LDL-C/HDL-C and apoAI/apoB were much worse discriminators than HDL-C or apoAI by themselves.
For all the statistical evaluations the following con-siderations must be empahsized.
1) The sensitivity can be increased to 1.0 with almost any variable just by moving the cut-off points to the right or to the left, but this goes on account of the specificity. We in our calculations have set the cut-off values such that the error rate, which is the sum of false negatives and false positives, reached a mini-mum.
2) The models which are calculated may be optimized by limiting the mumber of parameters, the laboratory costs, the availability of certain tests (antibodies) and so one. Thus with a large number of measured para-mters one is rather flexible by choosing several diffe-rent combinations with only limited loss of sensitivity and specificity.

3) The obtained models naturally need to be tested by new data to validate the results. This has been approached by the so called jackknife procedure (9). In our experiments, the apparent error rates matched very well the true error rate (8).

CONCLUSION

Due to the rather complex lipoprotein metabolism, the movement of lipids and apolipoproteins from one density class to another and the multifactorial ethiology of atherogenesis, the determination of one single blood parameter or only few of them will probably not allow in the future to provide a good measure for the atherosclerosis riks of single individuals. The inclusion of several parameters , however, greatly accounts for the complexity of the sytem and potentially allows with great accuracy the diagnosis of atherosclerotic diseases. Apo-Lp because of their active involvement in lipid metabolism need to be quantified in order to get insight in the dynamic system. This in fact proved to be true in all our studies in which by univariate analysis apo-Lp always were better discriminators for atherosclerosis than lipids. By multivariate analysis models were obtained using apo-Lp parameters which allowed a discrimination with highest accuracy.
In our studies we have also demonstrated that a differential diagnosis of various forms of vascular diseases may be possible in the future. Patients with peripheral vascular diseases exhibited rather high TG and probably IDL/CYM-remnant values accompanied with high TC, LDL-C and apoB. HDL-C and apo-A proteins were reduced. Lp(a) on the other hand seemed to be a very valuable discriminator for coronary atherosclerosis, which in combination with apoA & apoB yielded error rates of <10%.
Of particular interest were the results of the "stroke-study". The patients had exceptionally low HDL as well as apoAI and apoAII values but low normal TC and LDL-C concentrations. Thus by calculating the widely propagated atherosclerosis indices LDL/HDL-C or apoA/apoB, much worse discriminations between patients and controls were obtained as opposed to considering only HDL-C, HDL-PL or apoAI or apoAII.
It should be emphasized once more, that our studies must be considered as starting points for future work which necessarily needs to include other variables e.g. other apo-Lp or isoforms thereoff, parameters of hemostasis, platelet reactivity and the immune system. They also need to be verified by prospective studies which in the future may allow not only to diagnose individuals at increased risk with high accuracy by simple clinical chemical procedures, but also may provide further insight into the pathophysiological events

of atherogenesis.

REFERENCES

1. Hopkins, PN and Williams, RH (1981). A survey of 246 suggested coronary risk factors. Atherosclerosis, 40, 1-52
2. Kostner, GM (1983). Apolipoproteins and lipoproteins of human plasma: Significance for health and diseases. Adv. Lipid Res. 20, 1-44
3. Goldstein, JL and Brown, MS (1982).Lipoprotein receptors: genetic defense against atherosclerosis. Clin. Res. 30, 417-426
4. Krempler,F; Kostner, G; Bolzano,K and Sandhofer, F (1979). Lipoprotein Lp(a) is not a metabolic product of other apoB containing lipoproteins. Biochim. Biophys. Acta 575, 4911-4916
5. Rifkind BM et al. (1984). The lipid research clinics coronary primary prevention trial results. JAMA 251, 351-374
6. Kostner, GM; Avogaro, P; Cazzolato, G; Marth, E and BittoloBon G (1981). Lipoprotein Lp(a) and the risk for myocardial infarction. Atherosclerosis 38, 51-61
7. Pilger, E; Pristautz H; Pfeiffer, KH and Kostner GM (1983). Retrospective evaluation of risk factors for peripheral atherosclerosis by stepwise discriminant analysis.Arteriosclerosis 3, 57-63
8. Kostner GM; Marth E; Pfeiffer, KH and Wege H (1986). Apolipoproteins AI, AII and HDL-PL but not apoB are risk indicators for occlusive cerebrovascular disease. Eur. Neurol. 25, 346-353
9. Pfeiffer KP (1985). Stepwise selection and maximum likelihood estimation of smoothing factors of Kernel functions for nonparametric discriminant functions evaluated by different criteria. Comp. Biomed. Res. 18, 46-61

9
Genetic and non-genetic control of apoprotein
S. Eisenberg, D. Gavish, G. Friedman and
Y. Kleinman

In the last Symposium, we described findings of abnormal
lipoprotein systems in human subjects with dyslipoproteinemia,
predominantly hypertriglyceridemia (HTG) [1]. These studies [2,3]
can be summarized as follows: HTG states are associated with
excessive lipid transfer reactions [4]. The lipids that are
transferred are the hydrophobic cholesteryl ester (CE) and triglyceride (TG) molecules. The reaction thus causes excessive enrichment of VLDL with CE [5,6] while both LDL and HDL lose CE and
acquire TG [1,2,7]. Since acquired TG in LDL and HDL are hydrolyzed by plasma lipases [8,9], the particles are smaller and denser
than the normal lipoproteins. These observations suggested that
the metabolic fate of HTG-lipoproteins is abnormal [2]. For VLDL,
indeed, we showed that the less dense populations, VLDL-1 and
VLDL-II, contain 50-150% more CE molecules than present in LDL,
and pointed out that such particles cannot complete the
VLDL -> LDL conversion cascade [5]. Hence, in HTG, VLDL "remnant"
populations must be cleared from the plasma independently of the
LDL pathway. HTG-LDL is CE-poor, TG-rich, small and dense lipoprotein, and the cholesterol content of the LDL decreases with a
curvilinear relation to plasma TG levels. Such LDL's are expected
to be inefficient regulators of cellular metabolic activities that
depend on cholesterol influx, e.g., cholesterol synthesis and B,E
receptor protein activity. These postulates have been further
investigated in our laboratory during the last three years.

LDL has been isolated from the plasma of normo- and HTG-human
subjects and the same HTG-subjects during triglyceride lowering
therapy with bezafibrate (BZ) [2,10]. The HTG lipoprotein is
denser and smaller than N-LDL, is relatively enriched with protein
(predominantly apo B) and triglycerides and contains subnormal
amounts of free and esterified cholesterol. These abnormalities
are strongly and significantly related to the degree of triglyceridemia, and tend to revert towards normal when plasma TG levels
are reduced. In fibroblast cultures, abnormal metabolism of HTG-
LDL is clearly evident [10]. The first abnormality is defective
binding of HTG-LDL to the fibroblast B,E receptor. In upregulated

cells, specific binding of HTG-LDL is reduced by about 30%, and
the degree of binding of the HTG-LDL to the receptor reflects the
structural abnormalities of the lipoprotein. Consequently, we
observed decreased entry and degradation of the LDL by the cells.
A second abnormality is lower capacity of HTG-LDL to down regulate
cellular cholesterol synthesis and cellular B,E receptor activity

The reduced affinity of HTG-LDL to the B,E receptor is of
particular interest. To the best of our knowledge, this is the
first instance when abnormal metabolism of LDL is due to
reversible compositional and/or structural abnormalities of the
lipoprotein. Undoubtedly, this finding reflects conformational
changes of the apo B moiety that, in the HTG state, affect the
receptor recognition site on the B protein. Two studies were
performed in order to elucidate the mechanisms responsible for
defective binding of HTG-LDL to the B,E receptor. In the first
investigation, we compared the immunoreactivity of HTG-LDL (tested
with monoclonal antibodies to apo B) with the ability of the lipoprotein to bind to the fibroblast receptor [11]. Normal (N) and
LDL isolated from patients treated with bezafibrate (BZ) were
studied in parallel. When the LDL's are tested with an antibody
directed towards epitopes unrelated to the receptor recognition
site of apo B, all preparations (HTG, BZ and N) react similarly.
HTG-, but not BZ-LDL, however, exhibits reduced reactivity when
tested with monoclonals specific for epitopes at, or near, the
receptor recognition site of the apo B molecule. A strong and significant relationship is found between the degree of immunoreactivity of LDL's with the antibodies and their affinity to the
B,E receptor. Thus, it appears that abnormalities of HTG-LDL are
responsible for its decreased affinity towards the B,E receptor,
and that triglyceride lowering therapy restores the full ability
of the lipoprotein to interact with the receptor. In the second
investigation, we studied the biological reactivity of LDL's isolated from the plasma of patients with type I hyperlipoproteinemia
[12]. The plasma of these patients contains two LDL populations:
one (type I-LDL-1) is of normal density and size, while the second
(type I-LDL-2) consists of small size and dense LDL particles.
Both are enriched with TG and depleted of CE molecules. When tested in the fibroblast system, type I-LDL-1 binding and degradation
is about one half that of N-LDL; type I-LDL-2 metabolism is even
further reduced. These findings indicate that TG enrichment alone
can cause conformational changes at the receptor binding region of
apo B, and that the structural abnormalities further depress the
binding process.

The reduced ability of HTG-LDL to regulate cellular metabolic
activity is clearly due to the low number of cholesterol molecules
that enter the cells with the lipoprotein [10]. In the initial
study, we showed that the degree of regulation of cellular cholesterol synthesis is solely dependent on the influx of cholesterol
into the cells, irrespective of the type of LDL used. More recently, we demonstrated a similar phenomenon with regard to the regulation of LDL receptor activity (unpublished). Again, a very strong

correlation is found between the LDL-CE content and the capacity of the lipoprotein to regulate the LDL receptor activity. Noteworthy, correction of the compositional and structural abnormalities of the LDL by therapy, restored the full biological reactivity of the lipoprotein. It thus appears that in humans, the type of circulating LDL determines both total body cholesterol synthesis and B,E receptor activity.

Another mechanism responsible for non-genetic control of the metabolism of apo B-100 containing lipoproteins in humans is interaction and degradation of VLDL and IDL by cells. Experiments currently carried out in our laboratory focus on the role of IDL catabolism in regulating LDL formation through the VLDL ->IDL -> LDL cascade [13]. These experiments are conducted in cultured human skin fibroblasts and cultured human hepatoma cell line, Hep G-2. IDL has been isolated from the plasma of N and HTG human subjects. IDL of either source consists of spherical particles 270 A in diameter. The lipoprotein is TG and CE rich and contains apo B ($\approx$ 65%), apo E ($\approx$ 10%) and apo C ($\approx$ 25%). The apo E to apo B molar ratio is 2-3 mole/mole. In spite of the presence of apo E, the binding affinity of IDL to the B,E receptor is similar to LDL, and both are effective to the same extent in competitive displacement assays against ^{125}I-LDL. In cellular metabolism assays, the binding (at 37°C) of IDL to the receptor is similar to LDL but proteolytic degradation is about one half to one third. As well, the amount of cell associated IDL protein is less than that of LDL. These observations indicate that while IDL binds to the B,E receptor through high affinity processes, appreciable degradation of the IDL does not occur, unless other factors are present. The nature of such factors, either genetic or non-genetic, is currently being investigated.

Genetic defects (i.e., of the LDL (B,E) receptor gene) are responsible for pronounced elevation of plasma lipid and lipoproteins in relatively small number of individuals. The data described above indicate that non-genetic, environmental factors influence the distribution of plasma lipoprotein concentrations in a large number of subjects. We suggest that such non-genetic factors are responsible for the differences of lipoprotein levels and metabolism both within and between populations. It is these differences, we believe, that are the major cause of atherosclerotic diseases in the general population.

REFERENCES

1.   Eisenberg,S (1984). The molecular basis of plasma fat transport: effects of enzymes and lipid transfer proteins on the composition, structure and metabolism of plasma lipoproteins. In: Lenzi,S and Deskovich,GC (eds.) "Atherosclerosis and Cardio-vascular Diseases". pp.3-17 (Lancaster: MTP Press Ltd.)

2.   Eisenberg,S, Gavish,D, Oschry,Y, Fainaru,M. and Deckelbaum,RJ (1984). Abnormalities in very low, low and high density lipoproteins in hypertriglyceridemia. Reversal towards normal with bezafibrate treatment. J Clin Invest, 74, 470

3.   Gavish,D, Oschry,Y, Fainaru,M and Eisenberg,S (1986). Change in very low-, low-, and high-density lipoproteins during lipid lowering (Bezafibrate) therapy: Studies in Type IIA and Type IIB hyperlipoproteinemia. Europ J Clin Invest, 16, 61

4.   Eisenberg,S and Deckelbaum,R (1987). Intravascular lipoprotein remodelling: neutral lipid transfer proteins. Clin Biochem, In press

5.   Oschry,Y, Olivecronae,T, Deckelbaum,RJ and Eisenberg,S (1985). Is hypertriglyceridemic very low density lipoprotein a precursor of normal low density lipoproteins? J Lipid Res, 26, 158

6.   Eisenberg,S (1985). Preferential enrichment of large-sized very low density lipoprotein populations with transferred cholesteryl esters. J Lipid Res, 26, 487

7.   Deckelbaum,RJ, Granot,E, Oschry,Y, Rose,L and Eisenberg,S (1984). Plasma triglyceride determines structure-composition in low and high density lipoproteins. Arteriosclerosis, 4, 226

8.   Deckelbaum,R, Eisenberg,S, Oschry,Y and Olivecrona,T (1982). Reverse modification of human plasma low density lipoprotein toward triglyceride rich precursors: A mechanism for losing excess cholesterol ester. J Biol Chem, 257, 6509

9.   Deckelbaum,RJ, Eisenberg,S, Oschry,Y, Granot,E, Sharon,I and Bengtsson-Olivecrona,G (1986). Modeling of human plasma high density lipoproteins: Roles of neutral lipid exchange and triglyceride lipases. J Biol Chem, 261, 5201

10.   Kleinman,Y, Eisenberg,S, Oschry,Y, Gavish,D, Stein,O and Stein,Y (1985). Defective metabolism of hypertriglyceridemic low density lipoprotein in cultured human skin fibroblasts. J Clin Invest, 75, 1796

11.   Kleinman,Y, Schonfeld,G, Gavish,D, Oschry,Y and Eisenberg,S (1987). Hypolipidemic therapy modulates expression of apolipoprotein B epitopes on low density lipoproteins. J Lipid Res. In press

12.   Kleinman,Y, Oschry,Y., Berger,GMB and Eisenberg,S (1987). Familial lipoprotein lipase deficiency: abnormal lipoproteins and defective metabolism of low density lipoproteins in cultured human skin fibroblasts. Submitted for publication.

13.   Friedman,G, Gavish,D and Eisenberg,S (1986). Metabolism of human intermediate and low density lipoproteins by cultured Hep G2 cells. Arteriosclerosis, 6, 540a

10
The plasma metabolism of apolipoprotein A-IV
G. Ghiselli, R. Musanti and A.M. Gotto

INTRODUCTION

It is well known that net cholesterol efflux from the cells is operating only if a suitable acceptor is present in the media [1-3]. The rate of cholesterol efflux is either function of the rate of hydrolysis of the intracellular cholesteryl esters [3], and of the concentration of extracellular cholesterol acceptors [4]. The acceptor concentration may be a rate limiting step in poorly perfused tissues. Stein et al [5] have proposed that in human serum there are low molecular weight protein phospholipid complexes which can cross the endothelial barrier, in preference to lipoproteins, and promote cholesterol removal from peripheral tissues. The size of these complexes may be lower than 100,000 and would be thus circulating in VHDL or higher density plasma fractions. ApoA-I-phospholipids complexes are known to effectively promote cholesterol efflux [1,2,5]. Based upon the large degree of homology between apoA-I and apoA-IV structural organization [6], it has been suggested that apoA-IV-phospholipid complexes in LFF, are potential acceptors of tissue cholesterol [7]. Due to the conspicuous amount of apoA-IV in the lipoprotein free fraction (LFF) of plasma, the cholesterol efflux mediated by this apolipoprotein, free or complexed with phospholipids, may be large.

AN OVERVIEW OF APOLIPOPROTEIN A-IV

ApoA-IV has been first identified in rat plasma by Swaney et al [8]. It is a glycoprotein with molecular weight of 46,000 and its complete aminoacid sequence is known for rat and human [6,9]. In plasma and lymph, apoA-IV is polymorphic [10]. The chemical basis of this polymorphism is not known. The liver and the intestine are the major site of synthesis of apoA-IV in the rat [9]. In human, hepatic synthesis may be negligible [9]. Gordon et al [11] have shown that apoA-IV mRNA increases in the rat enterocytes during fat transport, supporting the idea of an increased synthesis of this apolipoprotein. Fat feeding in the rat [12] and human [13] slightly, but significantly, elevates plasma apoA-IV. In rat the concentration of LFF apoA-IV decreases during starvation, accounting for lower total plasma apoA-IV. With the aid of an anti-apoA-IV immunoaffinity column, Otha et al [14] have isolated from human plasma LFF, a complex of apoA-IV with phospholipids and cholesterol that also contains 30% of apoA-I as protein and another unrecognized protein. Sloop et al [7] have detected apoA-IV-lipid complexes in the peripheral lymph of dog, and their concentration increases in response to a cholesterol enriched diet. These complexes may or may not contain apoE, and it may be metabolically related to the plasma LFF-apoA-IV complexes. Steinmetz et al [15] have found that apoA-IV-phospholipid-cholesterol complexes are efficient substrate of LCAT and the enzyme displays maximal activity when acyl-saturated phospholipids are present. These results, together with the evidence later discussed, that the liver is the major site of catabolism of LFF-apoA-IV, lend support to the idea that apoA-IV may be involved in the cholesterol reverse transport shuttling cell cholesterol from the peripheral tissues to the liver. Lipoproteins abnormally enriched in apoA-IV have been observed in the plasma of subjects genetically deficient of apoE [16] and in others with chronic kidney failure [17] due to accumulation of cholesteryl ester-rich lipoproteins having the characteristics of chylomicron remnants. These observations suggest that apoA-IV may be also involved in the catabolism of the intestinal chylomicrons.

THE METABOLISM OF APOLIPOPROTEIN A-IV

We have investigated the plasma metabolism of apoA-IV in the human [18] and in the rat [19]. In rat we have also investigated the tissue site of catabolism of apoA-IV and the influence of fat absorption on its distribution in the mesentheric lymph. In human plasma [18], apoA-IV is mostly found in the lipoprotein free fraction of plasma (LFF). At least 20% is found associated with a subfraction of HDL of smaller size than HDL-3 based on molecular sieve chromatography. A much smaller fraction circulates with the triglyceride-rich lipoproteins. ApoA-IV distribution in plasma is similar in normolipidemic as well as hyperlipoproteinemic subjects, suggesting a relative independence of apoA-IV metabolism from major alteration in lipoprotein distribution and concentration. The functional significance of these findings was addressed with in vivo plasma turnover studies. For these studies, radioiodinated apoA-IV was added in vitro to fresh plasma and lipoproteins and LFF separated by molecular sieve chromatography. Radioiodinated apoA-IV-labeled HDL and LFF were then injected in normolipidemic subjects and the plasma drawn at later times, fractionated by chromatography for the determination of the radioactivity distribution. It was found that apoA-IV in LFF has a faster rate of catabolism than that of apoA-IV in HDL. On the other hand, apoA-IV in HDL had a turnover rate at least threefold higher than that of apoA-I and apoA-II, which are the major HDL apolipoproteins, suggesting major differences in their catabolism. In vivo, no transfer of radioactivity occurred between HDL and LFF, supporting the concept that apoA-IV is metabolically compartmentalized among these two pools in plasma. The results

94

also demonstrated that apoA-IV is one of the most actively synthesized apolipoproteins and its catabolism is very rapid. Interestingly, radioiodinated apoA-IV in LFF did not behave kinetically as a free protein since after injection it had a different behavior than that of the radioiodinated free apolipoprotein injected in other volunteers. This is consistent with the observation made by other investigators that complexes of apoA-IV and phospholipids of defined composition circulate in LFF.

In rat, the metabolism of apoA-IV is remarkably similar to that in human [19]. ApoA-IV in LFF had a faster catabolism than in HDL, and the residence time of apoA-IV in HDL was one-half that of apoA-I. Moreover, following injection of radioiodinated apoA-IV-labeled HDL and LFF, the radioactivity remained associated to the originally injected fraction. Further studies in this animal species have addressed the questions of the origin of apoA-IV pools in plasma and of the site of catabolism of apoA-IV in vivo. Chylomicrons from the mesentheric lymph were labeled by exchange in vitro with radioiodinated apoA-IV. When these were injected, the radioactivity rapidly transferred to the HDL but only minimally to LFF, suggesting that apoA-IV in intestinal chylomicrons is a precursor of the plasma HDL pool. These results could be mimicked in vitro by incubation of labeled chylomicrons with lipoprotein-lipase. Analysis of apoA-IV distribution in the mesentheric lymph by chromatography and radioimmunoassay, showed most of apoA-IV in LFF. It is thus conceivable that a large part of plasma LFF-apoA-IV is directly synthesized in this form by the intestine. Transfer of apoA-IV from the plasma compartment to the lymph is always minimal, even during active fat absorption. Further in vivo studies with radioiodinated or 14C-sucrose labeled apoA-IV in HDL and LFF showed that the liver is the major site of catabolism of apoA-IV. Similarly labeled human apoA-IV behaved in rat as the autologous protein. In fact, it disappeared from plasma at the same rate as rat apoA-IV and was rapidly catabolized in the liver. Binding studies [20] of complexes of rat apoA-IV and dimirystoyl-phosphatidyl choline (DMPC) of known stechiometry to highly purified plasma membranes of rat liver, suggest that a saturable and reversible binding site that displaying specificity for the ligand utilized is present on hepatic membranes. Binding could be virtually abolished by pretreatment of the membranes with pronase at the same concentration known to affect the binding of LDL to its receptor, suggesting the involvement of a membrane protein for binding. Such data corroborate the view that a specific mechanism is responsible for apoA-IV catabolism in the liver and are consistent with its rapid plasma catabolism.

SUMMARY

The data presented support the view that apoA-IV is ideally suited to serve in plasma as an agent capable of mediating reverse cholesterol transport. ApoA-IV-phospholipid complexes, which are a major secretory product of the intestine, have the potential to promote a net efflux of cellular cholesterol into the plasma compartment. Once enriched of cholesterol, the complexes become substrates for LCAT of which apoA-IV is an activator. Noteworthy, apoA-IV-lipid complexes in plasma do not transfer to or become part of larger lipoproteins. This may prevent futile cholesterol recirculation. Rather, they are directly, rapidly and specifically catabolized by the liver.

BIBLIOGRAPHY

1. Fielding, C.J. and Moser, K. (1982) J. Biol. Chem. 257:10955-10960.
2. Oram, J.F., Albers, J.J., Cheung, M.C., and Bierman, E.L. (1981) J. Biol. Chem. 256:8348-8356.
3. Daniels, R.J., Guertier, L.S., Parker, T.S., and Steinberg, D. (1981) J. Biol. Chem. 256:4978-4983.
4. Phillips, M.C., McLean, L.R., Stendt, G.W., and Rothblat, G.H. (1980) Atherosclerosis 36:409-422.
5. Stein, O., Fainaru, M., and Stein, Y. (1978) Biochim. Biophys. Acta 574:495-504.
6. Boguski, M.S., Elshourgaby, N., Taylor, J.M., and Gordon, J.I. (1984) Proc. Natl. Acad. Sci. USA 81:5021-5025.
7. Sloop, K.C., Dory, L., Krause, B.R., Castle, C., and Roheim, P.S. (1983) Atherosclerosis 49:9-21.
8. Swaney, J.B., Reese, H., and Eder, H.A. (1974) Biochem. Biophys. Res. Comm. 59:513-519.
9. Elshourbagy, N.A., Walker, D.W., Boguski, M.S., Gordon, J.L., and Taylor, J.M. (1986) J. Biol. Chem. 261:1998-2002.
10. Beisiegel, U. and Utermann, G. (1979) Eur. J. Biochem 93:601-608.
11. Gordon, J.L., Smith, D.P., Alpers, D.H., and Strauss, A.W. (1982) J. Biol. Chem. 257:8418-8423.
12. Dallinga-Thie, G.M., Groot, P.H.E., and van Tol, A. (1985) J. Lipid Res. 26:970-976.
13. Green, P.H.R., Glickman, R.M., Riley, J.W., and Quinet, E. (1980) J. Clin. Invest. 65:911-919.
14. Ohta, T., Fidge, N.H., and Nestel, P.J. (1984) J. Biol. Chem. 259:14888-14893.
15. Steinmetz, A. and Utermann, G. (1985) J. Biol. Chem. 260:2258-2264.
16. Ghiselli, G., Schaefer, E.J., Gascon, P., and Brewer, H.B. (1981) Science 214:1239-1241.
17. Nestel, P.J., Fidge, N.H., and Tan, M.H. (1982) N. Engl. J. Med. 307:329-333.
18. Ghiselli, G., Krishnan, S., Beigel, Y., and Gotto, A.M. Jr. (1986) 27:813-827.
19. Sherrill, B.C., Gotto, A.M. Jr., and Ghiselli, G. (1984) Arteriosclerosis 4:522A (Abstract).
20. Ghiselli, G., Crump, W.L., and Gotto, A.M. Jr. (1986) Biochem. Biophys. Res. Comm. 139:122-128.

11
Modified LDL in humans
P. Avogaro, G. Bittolo Bon and G. Cazzolato

Epidemiological experimental and clinical data support a primary atherogenic role for plasma low density lipoproteins (LDL) (1). The mechanism by which LDL are mostly cleared form the blood circulation is the LDL receptor pathway which is normally regulated by a feedbak mechanism thus preventing the accumulation of cholesterol esters in the cell (2). This pathway is altered in familial hypercholesterolemia (FH). The homozygous form of FH, in which LDL receptors are severely deficient (10%), occurs in only one subject out of every milion. Heterozygotes, with a consistent reduction of receptors (50%), represent one out of every 500 persons (3). Among patients with myocardial infarction under age 60 5% have a genetic defect of the LDL specific receptors (3). It happens therefore that coronary atherosclerosis, as well the others pictures of the clinical atherosclerosis, is mostly present in people having a normal receptorial system. The accumulation of cholesteryl esters in the foam cells, the peculiar trait of the atherosclerotic plaque, has to happen therefore through other pathways. Foam cells derive from two cellular sources: the arterial smooth muscle cells (SMC) and the monocytes-derived macrophages (MM) (4). The latter cells type, unlike many other cells, take up only a little amount of LDL by a receptor-mediated endocytosis mechanism, but have a distinct receptorial system that binds and degrades the more negatively charged LDL (5, 6). The incubation of cultured macrophages with LDL modified by acylation (acyl-LDL) results in a cholesteryl esters accumulation within the cells thus forming foam cells (5). The physiological significance of the acyl-LDL uptake system by macrophage is not known. "In vivo" moreover the acylation of plasma LDL seems unlikely (7). Two possible mechanisms by which the more negatively LDL can be produced "in vivo" at sites of incipient plaque have been reported. The interaction of LDL with malondialdehyde (MDA) release by aggregating platelets can lead to the formation of MDA-LDL that increase the cholesteryl ester deposition in cultured human MM (8). Moreover the interaction of LDL with endothelial cells also alters LDL (EC-LDL) thus allowing their uptake by the MM system (9). Furthermore experimental data have observed that LDL may exert their atherogenic properties by routes other than the interaction between LDL and its specific receptors. Several reports have actually demonstrated that LDL induce cytotoxicity (10), injury (11) or inhibition of proliferation (12) of cultured endothelial cells. Such toxicity needs the prsence of modified LDL and probably occurs as a result of the lipoprotein oxidation (10, 13). Since lipid peroxidation can occur under various pathological conditions (14, 15), the toxicity of peroxidized LDL observed "in vitro" may be related to an "in vivo" injury to the arterial wall. Modified LDL undergo relevant variations: a more negative electric charge and a faster electrophoretic run are the common denominators (8, 10, 13). In the case of EC-LDL also an increased hydrated density and a decrease in cholesterol and phosphatidilcholine content were recorded (13). We have observed that both the incubation of LDL with MDA (16) and treatment with O_2 (17) induce relevant variations of LDL apolipoprotein B with the appearence of higher molecular weight peptides and the change of their immunoreactivity. The "in vivo" correlate of modified LDL has not been yet identified, even if negatively charged LDL have been reported in human atherosclerotic lesions (18).

Through ion exchange chromatography we have been able to characterize a more electronegative subfraction of LDL in freshly prepared plasma LDL obtained from normal fasting subjects. The elution profile of LDL on ion exchange chromatography, as determined by optical absorbance at a wavelenght of 280 nm, reveals that the bulk of LDL proteins is followed by a more or less evident "shoulder" of proteins incompletely resolved from the major peak. With the optical measurements at a wavelenght of 254 nm, by which the presence of fatty acid conjugated dienes may be detected (19), a peak corresponding to the bulk of LDL proteins is followed by a second peak that corresponds to the protein "shoulder". The study of LDL proteins such obtained stresses the presence in the LDL bulk of the typical LDL apoprotein B (B-100) whereas in the LDL collected with a higher ionic strength, besides B-100, appear anti-apoB reactive peptides having a higher molecular weight. The more electronegative LDL have been found in normal subjects in an amount ranging from 5 to 20% of the total LDL; it contains more proteins and it is characterized by a low esterified/free cholesterol ratio and by a very low phospholipids content. This LDL subfraction shares many traits with MDA-LDL (8,

16), O$_2$ treated LDL (17) and EC-LDL (9, 13). These data support the possibility that this peculiar LDL is due to the effect of "in vivo" damage, possibly peroxidation, and that its plasmatic level may be crucial in atherogenesis.

REFERENCES

1. Kannel WB, Castelli WP, Gordon T and McNamara PM (1971). Serum cholesterol, lipoproteins and the risk of coronary heart disease. Ann Intern Med 74, 1

2. Goldstein JL and Brown MG (1977). Low density lipoprotein pathway and its relation to atherosclerosis. Annu Rev Biochem 46, 897

3. Goldstein JL and Brown MS (1983). Familial hypercholesterolemia. In: Stanbury JB, Wyngaarden JB, Fredrickson DS, Goldstein JL and Brown MS (eds.). "The metabolic basis of inherited disease. V". (McGraw Hill Co) p. 672

4. Ross R (1981). Atherosclerosis: a problem of the biology of arterial wall cells and their interactions with blood components. Arteriosclerosis 1, 293

5. Goldstein JL, Ho YK, Basu SK and Brown MS (1979). Binding site on macrophages that mediates uptake and degradation of acetylated low density lipoproteins, producing massive cholesterol ester deposition. Proc Natl Acad Sci USA 76, 333

6. Stein O and Stein Y (1980). Bovine aortic endothelial cells display macrophage-like properties towards acetylated 125I-labelled low density lipoproteins. Biochim Biophys Acta 620, 631

7. Goldstein JL and Brown MS (1982). Insights into the pathogenesis of atherosclerosis derived from studies of familial hypercholesterolemia. In: Carlson LA and Pernow B (eds.). "Metabolic risk factors in ischemic cardiovascular disease". (Raven Press, New York) p. 17

8. Fogelman AM, Shechter I, Seager J, Hokam M, Childs JS and Edwards PA (1980). Malondialdehyde alteration of low density lipoproteins leads to cholesterol ester accumulation in human monocyte-derived macrophages. Proc Nat Acad Sci USA 7, 2214

9. Henriksen T, Mahoney E and Steinberg D (1981). Enhanced macrophage degradation of low density lipoprotein previously incubated with cultured endothelial cells: recognition by receptors for acetylated low density lipoprotein. Proc Nat Acad Sci USA 78, 649

10. Hessler JR, Morel DW, Lewis JL and Chisolm GM (1983). Lipoprotein oxidation and lipoprotein-induced cytotoxicity. Arteriosclerosis 3, 213

11. Henriksen T, Evensen SA and Carlander B (1979). Injury to human endothelial cells in culture induced by low density

lipoproteins. Scand J Clin Lab Invest 39, 361

12. Schuh J, Novogzodisky A and Haschemeyer RH (1978). Inhibition of lymphocite mitogenesis by autoxidized low density lipoproteins. Biochem Biophys Res Comm 84, 763

13. Steinbrecher UP, Parthasazathy S, Leake DS, Witzum JL and Steinberg D (1984). Modification of low density lipoproteins by endothelial cells involves lipid peroxidation and degradation of low density lipoprotein phospholipids. Proc Natl Acad Sci USA 81, 3883

14. Nishigaki I, Hagihara H, Tusunekawa H, Maseki M and Yagi K (1981). Lipid peroxide levels of serum lipoprotein fractions of diabetic patients. Biochem Med 25, 373

15. Goto Y (1982). Lipid peroxides as a cause of vascular diseases. In: Yagi K (ed.) "Lipid peroxides in biology and medicine". (Academic Press Inc., New York) p. 295

16. Bittolo Bon G, Cazzolato G and Avogaro P (1983). Cjanges of apolipoprotein B molecular weight and immunoreactivity in malondialdehyde-modified low density lipoproteins. Artery 12, 74

17. Bittolo Bon G, Cazzolato G, Zago S and Avogaro P (1985). Effects of pantethine on in-vitro peroxidation of low density lipoproteins. Atherosclerosis 57, 99

18. Hoff HF (1979). LDL with altered surface charge: a new risk factor in atherogenesis? Artery 6, 178

19. Pryor WA, Castle L (1984). Chemical methods for detection of lipid hydroperoxides. In: Packer L (ed.) "Methods in Enzymology 105: oxigen radicals in biological systems". (Academic Press) p. 293

12
Clinical aspects of lipoprotein disorders

G. Crepaldi, E. Manzato, G. Baggio, S. Martini,
C. Gabelli, L. Previato and S. Zambon

Familial chylomicronemia (type I hyperlipoproteinemia) is a rare genetic disease due to the absence of the lipoprotein lipase activity. This genetic error involves either the extrahepatic lipoprotein lipase (lipoprotein lipase deficiency) or its obligatory co-factor, i.e. the apoprotein C-II (apo C-II deficiency). The clinical features of this disease, wich is usually diagnosed in infancy or childood, are hepatosplenomegaly, recurrent abdominal pain, pancreatitis, eruptive xanthomata and lipemia retinalis.

Lipoproteins, apoproteins, extrahepatic (LPL) and hepatic (HL) lipoprotein lipase activities were analyzed in 8 patients with familial LPL deficiency, in 2 patients with apo C-II deficiency, and in their first degree relatives (1). In both mutants severe hypertriglyceridemia was due to an accumulation of lipoproteins of density <1.006 g/ml. The LDL fraction was very reduced and abnormal in composition. Plasma apolipoprotein B levels were low and transported mainly in the VLDL fraction. Very low levels of cholesterol as well as apo A-I in HDL subfractions (HDL_2 and HDL_3) were also observed.

Only 3 out of the 24 first-degree relatives of 5 patients with LPL deficiency showed a small increase in plasma triglycerides, but 15 had low or low-normal LPL values. HL levels were normal in all subjects. The first-degree relatives of C-II deficiency patients showed normal levels of plasma lipids, LPL, and HL. Low LPL activities in the first-degree relatives of LPL deficiency patients might represent a biochemical marker for healthy carriers of LPL deficiency.

The plasma lipoproteins in these patients were further characterized by zonal ultracentrifugation under rate flotation conditions (2). Within the density range 1.006-1.063 g/ml 3 discrete LDL populations were described: IDL (d=1.006-1.019 g/ml),

LDL$_2$ (d=1.019-1.045 g/ml), and LDL$_3$ (d=1.045-1.063 g/ml). LDL$_3$ was never observed in normal subjects and was isolated by zonal ultracentrifugation as a single and discrete peak in all patients with chylomicronemia. HDL cholesterol levels were low and the HDL$_3$ flotation rate was lower than normal. LDL and HDL in these patients were cholesterol ester poor and triglyceride rich in comparison to normal lipoproteins.

Both in LPL deficiency and in apo C-II deficiency patients the plasma lipoprotein profile and the altered lipoprotein composition could be related to the impaired catabolism of triglyceride-rich lipoproteins caused by the absence of lipoprotein lipase activity.

The two patients (brother and sister of the same kindred) with apo C-II deficiency were characterized as regard clinical features, lipoproteins and apoproteins (3). The most important result of this study was the description of a new variant of apo C-II (apo C-II$_{Padova}$) with lower apparent molecular weight and more acidic isoelectric point (determined with two dimensional gel electrophoresis). Apo C-II levels quantitated by radioimmunoassay were 0.13 mg/dl for the male patient and 0.12 mg/dl for the female patient.

Moreover, the marked hypertriglyceridemia and the elevation of triglyceride-rich lipoproteins were corrected by the infusion of normal plasma or the injection of a biologically active synthesized 44-79 aminoacid residue peptide fragment of apo C-II. Genomic DNA of these 2 patients was analyzed with restriction enzymes and resulted normal (4, 5).

Familial hypercholesterolemia (FH) is a monogenic dominant disorder characterized by elevated plasma levels of LDL cholesterol and associated with the development of atherosclerosis and xanthomas. The genetic defect involves the LDL receptor.

At least 10 different mutations in the LDL receptor gene have been identified in homozygous and heterozygous FH patients. These allelic mutations can be divided into four classes: 1) the gene fails to specify the synthesis of a receptor protein, 2) the receptor sinthesized in the rough endoplasmic reticulum is not transported to the Golgi apparatus and thus does not undergo the carbohydrate processing reactions, 3) the receptor is synthesized, processed, and transported to the cell surface but fails to bind LDL, 4) the receptor is normally processed but fails to cluster in coated pits and does not internalize receptor-bound LDL.

The lack of receptor activity in FH results in the impaired LDL catabolism. However in FH patients there is also an overproduction of LDL. This disease is characterized by biochemical and clinical variability depending upon the heterozygous or homozygous state (gene-dose effect).

In FH patients the receptor-independent cholesterol metabolism (scavenger pathway) mediated by macrophages is increased: this compensatory mechanism has a dangerous effect since the accumulation of cholesteryl esters in macrophages can trasform them in foam cells.

A great number of patients with elevated plasma cholesterol is affected by **polygenic hypercholesterolemia** which is a multifactorial disease strongly influenced by environmemt factors, mainly by diet.

A third metabolic disease involving LDL is the **hyperapobetalipoproteinemia** which is characterized by an abnormal increase of apoprotein B in the LDL fraction. This disease is reported to be particularly associated with coronary heart disease.

Dysbetalipoproteinemia is a qualitative alteration of plasma lipoproteins present in subjects with apo E2/2 phenotype. This phenotype is found in 1% of the population. E2/2 homozygous subjects present reduced LDL levels and accumulation in plasma of remnants and apo E-HDL. As regard to the risk of vascular disease it is not yet clear if dysbetalipoproteinemia is a true disease or a "benefit".

Type III hyperlipoproteinemia is a rare familial disease occuring in 1-5/5000 in the population. Genetic, epidemiological, biochemical, and nutritional data are in agreement suggesting that type III is a multifactorial disorder. It is often associated with xanthomatosis, overweight, diabetes mellitus, hyperuricemia and coronary as well as peripheral atherosclerotic vascular disease. Type III hyperlipoproteinemia is usually manifested after the third decade of life in men and after the menopause in women. More than 85% of type III patients are E2/2 homozygous, other type III patients are E2 heterozygous or homozygous for rare apo E mutants. The common defect is a reduced binding affinity of apo E to the apo E receptor. This defect results in accumulations of abnormal remnant particles, in particular the ß-VLDL (an apo E rich VLDL with ß electrophoretic mobility) which is easily identified as a broad beta band in the lipoprotein electrophoresis.

Lipid and lipoprotein levels in type III are easily modified by dietary treatment and other exogenous factors.

Abnormally high plasma triglyceride levels are due to several different causes. Two genetic diseases (i.e. familial hypertriglyceridemia and familial multiple type hyperlipidemia or combined hyperlipidemia) are probably responsible for a large number of **primary hypertriglyceridemias**. These diseases produce different hyperlipoproteinemias which are classified as type IIa, IIb, IV, and V according to the WHO classification (6).

The prevalence of atherosclerotic vascular complications in

patients with type IIa, IIb, IV and V is particularly high. The prevalence of coronary and peripheral artery disease was studied in 280 patients with different types of primary hyperlipoproteinemia in our Lipid Clinic. The prevalence of coronary disease was 45% in type IIa, 47% in type IIb, 38% in type IV, and 17% in type V patients. On the other hand, the prevalence of peripheral vascular disease was higher in hypertriglyceridemic patients (21% in type IIb and 20% in type V) than in patients with hypercholesterolemia (9% in type IIa). Type IIb patients seem to be at very high risk of atherosclerotic complications (7).

The relationships between elevated plasma triglyceride levels and vascular complications are still under discussion. To better elucidate this topic it could be particularly useful to study the alterations of plasma lipoproteins in hypertriglyceridemia. Two pre-ß bands are frequently observed in the lipoprotein electrophoresis, in normals and hyperlipidemics. The slow and fast pre-ß were isolated by ultracentrifugation in zonal rotor and the slow band resulted to have a lower flotation coefficient than the fast one. Both fractions contained only apo B-100, while the slow fraction was rich in apo E and apo C-III. The slow pre-ß fraction has physicochemical properties quite similar to the remnants particles and could be important in relation to the atherogenesis process (8).

As reported in type I patients, LDL concentration in type V patients is extremely reduced, and LDL particles are heterogeneous. In these patients we have isolated: LDL_2 (d=1.019-1.045 g/ml) and LDL_3 (d=1.045-1.063 g/ml). LDL_2 and LDL_3 have ß mobility in agarose gel electrophoresis, and their diameters are inversely related to their densities. LDL_2 and LDL_3 of hypertriglyceridemic subjects are rich in triglycerides, poor in cholesterol, and contain only apo B-100. The LDL heterogeneity in type V patients could be important in evaluating the atherogenic risk of hypertriglyceridemia (9).

The lipoprotein modifications in patients with primary type V hyperlipoproteinemia were analyzed during dietary treatment. After 30 days of balanced isocaloric diet mean serum triglycerides fell from 2253 ± 1329 (mean$\pm$SD) to 251 ± 151 mg/dl. At the same time chylomicrons and Sf > 100 VLDL disappeared, LDL cholesterol concentration increased (from 61 ± 31 to 159 ± 44 mg/dl) and the LDL heterogeneity disappeared. The HDL cholesterol remained abnormally low throughout the study and no HDL_2 were observed at any time (10).

Several diseases can produce alterations of lipoprotein metabolism. The most common **secondary hyperlipoproteinemias** characterized by increased LDL levels are observed in hypothiroidism, nephrotic syndrome, cholestasis, while increased VLDL levels are often observed in diabetes, chronic renal failure, alcoholism, Cushing syndrome, acromegaly, paraproteinemias.

It has been well documented that the characteristic elevation of unesterified cholesterol and phospholipids in patients with **cholestasis** is due to the presence of a LDL (d=1.019-1.063 g/ml) with abnormal composition and properties. This lipoprotein is designated lipoprotein-X or LP-X (11). In native bile lipids are organized in the form of a lipoprotein carrying albumin as apoprotein. Bile-lipoprotein can be converted into "LP-X-like" material in vitro by adding albumin or serum to native bile. The LP-X-like material formed in vitro has physicochemical characteristics similar to LP-X isolated from serum. LP-X can be converted into bile-lipoprotein-like particles by adding bile salts to a LP-X positive serum (12). Furthermore, experimental anastomosis of the common bile duct to the vena cava is followed after a few hours by the appearance of LP-X. These facts strongly suggest that bile lipoprotein is a precursor for LP-X and that it refluxes into the plasma under cholestatic conditions.

LP-X can be easily visualized by agar gel electrophoresis. The determination of the presence of LP-X represents a diagnostic test in the differential diagnosis of liver disease (13).

Secondary hyperlipoproteinemias are frequently due to the **diabetes mellitus.** Serum lipid and lipoprotein levels were evaluated in 50 insulin-treated diabetic out-patients and in 46 normal volunteers. In these groups metabolic evaluation was carried out by assaying fasting plasma glucose, glucose in urine and glycosylated hemoglobin (G-HbA$_1$). No differences were observed in the lipid and lipoprotein patterns between diabetic patients and normals. HDL values were significantly lower in males (diabetics and normals) as compared to females, but no differences between the diabetic and the normal group were observed. G-HbA$_1$ was significantly correlated to fasting plasma glucose and glucose in urine, but also to serum and VLDL triglycerides. Fasting plasma glucose too was correlated to triglyceride levels. Moreover, a negative correlation was found between HDL cholesterol and triglycerides. These results show that well controlled insulin-treated diabetics do not have altered lipid and lipoprotein levels (14).

A retrospective study on 349 hospitalized diabetics demonstrated that only 13% of the patients were affected by macroangiopathy, 24% were affected by microangiopathy, and 33% by peripheral neuropathy. Some factors were significantly correlated to macroangiopathy: age, maleness, cigarette smoking, diastolic blood pressure, hyperglycemia, diabetes duration and insulin treatment. Hypercholesterolemia and hypertriglyceridemia, even if present, were not correlated to macroangiopathy (15).

The **treatment** of primary hyperlipoproteinemias begins with a dietary intervention (which is the only one possible in type I). Aim of the dietary treatment is a reduction of dietary fat, reduction of dietary cholesterol, balanced supply of poly-, mono-, and saturated fatty acids. In some patients it is also necessary to reduce the caloric intake and to avoid alcohol. The pharmacological treatment of the primary hyperlipoproteinemias should be chosen on the basis of the lipid disorder: bile sequestrant resins and HMGCoA reductase inhibitors are the first choice drugs in hypercholesterolemia, while fibrate analogs and nicotinic acid derivatives are useful both in hypercholesterolemia and in hypertriglyceridemia. The hypolipidemic effect of these drugs should be evaluated in each patient since some subjects could be more resistant to one drug than to another.

REFERENCES

1. Fellin, R, Baggio, G, Poli, A, Augustin, J, Baiocchi, MR, Baldo, G, Sinigaglia, M, Greten, H, Crepaldi, G (1983). Familial lipoprotein lipase and apolipoprotein C-II deficiency. Atherosclerosis, 49, 55
2. Manzato, E, Marin, R, Gasparotto, A, Baggio, G, Fellin, R, Crepaldi, G (1984). The plasma lipoproteins in familial chylomicronemia. J Lab Clin Med, 104, 778
3. Baggio, G, Manzato, E, Gabelli, C, Fellin, R, Martini, S, Baldo-Enzi, G, Verlato, F, Baiocchi, MR, Sprecher, DL, Kashyap, ML, Brewer, HB, Crepaldi, G (1986). Apolipoprotein C-II deficiency syndrome. J Clin Invest, 77, 520
4. Fojo, SS, Law, SW, Sprecher, DL, Gregg, RE, Baggio, G, Brewer, HB (1984). Analysis of the apo C-II gene in apo C-II deficient patients. Biochem Biophys Res Commun, 124, 308
5. Humphries, SE, Williams, L, Myklebost, O, Stalenhoef, AFH, Demacker, PNM, Baggio, G, Crepaldi, G, Galton, DJ, Williamson, R (1984). Familial apolipoprotein CII deficiency: a preliminary analysis of the gene defect in two independent families. Hum Genet, 67, 151
6. Beaumont, JL, Carlson, LA, Cooper, GR, Fejfar, Z, Fredrickson, DS, Strasser, T (1970). Classification of hyperlipidaemias and hyperlipoproteinaemias. In: Bull Wld Hlth 43: 891-53.
7. Crepaldi, G, Fellin, R, Briani, G, Baggio, G, Manzato, E, Veronese, R (1977). Prevalence of coronary artery disease and peripheral artery disease in patients with different types of primary hyperlipidemia. Atherosclerosis, 26, 593

8. Manzato, E, Pagnan, A, Ziron, L, Gasparotto, A, Braggion, M (1984). Double pre-beta lipoprotein. Isolation and characterization of the two population of very low density lipoproteins by zonal ultracentrifugation. Arteriosclerosis, 4, 598

9. Manzato, E, Gasparotto, A, Marin, R, Baggio, G, Baldo, G, Crepaldi, G (1984). Characterization with zonal ultracentrifugation of low-density lipoproteins in type V hyperlipoproteinemia. Biochim Biophys Acta, 793, 365

10. Manzato, E, Marin, R, Gasparotto, A, Baggio, G, Martini, S, Gabelli, C, Crepaldi, G (1986). Lipoprotein modifications during dietary treatment in patients with primary type V hyperlipoproteinaemia. Europ J Clin Invest, 16, 149

11. Manzato, E, Fellin, R, Baggio, G, Walch, S, Neubeck, W, Seidel, D (1976). Formation of lipoprotein-X. Its relationship to bile compounds. J Clin Invest, 57, 1248

12. Baggio, G, Muller, P, Wieland, H, Niedmann, PD, Seidel, D (1978). Influence of bile acids and free fatty acids on physicochemical properties of LP-X. Res Exp Med 172, 211

13. Fellin, R, Manzato, E, Zotti, S, Baggio, G, Briani, G, Rugge, M (1978). Lipoprotein-X and diagnosis of cholestasis: comparison with other biochemical parameters and liver biopsy. Clin Chim Acta, 85, 41

14. Fedele, D, Fellin, R, Lapolla, A, Baggio, G, De Romedi, F, Frigato, F, Crepaldi, G (1982). Serum lipid and lipoprotein levels and metabolic control in insulin-treated diabetics. Acta Diabetol Lat, 19, 151

15. Fedele, D, Tiengo, A, Bertotti, P, Crepaldi, G (1982). Macroangiopatia e parametri clinico-metabolici nella malattia diabetica. Studio retrospettivo su 349 diabetici ricoverati in ambiente ospedaliero. Giorn Arterioscl, 7, 277

FIXED VERSUS DYNAMIC STENOSIS: POSSIBLE CAUSES AND THERAPEUTIC APPROACHES

13
Fixed versus dynamic stenosis: possible causes and therapeutic approach
A. Maseri

In my opinion the major effect of the revival of coronary spasm (1) was the stimulus to begin to look at coronary artery disease as a much more varied and dynamic process than the static and rather stale picture we were presented with at medical school.

Transient acute myocardial ischaemia can be brought about by a variety of causes (2): rarer causes are represented by extracoronary causes (such as for example aortic stenosis) and small coronary vessels disease; I believe that forms of small vessel disease do exist, they seem to be benign, but we do not know enough about them; the extent of our knowledge about small vessel disease is concisely summarised by the term proposed by some authors (3,4): Syndrome X. Two causes of ischaemia are by far the most frequent and most important: excessive increase of myocardial demand in the presence of fixed stenosis, or sudden impairment of coronary blood flow caused by transient obstructions of epicardial coronary arteries. These causes of ischaemia most often coexist in variable combination, or concur to cause ischaemia, in the same patient.

The causes of dynamic stenoses are listed below:
1. "Physiological" response of coronary smooth muscle
   to constrictor stimuli in the presence of a subintimal
   pliable plaque.
2. Hyperresponse to constrictor stimuli or abnormal
   stimuli resulting in total or subtotal occlusion of a
   segment of coronary artery.
3. Intravascular plugging by platelets and thrombus.
4. Combination of causes 3 + 1 or 3 + 2 or 2 + 3.

Intravascular plugging by platelet aggregates and thrombosis probably plays a major role in unstable angina resistant to medical therapy most likely in combination with increased vasomotor tone or with spasm.

Spasm is typically recognised in variant angina, which is a rare syndrome. A "physiological" increase of coronary smooth muscle tone is likely to play the major role in determining the variability of exercise tolerance and episodes of spontaneous ischaemia in patients with chronic stable angina.

111

A number of features distinguish spasm from "physiological" coronary constriction. "Physiological" coronary constriction represents a normal response:

Vasoconstrictor stimuli produce a rather predictable and uniform but small reduction of calibre in epicardial coronary arteries. This effect depends on vascular basal tone, reactivity and compliance. The effect of "physiological" smooth muscle constriction is magnified by the presence of a subintimal plaque (5).

A major distinctive feature between physiological coronary constriction and spasm is demonstrated by a classical study on unselected patients with chronic stable angina by Brown et al (6). During handgrip the calibre of both normal and stenotic segments is reduced on average by about 10% and transtenotic resistance increased by about 40%. Conversely following GTN both normal and stenotic segments dilate about 20% and transtenotic resistance decreases by about 20%. Thus on the average transtenotic resistance appears to vary by as much as 60%; obviously in some patients it may vary more, in others less. This behaviour, observed in a group of unselected patients is indicative of a common type of response, hence "physiological", quite at variance with the rarity of coronary artery spasm at least of the kind seen in variant angina. Subsequent studies by Lictlen et al (7) indicate that eccentric but not concentric lesions can vary their calibre. Post mortem studies indicate that about 75% of stenoses are eccentric (8).

Changes of transtenotic resistance of the magnitude observed by Brown and coworkers (6) can well account for important variations of the ischaemic threshold. They may well explain the observations made during ambulatory monitoring in patients with chronic stable angina. A number of studies from other groups and from our own indicate that most ischaemic episodes recorded during ordinary daily life develop at levels of heart rate and of heart rate blood pressure product much lower than those tolerated at other times of the day without any signs of ischaemia (9-14). How can these findings be explained?

It is apparent that these observations are rather difficult to reconcile with the traditional view that the impairment of coronary flow reserve caused by coronary occlusions is fixed: (the result of the balance between severity of a critical stenosis and of the development of collaterals). The very wide variability of the ischaemic threshold often observed during ambulatory monitoring in many patients with chronic stable angina appears more compatible with a modification of this traditional concept of fixed residual coronary flow reserve, whereby residual coronary flow reserve is not fixed during the 24 hours as it is modulated by changes of resistance at the site of the flow limiting stenoses. Thus occasionally flow may be dramatically reduced to produce ischaemia at rest, or coronary flow reserve may be only moderately reduced so that ischaemia develops only in coincidence with moderate efforts, well tolerated on other occasions. Also in this scheme efforts greater than a rather predictable level are never tolerated but smaller efforts may or may not cause ischaemia depending on the simultaneous behaviour of coronary flow reserve (14).

We were able to document a number of features which suggest that the changes of vasomotor tone responsible for this wide variability of residual coronary flow reserve in chronic stable angina are different from spasm, at least in the form that is most commonly seen in variant angina.

Patients with chronic stable angina may have a positive ergonovine test but never with ST elevation or coronary occlusion (15); often have a positive cold pressor test but never a positive hyperventilation test (16); have predominantly diurnal ischaemic episodes (17).

An even clearer indication that spasm, as typically seen in variant angina, is different from the "physiological" changes in coronary vasomotor tone seen in normal patients and in chronic stable angina is provided by the results of a series of studies on the pathogenetic mechanisms of spasm that we have performed during recent years in patients with variant angina. We tried to assess the role of triggering factors (18) by attempting to prevent the development of spasm by a number of drugs but we had a series of negative results (19-22). Although the reasons can be multiple, this series of negative results is also compatible with a dominant role of an aspecific local hyperreactivity to a variety of constrictor stimuli. A recently completed study in our institution appears to support this possibility rather strongly (23).

Several patients with variant angina were positive to more than one type of constrictor stimulus known to act on different receptors. Ergonovine was by far the most powerful spasmogenic stimulus and the other tests were more often positive when ergonovine was positive at low dose.

The results of intracoronary injection of ergonovine (24) indicate that only the spastic segment hyperreacts to ergonovine but not the proximal segment of the same branch nor the other branches which behave like the arteries in control patients with 10-20% reduction of diameter (a physiological response). Thus total occlusion of a coronary artery segment represents a local hyperresponse to the same dose of agent which causes only physiological constriction in other branches or in other patients.

Therefore in this interesting human model of disease that is variant angina in its most typical form:
- Spasm can be caused by a variety of constrictor stimuli acting on different receptors. This is compatible with a local aspecific alteration of a segment of the arterial wall which makes it hyperreactive.
- The documented persistance of spasm (off therapy) for 6 - 48 months in 10/28 patients suggests that the local vascular alteration may be chronic and stable.

The concept of a local vascular abnormality that can cause coronary segments to become occluded in response to constrictor stimuli which produce only a modest constriction in other branches might be extrapolated.

If we reexamine now the varied causes of active dynamic stenoses we could entertain the possibility that mural or intraintimal white thrombus formation may be associated with only moderate constriction or with occlusive spasm depending on the local reactivity of the smooth muscle. If this hypothesis is valid, then a local hyperreactivity of the coronary smooth muscle might play a role in the very early phase of coronary artery occlusion; subsequently, when the artery segment is totally occluded a red thrombus or clot is likely to form especially in diseased arteries and can maintain a total occlusion, also when a spasm is relieved. The 20% incidence of positive ergonovine tests in patients with recent infarction observed by Bertrand et al (25) would lend support to the hypothesis that a local coronary artery hyperreactivity is frequent in acute myocardial infarction.

The rarity of acute coronary occlusion in the life of patients with even severe coronary atherosclerosis compared with the frequent finding of plaque fissures in patients dying of non-cardiac death suggest that a combination of local alterations (plaque fissure, increased susceptibility to constrictor stimuli or vice versa) together with displacement of the local thrombotic – thrombolytic equilibrium towards thrombosis may often be required to initiate occlusion and clot formation (26).

REFERENCES

1. Maseri, A (1981). The revival of coronary spasm. Am J Med, 70, 752.
2. Maseri, A (1983). The changing face of angina pectoris: practical implications. Lancet, I, 746.
3. Opherk, D, Zebe, H, Weihe, E et al (1981). Reduced coronary dilatory capacity and ultrastructural changes of the myocardium in patients with angina pectoris but normal coronary arteriograms. Circulation, 63, 817.
4. Cannon, RO, Watson, RM, Rosing, DR et al (1983). Angina caused by reduced vasodilator reserve of the small coronary arteries. J Am Coll Cardiol, I, 1359.
5. MacAlpin, RN (1980). Contribution of dynamic vascular wall thickening to luminal narrowing during coronary arterial constriction. Circulation, 61, 296.
6. Brown, BG, Bolson, E, Petersen, RB et al (1981). The mechanisms of nitroglycerin action: stenosis vasodilatation as a major component of the drug response. Circulation, 69, 1089.
7. Rafflenbeul, W, Lichtlen, PR (1983). Quantitative coronary angiography: evidence of a sustained increase in vascular smooth muscle tone in coronary artery stenoses. In: Kaltenbach, M, Bussmann, WD, Kober, G, and Schneider, W (eds). "Nitrates IV Cardiovascular Effects". Z Kardiol, 72, 87.
8. Vlodaver, Z, and Edwards, JE (1971). Pathology of coronary atherosclerosis. Prog Cardiovasc Dis, 14, 256.
9. Schang, SJ, and Pepine, CJ (1977). Transient asymptomatic ST segment depression during daily activity. Am J Cardiol, 39, 396.
10. Selwyn, AP, Fox, K, Eves, M et al (1978). Myocardial ischaemia in patients with frequent angina pectoris. Br Med J, 2, 1594.
11. Deanfield, JE, Maseri, A, Selwyn, AP, Ribeiro, P, Chierchia, S, Krikler, S and Morgan, M (1983). Myocardial ischaemia during daily life in patients with stable angina: its relation to symptoms and heart rate changes. Lancet, II, 753.

12. Chierchia, S, Gallino, A, Smith, G, Deanfield, J, Morgan, M, Croom, M and Maseri A (1984). The role of heart rate in the pathophysiology of chronic stable angina. Lancet, II, 1353.
13. Cecchi, AC, Dovellini, EV, Marchi, F et al (1983). Silent myocardial ischemia during ambulatory electrocardiographic monitoring in patients with effort angina. J Am Coll Cardiol, 1, 934.
14. Maseri, A, Chierchia, S, Kaski, JC (1985). Mixed angina pectoris. Am J Cardiol, 56, 30E.
15. Crea, F, Davies, G, Romeo, F, Chierchia, S, Bugiardini, R, Kaski, JC, Freedman, B and Maseri A (1984). Myocardial ischemia during ergonovine testing: different susceptibility to coronary vasoconstriction in patients with exertional and variant angina. Circulation, 69, 690.
16. Crea, F, Davies, G, Chierchia, S, Romeo, F, Bugiardini, R, Kaski, JC, Freedman, B and Maseri A (1985). Different susceptibility to myocardial ischemia provoked by hyperventilation and cold pressor test in exertional and variant angina pectoris. Am J Cardiol, 56, 18.
17. Chierchia, S, Berkenboom, G, Deanfield, J, Morgan, M and Maseri, A (1982). Holter monitoring in classical and variant angina: a clue to different pathogenetic mechanisms. Clin Sci, 63, 39p.
18. Maseri, A, Parodi, O, Severi, S and Pesola, A (1976). Transient transmural reduction of myocardial blood flow, demonstrated by thallium-201 scintigraphy, as a cause of variant angina. Circulation, 54, 280.
19. Chierchia, S, De Caterina, R, Crea, F, Patrono, C and Maseri, A (1982). Failure of thromboxane A_2 blockade to prevent attacks of vasospastic angina. Circulation, 66, 702.
20. Chierchia, S, Patrono, C, Crea, F, Ciabattoni, G, De Caterina, R, Cinotti, GA, Distante, A and Maseri, A (1982). Effects of intravenous prostacyclin in variant angina. Circulation, 65, 470.
21. Chierchia, S, Davies, G, Berkenboom, G, Crea, F, Crean, P and Maseri, A (1984). Alpha-adrenergic receptors and coronary spasm: an elusive link. Circulation, 69, 8.
22. Freedman, SB, Chierchia, S, Rodriguez-Plaza, L, Bugiardini, R, Smith, G and Maseri A (1984). Ergonovine-induced myocardial ischemia: no role for serotonergic receptors? Circulation, 70, 178.
23. Kaski, JC, Crea, F, Meran, D, Rodriguez, L, Araujo, L, Chierchia, S, Davies, G and Maseri, A (1986). Local coronary supersensitivity to diverse vasoconstrictor stimuli in variant angina. Circulation, 74, 1255.
24. Hackett, D, Chierchia, S, Davies, G and Maseri A (1986). Intracoronary ergonovine in variant angina pectoris. Clin Sci, 70(13), 1p.
25. Bertrand, ME, La Blanche, JM, Tilmant, PY et al (1983) (1983). The provocation of coronary arterial spasm in patients with recent transmural myocardial infarction. Eur Heart J, 4, 532.
26. Maseri, A, Chierchia, S, and Davies, G (1986). Pathophysiology of coronary occlusion in acute infarction. Circulation, 73, 233.

14
The epicardial coronary arteries at necropsy in acute myocardial infarction
W.C. Roberts

This paper focuses on the findings in the major epicardial coronary arteries in acute myocardial infarction (AMI).

CORONARY ARTERIAL LUMINAL NARROWING

AMI, in the absence of severe, i.e. >75% cross-sectional area (XSA), luminal narrowing of one or more epicardial coronary arteries is extremely rare. Patients with hypertrophic cardiomyopathy and idiopathic dilated cardiomyopathy at necropsy may have transmural left ventricular (LV) scars and the epicardial coronary arteries may be normal or near normal[1]. The finding of normal or near-normal coronary arteries at necropsy, however, in a patient with transmural LV scarring does not indicate that all coronary arterial lumens were normal or near normal at the time of AMI. Many patients have been reported with "myocardial infarction and angiographically normal coronary arteries"[2]. With a few exceptions, however, the coronary angiogram was not performed at the time of AMI, but weeks or months later. To my knowledge, coronary angiography performed at the time of AMI has always demonstrated at least one major coronary artery to be severely narrowed or totally occluded. It is well-recognized that coronary thrombi or emboli may lyse, recanalize or retract along one side so that coronary angiography weeks or months after AMI may show an angiographically normal coronary tree[2]. Coronary spasm in the absence of fixed coronary narrowing has never been demonstrated to be the cause of AMI[3]. Thus, although transmural LV scarring may be observed at necropsy in the absence of severe fixed narrowing of one or more major epicardial coronary arteries, the presence of a normal coronary tree or one without significant narrowing has not been demonstrated at the time of AMI. Consequently, it is most reasonable to believe that severe narrowing of one or more major epicardial coronary arteries is a necessity for AMI to occur.

Although severe narrowing of a coronary artery in the absence of underlying atherosclerotic plaque may be produced entirely by a thrombus or embolus, such an occurrence is rare and will not be discussed further here.

CORONARY ARTERIAL ATHEROSCLEROSIS

With certain exceptions, mentioned above, AMI occurs only when there exists considerable quantities of atherosclerotic plaque within the lumens of one or more major epicardial coronary arteries. Over 95% of necropsy patients with fatal transmural (involvement of more than the inner one-half of the LV wall) AMI have >75% XSA luminal narrowing by atherosclerotic plaque alone of two or more of the four major (left main, left anterior descending (LAD) left circumflex (LC) and right) epicardial coronary arteries[4]. Of 27 patients with fatal AMI studied by Roberts and Jones[4], all had >75% XSA narrowing by plaque in two or more of the four major coronary arteries: three patients (11%) had this degree of narrowing in all four major arteries ("quadruple vessel disease"), 14 (52%) had three arteries so narrowed ("triple vessel disease") and ten (37%) had two arteries so narrowed ("double vessel disease"). Of the possible 108 major coronary arteries in the 27 patients, 74 (69%) were narrowed >75% in XSA at some point by atherosclerotic plaque alone, an average of 2.7 of 4 arteries per patient. With the exclusion of the left main artery, 71 (88%) of the other 81 major arteries were severely (>75% XSA) narrowed at some point by atherosclerotic plaque (average 2.6 of 3 coronary arteries per patient). Similar observations had been made years earlier by Saphir and associates[5], Blumgart et al.[6], and Yates et al.[7] who found "complete occlusions" of usually two major epicardial coronary arteries in patients with fatal AMI studies at necropsy.

Determination of the maximal degree of narrowing at any point in a major coronary artery has proven to be useful in evaluating patients clinically with symptoms of myocardial ischaemia. The one, two-, three- or four-vessel disease approach, however, provides limited information on the extent of the coronary arterial atherosclerotic process. In recent years my colleagues and I have examined the four major coronary arteries at necropsy by what we have called the quantitative approach. Each of the four major coronary arteries are excised intact from the surface of the heart. If calcific deposits are present, the arteries are decalcified and then each major artery is divided into 5-mm long segments, the cut being at right angles to the longitudinal axis of the artery. An average of 54 5-mm segments are examined from each heart because in the adult human heart the sum of the lengths of the four major coronary arteries is about 27 cm (right = 10 cm; left main = 1 cm; LAD = 10 cm and LC = 6 cm). Because each 1 cm is divided into two 5-mm segments, about 54 segments are available for each heart. The amount of XSA narrowing in each 5-mm segment is categorized into five groups: 0-25%; 26-50%; 51-75%; 76-95% and 96-100%. The 5-mm segments are graded by examination of a histological section stained by the Movat method and prepared from each segment. The internal elastic membrane serves as the normal demarcation line.

Examination of the numerous 5-mm segments has demonstrated that the atherosclerotic process among patients with fatal AMI not only produces severe narrowing but that the atherosclerotic process is diffuse and extensive. Indeed, among these patients a normal 5-mm segment is rarely encountered by microscopic examination. Of the 1,403 5-mm segments examined in the 27 patients with fatal transmural AMI[4], 484 (34%) were narrowed 76-100% in XSA by plaque (3% of the 484 segments were narrowed 96-100%); 528 segments (38%) were narrowed 51-75%; 319 (23%), 26-50%, and 72 (5%), 25% or less in XSA by plaque alone[4]. The mean percent of 5-mm segments of right, LAD and LC coronary arteries at each of the five levels of narrowing was similar in the proximal and distal halves. Thus, among these 27 victims of AMI, 95% of the entire lengths of the four major coronary arteries were narrowed 26-100% in XSA by atherosclerotic plaque or only 1 in 20 5-mm segments of a major coronary artery even approached normal.

The amount of severe coronary arterial narrowing by atherosclerotic plaque in fatal AMI is greater in necropsy patients with transmural anterior wall infarcts compared to those with posterior (a term preferable to "inferior") wall infarcts. Brosius and I[8] determined the percentage of XSA narrowing by atherosclerotic plaque in each 5-mm segment of the four major epicardial coronary arteries in 22 patients with their first (and only) anterior wall AMI and in 28 patients with their first (and only) posterior wall AMI. Although the percentage of coronary arteries narrowed at some point 76-100% in XSA by plaque was similar in both groups (74%-vs-75%); mean 3.0 of 4 coronary arteries per patient), quantitatively the amount of narrowing was different. Of 1,166 5-mm coronary segments in the 22 patients with anterior wall AMI, 23% were narrowed 76-100% in XSA by plaque alone, and of the 28 patients with posterior wall AMI, 39% were so narrowed (p<.001). The extent of the severe coronary narrowing, however, varied greatly among the individual patients. Among the 22 anterior wall AMI patients, 4-61% of the 5-mm segments were narrowed 76-100% by plaque, and of the posterior wall AMI patients, 18-71% of the segments were similarly narrowed.

Most physicians, I suspect, believe that patients with anterior wall AMI have severe narrowing of the LAD coronary artery by atherosclerotic plaque with less severe narrowing of the dominant posterior coronary artery, and that patients with posterior wall AMI have severe narrowing of the right or LC coronary artery (or both) with less narrowing of the LAD coronary artery. The data collected by Brosius and me do not support this belief[8]. In all 22 patients with anterior AMI, the LAD artery was narrowed 76-100% by plaque, but in 20 of these 22 patients the dominant posterior coronary artery (right in 86%) also was severely narrowed by plaque. In all 28 patients with posterior AMI, both the dominant posterior (right in 93%) and the LAD coronary arteries were narrowed 76-100% by plaque. The mean percent of 5 mm segments of LAD narrowed 76-100% in XSA by plaque was greater than that of either the "dominant" posterior or "other" posterior coronary artery in the 22 patients with anterior AMI (30%-vs-21%, p<0.05). Among the 28 patients with posterior AMI, however, the percent of 5 mm segments narrowed 76-100% in XSA did not differ among the LAD, dominant posterior (right in 93%) or other posterior (LC in 93%) coronary artery. Thus, why some patients with severe coronary atherosclerosis have anterior wall AMI and others have posterior wall AMI cannot be explained by the amount of luminal narrowing by atherosclerotic plaque in either the anterior or posterior perfusing coronary arteries.

CORONARY ARTERIAL THROMBOSIS

Views on the frequency of, and the significance of, coronary arterial thrombi in patients with AMI have varied. The facts are these[9-11]:

(1) thrombus is observed at necropsy in a coronary artery in 50-80% of patients with fatal transmural AMI;

(2) when present, the thrombus always is located in the coronary artery responsible for perfusing the area of LV myocardium which is necrotic;

(3) the larger the area of myocardial necrosis, the greater the likelihood of finding a coronary thrombus at necropsy;

(4) the thrombus is usually short (<2 cm long);

(5) the thrombus nearly always is located in the proximal one-half of the LAD or LC coronary arteries, but the distal half of the right coronary artery is frequently its location when this artery is involved;

(6) the thrombus is virtually always superimposed on underlying atherosclerotic plaque;

(7) the area of the coronary lumen occupied by thrombus is usually much less than that occupied by underlying atherosclerotic plaque.

For years coronary thrombosis was considered the cause of AMI and indeed for years AMI clinically was called "coronary thrombosis". The idea, of course, was that the lumen of a coronary artery was suddenly occluded by a thrombus, and blood thereafter was unable to perfuse LV myocardium distal to the thrombus with resulting LV myocardial necrosis. This idea was reinforced by the observation that the thrombus was always located in the coronary artery responsible for perfusing the area of myocardium which now was necrotic. In the 1960s and early 1970s, however, the concept that coronary thrombus was the precipitator of AMI was questioned and the view was presented that the coronary thrombus was the consequence of the AMI rather than the cause of it. Support for the "secondary" thesis was derived from the observation that the coronary thrombus appeared "younger" than the area of myocardial necrosis and that coronary thrombi were observed most often in the patients who had been in cardiogenic shock. Because cardiogenic shock occurs almost entirely in the patients with large infarcts compared to those with small infarcts, the frequency of coronary thrombus was observed to be much higher in the patients with the larger infarcts. Flow of blood in the coronary arteries presumably is much "slower" in the patients with, compared to those without, shock; relative stasis is increased, and clot formation, therefore, is more likely.

The secondary thesis of coronary thrombus in AMI appeared to be gaining advocates until the introduction of intracoronary (later intravenous) streptokinase therapy for AMI. Use of thrombolytic therapy required coronary angiography during the first few hours after onset of AMI. Injection of contrast material usually showed total occlusion of the coronary artery corresponding to the electrocardiographic location of the AMI. When the intracoronary streptokinase infusion produced opening of the coronary artery at the site of previous occlusion, it was therefore assumed that a thrombus was responsible for the final occlusion. Residual narrowing (by underlying atherosclerotic plaque), however, was nearly always apparent after the superimposed filling defect, presumably a thrombus, was lysed. Thus, today the view that coronary thrombus does play the primary role in precipitating AMI has returned. We must all be cautious, however, in diagnosing coronary thrombus by contrast material. (What is and is not thrombus is debated even at necropsy at times.) Another factor supporting the primary role of coronary thrombus in precipitating AMI is the observation at surgery within a few hours after onset of AMI of a thrombus in the "infarct vessel". How one distinguishes, however, a true thrombus, which is only 2 or 3 hours old and therefore only loosely adherent, from a nonadherent blood clot (not a true thrombus) has not been resolved.

Irrespective of whether it precipitates or follows AMI, coronary thrombus is considerably less important than is the underlying atherosclerotic plaque. Some patients have transmural AMI without identifiable coronary thrombus by any means. The amount of coronary luminal area occupied by thrombus compared to the amount occupied by underlying plaque is small. Brosius and I[10] examined histological sections of coronary arteries containing thrombi in 54 necropsy patients with transmural AMI. The 54 coronary arteries in the 54 patients were narrowed 33-95% (mean 81) in XSA by atherosclerotic plaque alone at the site of the thrombus (occlusive in 47 and non-occlusive in 7) and from 26 to 98% (mean 75) within the 2 cm portion of artery distal to the distal site of attachment of the thrombus. Of the 54 arteries, 52 (96%) were narrowed 76 to 98% in XSA by atherosclerotic plaque alone at or immediately proximal or distal to the thrombus and 26 (48%) were narrowed 91-98% by plaque alone. The thrombi were 0.1-6.0 mm^2 (mean 1.4) in XSA_2 and the underlying atherosclerotic plaques were 3.0-21.0 mm^2 (mean 9). Thus, among necropsy patients with transmural AMI, coronary thrombi occur at sites already severely narrowed by atherosclerotic plaques.

Although their importance in precipitating AMI can be questioned or minimized, coronary thrombi may play a major role in the development of the atherosclerotic plaque in the first place. Several observations suggest the atherosclerotic plaques result, at least in part, from the organization of thrombi[12]:

(1)   The presence of known components of thrombi - namely fibrin and platelets - within atherosclerotic plaques.
(2)   The occurrence of known components of atherosclerotic plaques - namely foam cells, cholesterol clefts, pultaceous debris, calcium - in organized haematomas or known thrombi wherever they occur in the body.
(3)   The presence of multiple channels in lumens - a recognized consequence of organization of pulmonary thromboemboli. Such multiluminal channels are found in about 7% of 5-mm segments of coronary arteries in patients with fatal coronary events[13].
(4)   The major component of the complicated atherosclerotic plaque, i.e. those capable of causing significant luminal narrowing, in the coronary arteries of patients with fatal coronary heart disease is fibrous tissue or collagen, not lipid. Often the "density" of the fibrous tissue obstructing the coronary lumen is different in different portions of a plaque, and these subunits may be demarcated by distant elastic lamellae. These subunits suggest that thrombus is deposited at different times and that the "density" of the resulting fibrous tissue may be determined by the composition of the initial thrombus, i.e. whether platelets or fibrin predominated.
(5)   Experimentally induced thrombi under proper conditions may be transformed into atherosclerotic plaques closely resembling those observed in human coronary arteries.

These factors do not prove that thrombosis is the cause of atherosclerosis, but together they strongly suggest that organization of thrombi plays a major role in the development of the complicated atherosclerotic plaque. Most serious students of the morphology of the arterial plaque presently support, in whole or in part, the thrombogenic origin of atherosclerosis. Because the clotting factors in the blood appear to be similar in all population groups and because symptomatic atherosclerosis develops only in the population groups with total blood cholesterol levels >150 mg/dl, the latter also play a role in the development of the plaque. Cholesterol may exert its effect, however, more by its ability to alter the clotting mechanism than by its ability to infiltrate the arterial wall.

REFERENCES

1. Maron BJ, Epstein SE, Roberts WC. Hypertrophic cardiomyopathy and transmural myocardial infarction without significant atherosclerosis of the extramural arteries. Am J Cardiol 1979; 43: 1086-1102.
2. Arnett EN, Roberts WC. Acute myocardial infarction and angiographically normal coronary arteries. An unproven combination. Circulation 1976; 53: 395-400.
3. Roberts WC, Curry RC, Jr, Isner JM, Waller BF, McManus BM, Mariani-Constantini R, Ross AM. Sudden death in Prinzmetal's angina with coronary spasm documented by angiography. Analysis of three necropsy patients. Am J Cardiol 1982; 50: 203-210.
4. Roberts WC, Jones AA. Quantification of coronary arterial narrowing at necropsy in acute transmural myocardial infarction: analysis and comparison of findings in 27 patients and 22 controls. Circulation 1980; 61: 786-790.
5. Saphir O, Priest WS, Hamburger WW, Katz LN. Coronary atherosclerosis, coronary thrombosis and the resulting myocardial changes. An evaluation of their respective clinical pictures including the electrocardiographic records based on the anatomical findings. Am Heart J 1935; 10: 567.
6. Blumgart HL, Schlesinger MJ, Davis DK. Studies on the relation of the clinical manifestations of angina pectoris, coronary thrombosis, and myocardial infarction to the pathologic findings with particular reference to the significance of the collateral circulation. Am Heart J 1940; 19: 1.
7. Yater WM, Traum AH, Brown WC, Fitzgerald RP, Geisler MA, Wilcox BB. Coronary artery disease in men 18-39 years of age. Report of 866 cases; 450 with necropsy examination. Am Heart J 1948; 36: 334-372, 481-526, and 683-722.
8. Brosius FC, III, Roberts WC. Comparison of degree and extent of coronary narrowing by atherosclerotic plaque in anterior and posterior transmural acute myocardial infarction. Circulation 1981; 64: 715-722.
9. Roberts WC, Buja LM. The frequency and significance of coronary arterial thrombi and other observations in fatal acute myocardial infarction. A study of 107 necropsy patients. Am J Med 1972; 52: 425-443.
10. Brosius FC, III, Roberts WC. Significance of coronary arterial thrombus in transmural acute myocardial infarction. A study of 54 necropsy patients. Circulation 1981; 63: 810-816.
11. Roberts WC. Coronary thrombosis and fatal myocardial ischaemia. Circulation 1974; 49: 1-3.

12. Roberts WC. Does thrombosis play a major role in the development of symtom-producing atherosclerotic plaques? Circulation 1973; 48: 1161-1166.
13. Virmani R, Roberts WC. Extravasated erythrocytes, iron and fibrin in atherosclerotic plaques of coronary arteries in fatal coronary heart diseases and their relation to luminal thrombus: frequency and significance in 57 necropsy patients and in 2958 5-mm segments of 224 major epicardial coronary arteries. Am Heart J 1983; 105: 788-797.

15
Perspectives in the management of acute myocardial infarction
F. Mauri, A. Roghi and F. Rovelli

INTRODUCTION

The primary objective of the treatment of acute myocardial infarction (AMI),with sudden and unexpected death essentially eliminated by the preventive approach to the ventricular arrhythmias,is now the other major complication of AMI:pump failure.Although advances have been made in the treatment of heart failure,it remains the primary cause of in-hospital death from AMI.The extent of ischemic necrosis correlates well with the degree of pump failure and with mortality.Over the last 15 years,intervention trials to reduce infarct size and mortality during the acute phase of AMI have been performed with beta-blockers,calcium antagonists and thrombolytic drugs.
A review of these trials is essential to understand their limits and to suggest perspectives of treatment.(1)

BETA-BLOCKERS

A review of three large randomised studies on beta-blockers in AMI (Goteborg Metoprolol Trial (2),MIAMI (3), ISIS-1 (4)),suggest that this treatment can decrease infarct size and reduce the incidence of ventricular arrhythmias.In addition,beta-blockers reduce early in-hospital reinfarction.Examination of all available randomised trials,involving over 27.000 patients,suggests that beta-blockers reduce early mortality by about 14%,but only half of all patients admitted to the coronary care units (CCUs) have been eligible for such treatment.
A review of fatal and non-fatal events in these trials suggests that treatment reduces mortality in the first week by about 15%,but the low vascular mortality of these patients (3.8 treated group vs 4.57 control group), suggests a strong pre-selection of patients with a lower mortality rate than expected (10-12%).In the MIAMI study,

Table 1. Trials on AMI: number of patients,contraindica-
tions,time from the onset of symptoms,time of
mortality rate assessment,mortality rate.
T.=treated, C.= controls

TRIAL	ELIGIBLE	ENROLLED		CONTR.	ONSET TIME		MORTALITY	
					SYMPT.	ASS.M.	T.	C.
	n	n	%	%	h	days	%	%
GOTEBORG	2802	1395	49.7	28	48	11	4.2	5
MIAMI	26439	5778	21.9	38	24	14	4.3	4
ISIS-1	?	16027	-	-	12	7	3.9	4
DANISH	7415	3498	47.1	37	no limits	21	9.5	8
GISSI	31826	11806	37.1	13	12	14-21	10.7	13
ISAM	3344	1741	57.1	-	6	21	6.3	7

a retrospective subgroup analysis indicated that all the
observed reduction in mortality was among patients defined at high risk (age over 60,female,electrocardiographic
signs of AMI on admission,diabetes,previous myocardial
infarction,angina pectoris,hypertension,congestive heart
failure),but other trials as ISIS,with a larger randomised population,have not confirmed these findings:this
suggests that identification of subgroups of patients is
unlikely to be possible in trials that are scarcely large
enough on their own to determine the overall effect of
treatment.
However,there is increasing evidence that in AMI,with
early intravenous infusion (iv) of beta-blockers,is possible to reduce cumulative enzyme release and the electro
cardiographic evolution (5),suggesting a significative
reduction of infarct size (about 20%).
These studies also provide evidence of reduction of ventricular arrhythmias:striking effects on ventricular fibrillation have been seen;Goteborg Trial observed a reduction of ventricular tachicardia of .9% vs 2.4%;also
ventricular fibrillation was reduced (2% vs 3.7%).Data on
cardiac arrests in hospital suggests that early iv treatment might produce a reduction of about 15% in the odds
of cardiac arrest.
A review of reinfarction in hospital in ISIS-1,MIAMI and
Goteborg,suggests a reduction by about 18% of this event.

In addition,these studies provide indirect evidence that early iv treatment with beta-blockers in unstable angina is effective in prevention of AMI.

CALCIUM ANTAGONISTS

Experimental evidence of calcium antagonists efficacy in reducing infarct size and clinical evidence of their activity as vasodilators and on coronary spasm,favour the theoretical use of these drugs in the early hours of AMI. Intervention trials during the acute phase of AMI have been performed with calcium antagonists verapamil,nifedipine and diltiazem (6,7,8).

The Danish Multicenter Study Group on Verapamil in Myocardial Infarction (6) is the only randomised large scale intervention study on verapamil:3498 patients were enrolled (47% of eligible population),while 37% of all patients admitted met the exclusion criteria (shock,hypotension,heart failure,bradycardia,atrioventricular block, valvular or congenital heart disease,beta-blockers treatment).After three weeks from the onset of symptoms the mortality rate was sligthy higher in the verapamil group (9.48 vs 8.06),although this difference is not statistically significant.Even after six and twelve monthes no significative differences were found in the mortality rate of the two groups.In this trial 40% of patients were enrolled after 6 hours from the onset of symptoms: contrary to expectations,no differences were found in the mortality rates in patients with a duration of symtoms up to six hours.Paradoxically,the mortality rate was significantly reduced in the verapamil group of patients with a duration of symptoms between 6 and 24 hours,suggesting the unlikely hypotesis that very early intervention do not change the prognosis of AMI.

We need further large,randomised studies to evaluate the effects of calcium antagonists in AMI.

THROMBOLYTIC TREATMENT

An occlusive or near-occlusive thrombus overlying or adjacent to an atherosclerotic plaque in a coronary artery appears to be the cause of most transmural infarcts: therefore,reperfusion of the ischemic zone by the promt dissolution of the thrombus with a thrombolytic agent is a logical approach to the reduction of infarct size.Numerous studies (11) clearly suggested that the administration of Streptokinase (SK) via a coronary catheter is effective in lysing the offending thrombus in about 75% of cases,but this therapeutic approach needs an operational setting not easy achievable in all CCUs and is very expensive.

The trial of the Italian Group for the Study of Streptokinase in Infarct (GISSI) (9),which enrolled a central
randomised population of 11.712 patients with AMI,admit-
ted to 176 CCUs within 12 hours from the onset of symptoms (50% within three hours),clearly suggests that:

(1) Intravenous infusion of 1.5 million units of SK
over 60 minutes reduces in-hospital mortality (10.3 vs
13%,p 0.0002);

(2) The decrease of mortality is most streaking in
patients treated early,overall in those treated within
three hours from the onset of symptoms (9.2 vs 12%,
p 0.0005);

(3) A data generated analysis of the 1277 patients
randomised within 1 hours from the onset of pain suggests
that the very early treatment reduces in-hospital mortality by about 47%;

(4) The release of creatinine Kinase MB was studied
in 7632 patients (3568 SK group,4064 control group) with
serial blood samples: the time of peak CK-MB was significant earlier in patients of SK group than control group
and the morphology of the obtained curves was clearly
different in the two groups,suggesting an infarct size
reduction in those treated with SK (overall in the early
treated patients);

(5) The result of the follow-up (6-12 monthes) demonstrate that a significant reduction of mortality is
still present;

(6) The adverse reaction of SK (major bleeds or
others), proved to have a lower incidence than expected;

(7) The incidence of reinfarctions is significantly
increased (doubled) in the SK group,and this opens important questions about the correct therapeutic approach
after thrombolysis.

PERSPECTIVES

GISSI trial confirms that with a safe tretment which
needs a simple operational setting achievable in all
CCUs,is possible to change the natural history of AMI:
the question remains open whether any form of anticoagu-
lation or of antiplatlet therapy could prevent reocclu-
sion of opened infarct-related arteries and/or reinfarction.

An other important question is about prevention of ischemic and reperfusion myocardial damage.There is increasing
evidence that reperfusion is a very powerful salvaging a-
gent in reversibly ijured cells,but it can also accelera-

GISSI: RELATIVE RISK SK/C IN RELATION TO TIME FROM ONSET OF SYMPTOMS AND TREATMENT.

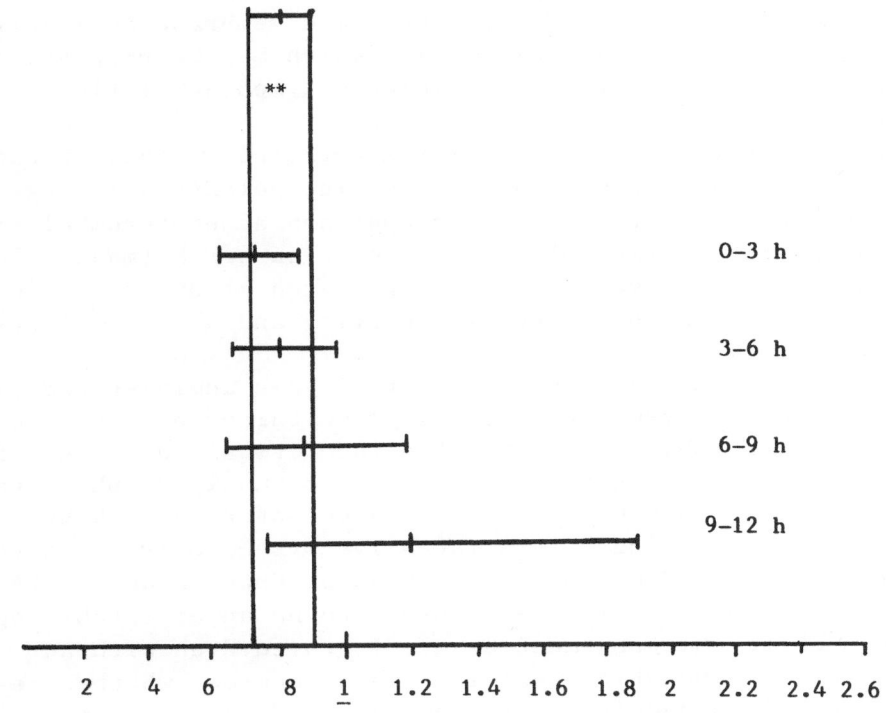

```
**



                                                    0-3 h



                                                    3-6 h



                                                    6-9 h


                                                    9-12 h




    2    4    6    8   1   1.2  1.4  1.6  1.8  2   2.2  2.4 2.6
```

** = confidence limit
SK = treated with streptokinase
C = controls

te destruction in cells which are already dead at time
of reflow (12),depending on the severity and duration of
ischemia.Reperfusion in the early stages of ischemia,
with cellular structures and pathways of electron transport and oxidative phosphorilation still intact,should
result in a prompt resumption of contractile activity,
without significative cellular damage.After a prolonged
period of ischemia (whose length is difficult to establish in man,since often the beginning of ischemia can
not be exactly identified),myocardial reperfusion do not
let to cellular function restablishment:on the contrary,
it produce lactate and CPK release in coronary venous
circulation,with massive tissue and mithocondrial calcium overload and further decline in mithocondrial fun-
ction.Myocardial ischemia reduces the activity of enzymes as superoxide dismutase and glutathione peroxidase

which are important difensive mechanisms against activated metabolites of oxigen:reperfusion could produce
oxygen radicals above the neutralizing capacity of the
cells,leading to the peroxidation of membrane lipids.
This in turn results in an increased membrane permeability and mithocondrial alteration which may be responsable
of large efflux of intracellular enzymes and influx of
calcium.(13)
Trials in progress with calcium-antagonists,anti-oxidant
agents,antiplatlets drugs and anticoagulants will suggest the correct therapeutic approach after thrombolysis.
The potential risk of adverse reaction of SK (major bleeds or others),stimulated the research of others lytic
agents with a more specific activity and a lower aller-
gic reactivity.
Tissue plasminogen activator (tPA),when administered intravenously,lyses approximately two-thirds of recent coronary thrombi (14);it has the theoretical advantage of
causing fibrinolytic activity predominantly at the site
of a fresh thrombus,and thus may be safer than SK by
virtue of causing a less intensive systemic lytic state
than that produced by intravenous SK.However,until tPA
will be fully available,SK seems to be an acceptable approach to AMI treatment,as GISSI proved.Even with an
ideal thrombolytic agent,it remains unclear whether mechanical revascularization by means of coronary angioplasty or by-pass surgery will be required following
successfull thrombolysis.A post-thrombolysis rational
therapeutic approach imposes the evaluation of the residual areas of myocardial ischemia and of coronary steno-
sis.Further studies are need on coronary artery by-pass
grafting after thrombolysis to assess long-term results.
Percutaneous transluminal coronary angioplasty (PTCA)
appears to be a reasonable approach to therapy (15),if a
severe obstruction persists.The necessity of having a
well-trained angiography team "stand-by" at all times
limits this approach to a small fraction of patients
with AMI,although in single cases PTCA could be carried
out within few days from the onset of symptoms,following
thrombolytic therapy.
At present, it is advisable to restrict an aggressive
therapeutic approach of AMI to selected patients.
In our experience,patients with AMI without contraindications (recent bleedings,cerebrovascular accidents,sur-
gical procedures,trauma or invasive procedures,uncon-
trolled hypertension,previous treatment with SK) are

treated with SK,then with heparin followed by oral anti-
coagulants.All drugs utilized in the acute phase of infarction to reduce the necrotic area and to protect i-
schemic myocardium (beta-blockers,calcium-antagonists,
nitrates) are,if possible,discontinued to evaluate the
residual myocardial ischemia.If ischemia persists,pa-
tients are submitted to coronarography and eventually to
PTCA or by-pass surgery.
At present this is our policy which could be proposed to
almost all CCUs for its feasibility.Actually,considering
the high number of patients affected by AMI,the most important problem is to identify a therapeutic approach
effective in all circumstances,feasible in the majority
of Cardiac Departments.

REFERENCES

1.   Yusuf S,Peto R,Lewis J,Collins R,Sleigh P (1985).
Beta-blockade during and after myocardial infarction:an
overview of the randomised trials.Prog Car Dis,27:335-71
2.   Herlitz J,Elmfeldt D,Holmberg S,Malek I,Nyberg G,
Pennert K,Ryden L,Swedberg K,Vedin A,Waagstein F,
Waldenstrom I,Wedel H,Wilhelmsen L,Wilhelmsson G,
Hjalmarson A (1984).Goteborg Metoprolol Trial:Mortality
and Causes of Death.Am J Cardiol,53:9D:14D
3.   The MIAMI trial research group:Metoprolol in acute
myocardial infarction (MIAMI).A randomized placebo-controlled international trial (with discussants) (1985).
Eur Heart J,6:199-226.
4.   ISIS-1 (First International Study of Infarct Survival) Collaborative Group:Randomised Trial of Intravenous
Atenolol Among 16027 Cases of Suspected Acute Myocardial
Infarction (1986).Lancet,july 12:57-66
5.   Yusuf S,Sleigh P,Rossi PRF,et al.(1983).Reduction in
Infarct Size,Arrhythmias,Chest Pain and Morbidity by
Early Intravenous Beta-Blockade in Suspected Acute Myocardial Infarction.Circulation,67:32-41
6.   Verapamil in Acute Myocardial Infarction:The Danish
Study Group on Verapamil in Myocardial Infarction (1984).
Eur Heart J,5:516-528
7.   Pearle DL (1984).Nifedipine in Acute Myocardial In-
farction.Am J Cardiol,54:21E-23E
8.   Gibson RS,Boden WE,Theroux P,Strauss HD,Peatt GM et
al.(1986).Diltiazem Reinfarction Study Group:Diltiazem
and Reinfarction in Patients with non-Q Wave Myocardial
Infarction.Results of a Double-Blind,Randomised Multicenter Trial.N Engl J Med,315:932-936
9.   GISSI (Gruppo Italiano per lo Studio della Strepto-

chinasi nell'Infarto Miocardico):Effectiveness of
Intravenous Thrombolytic Treatment in Acute Myocardial
Infarction (1986).Lancet,February 22:397-401.

10. The I.S.A.M. Study Group:A Prospective Trial of In-
travenous Streptokinase in Acute Myocardial Infarction:
Mortality,Morbidity and Infarct Size at 21 Days (1986).
N Engl J Med,414:1465-1471

11. TIMI Study Group: The Thrombolysis in Myocardial
Infarction.Phase I findings (1985).N Engl J Med,312:932-
936

12. Schaper W. (1984).Experimental infarcts and the
Microcirculation.In "Therapeutic approaches to Myocardial Infarct Size Limitation".p.79.(New York:Raven Press)

13. Ferrari R,Ceconi C,Curello S,Bigoli MC,Raddino R,
Albertini A,Visioli O,(1984).Reversible and Irreversible
Ischemic Damage:Importance of Energy Metabolism.G Ital
Cardiol 14/2:867-874

14. Verstraete M,Bernard R,Bory M et al. (1985).Rando-
mised Trial of Intravenous Recombinant Tissue-Type Plasminogen Activator Versus Intravenous Streptokinase in
Acute Myocardial Infarction.Lancet,i:842-847

15. Meyer J,Merx W,Schmitz H,Erbed R,Dorr T.K.,Lambertz
H et al. (1982).Percutaneous Transluminal Coronary Angioplasty Immediately After Intracoronary Streptolysis
of Transmural Myocardial Infarction.Circulation vol.66:
905-912

16
Atherosclerosis and ischaemic heart disease: surgical solutions

A. Pierangeli, G. Marinelli, F. Dozza, B. Turinetto
and V. Pierangeli

SUMMARY

From July 1974 to December 1985 868 patients with coronary artery disease underwent surgery at the Cardiosurgical Department of the University of Bologna.

One or two vessels disease was present in 31,8%, three or more vessels disease in the remaining 68,2%.

Early mortality was 7% and late mortality 5%.

Surgical results are analized in relation to the kind of operation (elective, urgent, emergency), the EF, the LVEDP, the number of distal anastomosis, the type of rivascularization (complete of incomplete) and the ventricular score.

INTRODUCTION

Optimal treatment of ischemic heart disease is still object of discussion since in 1967 Favaloro introduced routine coronary artery by-pass surgery for treatment of coronary arteries stenosis.

As the matter of facts the surgery represents one possible solution to this disease which accounts as the mayor cause of mortality in occidental countries.

The aim of this work is to evaluate short and long term surgical results in relation to the kind of operation (elective, urgent, emergency) to some functional parameters (left ventricular score, EF, LVEDP) to the number of distal anastomosis and to the type of rivascularization (complete, incomplete).

MATERIAL AND METHOD

From July 1974 to December 1985 994 patients underwent myocardial rievascularization at the Cardiosurgical Institute of the University of Bologna. 868 had isolated coronary artery by-pass graft (CABG); in 126 associated procedures like left ventricular aneurysmectomies, valvular replacements, ASD closure and carotid thromboendo-arterectomies were performed as well.

In this study only isolated CABG patiets are considered: in 791 the operation was electivly done in 53 urgent and in 23 as emergency.

The early mortality was 4,7% (41 pts), in great majority (32 pts.) due to peri- or post-operative myocardial infarction.

The late mortality was 5% (43 pts.): 14 died for AMI, 2 for hepatitis, 6 for neoplastic disease and 19 for unknown reasons.

Table I

N. patients: 868

Age: $\begin{cases} \text{min.} \quad 33 \text{ years} \\ \text{max.} \quad 75 \text{ years} \end{cases}$ $\overline{56,1} \pm 7,8$

Sex: $\begin{cases} \text{O} \quad 766 \text{ pts.} \\ \text{O} \quad 102 \text{ pts.} \end{cases}$

N. vessels diseased: $3 \pm 1,2$ (1   8)

N. By-pass: $2,6 \pm 1,2$ (1   9)

Type of rivascular.: $\begin{cases} \text{complete} \quad 586 \text{ pts}(68,1\%) \\ \text{incomplete} \quad 275 \text{ pts}(31,9\%) \end{cases}$

Type of graft: $\begin{cases} \text{saphenous v.} \quad 828 \text{ pts}(95,6\%) \\ \text{mammary a.} \quad 38 \text{ pts. } (4,4\%) \end{cases}$

Kind of operation:	Elective	Urgent	Emergency
N. pts.	791	53	23
Early mortality	36 (4,6%)	6 (11,3%)	1 (4,3%)
Late mortality	37 (4,7%)	4 (7,5%)	2 (8,7%)

The clinical results have been good; as shown in Table II after surgery more than 90% of the patients are in CCS 1 or 2.

Table II

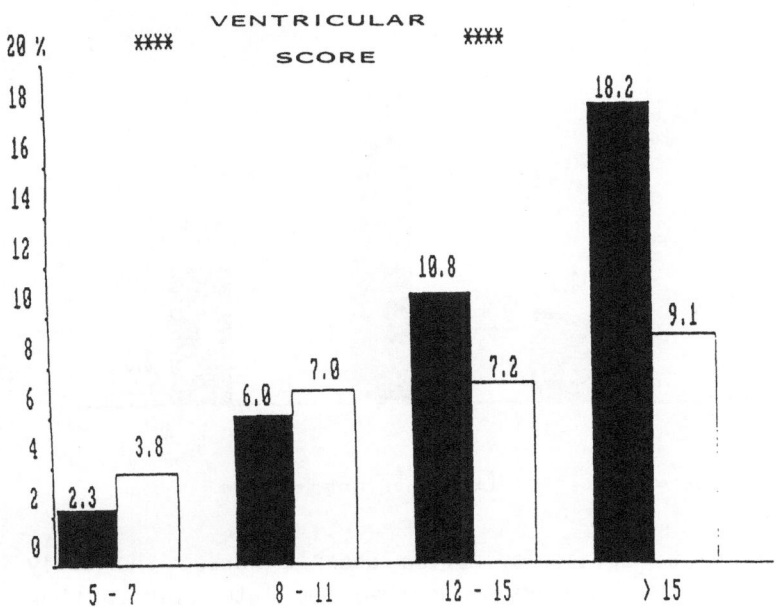

The statistical analysis of the factors correlated to the early and late mortality has been carried out by the Student t- test and by the χ square method.

RESULTS

Early prognosis is worse in patients operated on urgent or emergency situations whereas the late one doesn't seem modified.

The global results are unfavorably affected by the presence of an EF $<$ 50% and a LVEDP $>$ 15 mmHg even if the difference is not statistically significative.

The early and late mortality are strictly correlated to the coronary score with an almost linear rate (p $<$ 0.001).

Table III

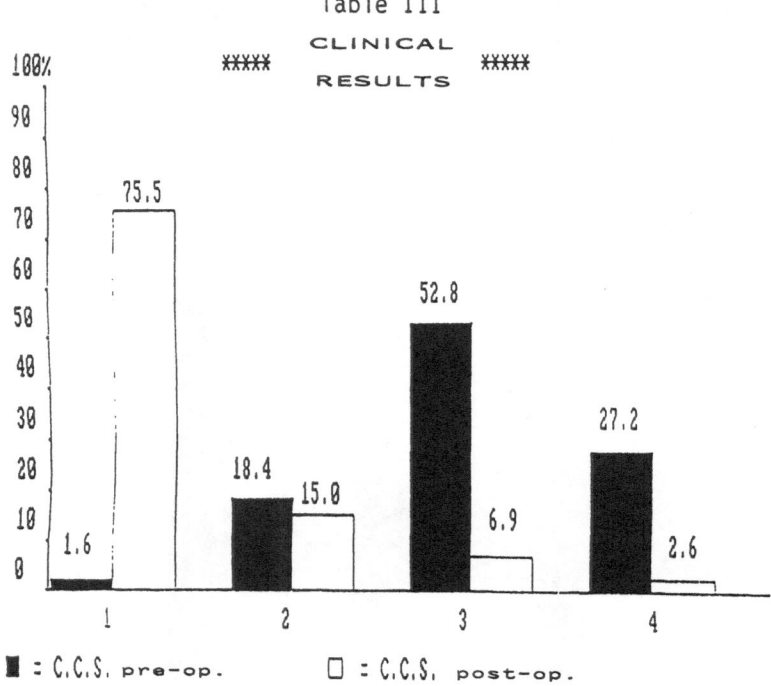

CLINICAL RESULTS

■ = C.C.S. pre-op.   □ = C.C.S. post-op.

Incomplete revascularization doesn't worsen the early outcome and doesn't seem to improve the late results when compared to the complete revascularization.

CONCLUSIONS

The actual treatment of the ischemic heart disease is based upon three different possibilities:
1) medical treatment;
2) coronary angioplasty (PTCA) and
3) coronary artery by-pass surgery.

It is reported in numerous studies (Cass V.A. Coop S. ECSS) that in well selected subgroups of patients like those with left main[6-11] trunk stenosis, with triple vessels disease, with isolated stenosis of the LAD highly located[12], particularly in the young people, or with angina refractory to the medical treatment there is no doubt that the CABG is the best available treatment as far as the clinical results and the survival are concerned[9].

The operative risk seems to be better correlated to the left ventricular contractility which is directly or indirectly evaluated by some parameters like the EF, the

LVEDP and the coronary score than to the anatomy of the coronaries.[1-2-3-4-5-13]

The extent of the coronary arteries disease even in our experience seem to effect mostly the long term survival particularly in case of multiple lesions in young patients or in case of left main trunk disease.

The clinical results as far as the "angina" is concerned are very good and anyway superior to the medical treatments.[2-3-9]

Unfortunately the CABG doesn't modify the evolution of the artheriosclerosis: after 10 years a progression of the disease is discovered in the native circulation of 50% of the patients.

Therefore the CABG is an excellent "palliative" treatment for the coronary artetry disease; the operation in any case carries an higher operative[7-8-10] risk and a smaller probability of long term success.

BIBLIOGRAPHY
1.   Brandt III, B, Wright, CB, Doty, DB, Rossi, NP and Ehrenhaft, JL (April 1980). Surgical treatment of left main coronary artery disease: operative risk. Surgery, 436, 440, vol.87, n.4.
2.   European coronary surgery study group. Prospective randomized study of coronary artery bypass surgery in stable angina pectoris: a progress report on survival (1982). Circulation 11, 65.
3.   Foster, ED, Fisher, LD, Kaiser, GC and Myers,WO (1984). Comparison of operative mortality and morbidity for inital and repeart coronary artery bypass grafting: the coronary artery surgery study (CASS). Registry experience. Ann Thorac Surg 38, 563.
4.   Kirklin, JW, Kouchoukos, NT, Blackstone, EH and Oberman, A (1979). Research related to surgical treatment of coronary artery disease. Circulation, 60, n.7.
5.   Kennedy, JW, Kaiser, GC, Fisher, LD, Fritz, JK, Mysers, W, Mudd, JG and Ryan, TJ (1981). Clinical and angiographic predictors of operative mortality from the collaborative study in coronary artery surgery (CASS). Circulation, 63, n.4
6.   Jones, EL, King III, SB, Craver, JM, Douglas, JS Jr, Kaplan, JA, Morgan, EA, Brown, CM, Bradford, JM and Hatcher, CR Jr (1980). The spectrum of left main coronary artery disease. J Thorac Cardiovasc Surg, 79, 109-116.

7.   Loop, FD (July 1981). On reoperations. The Annals of Thoracic Surgery, 4, 5, vol. 32, n.1.

8.   Loop, FD, Cosgrove, DM, Kramer, JR, Lytle, BW, Taylor, PC, Golding, LAR and Groves, LK (May 1981). Late clinical and arteriographic results in 500 coronary artery reoperations. The Journal of Thoracic and Cardiovascular Surgery, 675, 685, vol. 81, n. 5.

9.   Loop, FD, Cosgrove, DM, Lytle, BW and Golding, LR (1981) Life expectancy after coronary artery surgery. The American Journal of Surgery, 665, 671. 10. Qazi, A, Garcia, JM, Mispireta, LA and Corso,PL (1981). Reoperation for coronary artery disease. The Annals of Thoracic Surgery, 16, 18, vol. 32, n. 1.

11.   Tahan, SR, Geha, AS, Hammond, GL, Cohen, LW and Langou, RA (1980). By-pass surgery for left main coronary artery disease. Reduced perioperative myocardial infarction with preoperative intra-aortic balloon counterpulsation. Br Heart, 191, 198.

12.   Tyras, DH, Kaiser, GC, Barner, HB, Codd, JE, Pennington, G and Willam, VL (1980). The rationale for operrative therapy of symptomatic single-vessel coronary artery disease. J Thorac Cardiovasc Surg, 80, 73, 78.

13.   Veterans administration coronary artery bypass surgery cooperative study group (1984). Elevenyear survival in the veterans administration randomized trial of coornary by-pass surgery for stable angina. N Engl J Med, 311, 1333.

PRESENT KNOWLEDGE AND PERSPECTIVES OF CALCIUM ENTRY BLOCKERS IN THE MANAGEMENT OF CORONARY ARTERY DISEASE

17
Effects of calcium antagonists and adrenergic antihypertensive drugs on cellular cholesterol metabolism

W. Krone, A. Klass, H. Nägele, B. Behnke and
H. Greten

INTRODUCTION

Hypertension and hyperlipidemia are major risk factors for coronary heart disease and atherosclerosis. Several studies have shown a decrease in cardiovascular disease by lowering blood pressure. However, there has been a failure to demonstrate a significant reduction in myocardial infarction, particularly in mildly hypertensive patients. Since many antihypertensive drugs alter plasma lipoprotein levels in an unfavourable way they may increase coronary risk and therefore offset the beneficial effects of lowering blood pressure. Other antihypertensive agents have few adverse or even beneficial effects on plasma lipoprotein levels (for review see 1). The mechanisms responsible for these drug effects have not been established. Furthermore it is not yet clear whether antihypertensive agents directly affect cellular lipid and cholesterol metabolism.

Increases of plasma lipid levels may be caused by an increased synthesis or a decreased catabolism of lipoproteins (for review see 2). The triglyceride-rich very low density lipoproteins (VLDL) which transports lipids of hepatic origin in plasma interact with lipoprotein lipase in capillaries, releasing most of their triglycerides. The VLDL return to the circulation as intermediate density lipoprotein. Some of these particles were taken up by the liver by interacting with the apo E and apo B, E receptors, others undergo further triglyceride hydrolysis and are converted to low density lipoproteins (LDL). The pathway of LDL involves high affinity binding to specific LDL receptors of the liver and extrahepatic tissues, internalization and lysosomal degradation. The resulting free cholesterol then suppresse endogenous cholesterol and LDL receptor synthesis and stimulates cholesterol ester formation, thereby regulating cholesterol homeostasis of the cell. Therefore, the activity of lipoprotein lipase and the number of lipoprotein receptors in the liver and extrahepatic tissues may determine the degradation and uptake of plasma lipoproteins. Brown and Goldstein have provided strong evidence that there is an inverse association between the plasma cholesterol levels and LDL receptor number (2). Several genetic, nutritional, hormonal and pharmacologic factors affect LDL receptor activity (3). While an increase is caused by a cholesterol low diet, insulin, thyroxin and bile acid-binding resins, recent studies from our laboratory have shown that catecholamines suppress LDL receptor activity (table 1), thus increasing plasma cholesterol concentrations. The action of calcium antagonists and antihypertensive adrenergic drugs at the cellular level, however, is not clear.

VLDL metabolism

Reduced lipoprotein lipase activity and decreased degradation of VLDL by the unspecific beta-blocker propranolol has been reported (5). In contrast the cardioselective beta-blocker metoprolol did not change (6) and the alpha-1-antagonist prazosin increased the enzyme activity (6). These results might partly explain why there is an increase of plasma triglyceride by propranolol, only a small effect by metoprolol and a decrease in triglycerides by prazosin (1).

LDL metabolism

Freshly isolated human mononuclear leukocytes have been useful cells for studying the regulation of cholesterol metabolism by lipoproteins (7), hormones (8) and drugs (9). Strong evidence has been provided that mononuclear leukocytes possess alpha-1 (10), alpha-2 (11) and beta-2 (12) adrenergic receptors. Studies from our laboratory have shown that cholesterol biosynthesis is regulated by catecholamines (13) which may act via alpha-2- (14) and beta-2- (15) adrenoceptors. Therefore mononuclear leukocytes were used to study the effects of the adrenergic antihypertensive drugs propranolol, clonidine, alpha-methyldopa, urapidil, indoramin and prazosin on cholesterol synthesis (15). The beta-blocker propranolol which per se had no effect on the pathway reversed the epinephrine induced inhibition of sterol synthesis. The central acting antihypertensives clonidine and alpha-methyldopa caused a marked suppression of sterol synthesis. In contrast the alpha-1-antagonists indoramin, prazosin and urapidil had no effect per se or on the epinephrine induced suppression of cholesterol synthesis. Catecholamines exert their action on sterol synthesis by stimulating adenylate cyclase as well as by processes

142

Table 1. Effects of calcium antagonists, beta-blockers and alpha-adrenergic antihypertensive drugs on LDL receptor activity and cholesterol biosynthesis rate in freshly isolated human mononuclear leukocytes. For comparison the effects of hormones, lipid lowering drugs and diets are shown which consistently led to parallel changes in both, LDL receptor activity and cholesterol biosynthesis rate.

Regulating factors	Effect on	
	LDL receptor	Cholesterol synthesis
Calcium antagonists		
Verapamil	↑	↑
Nifedipine	=	=
Beta-blockers		
Propranolol*	↑	↑
Alpha-adrenergic antagonists		
Indoramin*	n.d.	=
Prazosin*	n.d.	=
Urapidil*	n.d.	=
Clonidine	n.d.	↓
Alpha-Methyldopa	n.d.	↓
Hormones		
Epinephrine	↓	↓
Insulin	↑	↑
Thyroxin	↑	↑
Lipid-lowering drugs		
Cholestyramine	↑	↑
Diets		
Cholesterol-rich	↓	↓
Cholesterol-low	↑	↑

n.d. means not determined; *, in the presence of epinephrine; ↑, increase; ↓, decrease; =, no change.

143

that regulate calcium ion fluxes. Experiments were performed to define the effects of calcium channel blockers
on cholesterol synthesis in human mononuclear leukocytes.
The clacium antagonist verapamil at higher concentrations increased sterol synthesis while nifedipine had no
effect (17) . In the presence of propranolol, which caused a total beta-blockade, epinephrine, alpha-methyl-
norepinephrine and N-methyldopa produced a marked inhibition of sterol synthesis which may be mediated by
alpha-2-adrenergic receptors (17). This suppression
could be abolished by both, verapamil and nifedipine.
    We have recently shown that insulin stimulated and
catecholamines suppress LDL receptor activity, i.e. the
high affinity accumulation and degradation of LDL in
human mononuclear leukocytes (18). The unspecific beta-
blocker propranolol had no effect per se but reversed
the epinephrine induced suppression of LDL receptor activity. Further studies in our laboratory show that the
LDL receptor is also regulated by alpha-receptors (Krone
W., Nägele H., Behnke B., unpublished results). This has
been deduced from experiments in which the unspecific
alpha-blocker phentolamine in the presence of propranolol totally prevented the suppression of LDL receptor
activity caused by epinephrine. The action of alpha-
adrenergic antihypertensive drugs on the LDL-pathway remains to be established. The calcium antagonist verapamil and nifedipine have different effects per se on LDL
receptor activity in human mononuclear leukocytes. While
verapamil cuased a marked stimulation of the high affinity accumulation and degradation, nifedipine did not
affect the pathway (Krone W., Nägele H., Behnke B., unpublished results).

High density lipoprotein (HDL) metabolism

The mechanisms of changes of plasma HDL-levels caused by
antihypertensive drugs are not understood. A direct correlation between lipoprotein lipase activity and HDL levels have been described (19). Athletes tend to have
high lipoprotein lipase activities and high plasma HDL
concentrations (19). Catecholamines may alter HDL levels
since a decrease has been shown by treatment with the
beta-blocker propranolol and an increase by therapy with
terbutaline, a beta-agonist (20). A direct effect of
catecholamines on HDL metabolism has been postulated recently (21). These hormones may stimulate the activity
of cholesterol ester hydrolase resulting in an increased
cellular free cholesterol concentration. This may induce
HDL binding activity at tne cell surface and enhance efflux of cholesterol from cells leading to an increased
HDL level in plasma.

DISCUSSION AND SUMMARY

Calcium antagonists and antihypertensive alpha-adrenergic and beta-adrenergic drugs may cause changes in plasma lipoprotein levels. Different mechanisms by which these antihypertensive agents affect cellular lipid metabolism have been proposed (1). The activity of lipoprotein lipase which determines the catabolism of VLDL is decreased by the beta-blocker propranolol and increased by alpha-1-antagonists (11). The plasma cholesterol or LDL level is inversely associated with the number of LDL receptors. Catecholamines suppress the LDL receptor activity thus leading to an increase in plasma cholesterol concentration. The calcium antagonist verapamil and the beta-blocker propranolol may increase LDL receptor activity either per se or by its antagonizing effect on the catecholamine action. The metabolism of HDL may be affected directly by catecholamines which might increase HDL activity, thereby enhancing efflux of cholesterol from cells.

Catecholamines inhibit cholesterol biosynthesis in extrahepatic cells. The effects are mediated by alpha-2- and beta-2-adrenergic receptors. Accordingly, the alpha-2-agonists clonidine and alpha-methyldopa mimicked and propranolol opposed the catecholamine action. In contrast the alpha-1-antagonists indoramin, prazosin and urapidil had no effect on cholesterol synthesis. These results in vitro may explain at least partly that an antihypertensive therapy with calcium channel blockers, unspecific beta-blockers and alpha-1-antagonists may produce no changes or even a decrease in plasma LDL levels. Nevertheless more work has to be done to elucidate the mechanisms whereby these agents cause plasma lipid changes. In particular, research should focus on how agents act on cholesterol metabolism at the cellular level. By a better understanding of the molecular mechanisms of drug action it may soon be possible to provide a scientific answer to the question which antihypertensives may have no adverse or even beneficial effects on the development of atherosclerosis and should therefore be preferred in the treatment of hypertension.

REFERENCES

1. Krone, W, Müller-Wieland, D, and Greten, H (1984). Antihypertensive Therapie und Fettstoffwechsel. Klin Wochenschr, 62, 193
2. Brown MS, and Goldstein, JL (1986). A receptor-mediated pathway for cholesterol homeostasis. Science 232, 34
3. Brown MS, Kovanen, PT and Goldstien, JL (1981). Regulation of plasma cholesterol by lipoprotein receptors. Science 212, 628

4. Krone, W, Müller-Wieland, D, Nägele H, Behnke, B and Greten, H (1985). Adrenergic antihypertensive drugs affect LDL receptor activity and cholesterol snythesis - atherogenic factor in diabetes? Diabetes Reséarch and Clinical Practice (Suppl), 1, 319

5. Tanaka, N, Sakaguchi, S, Oshiga, K et al. (1976). Effect of chronic administration of propranolol on lipoprotein composition. Metabolism, 10, 1071

6. Ferrera, LA, Moratta, T, Rubba, P et al. (1986). Effects of alpha-adrenergic and beta-adrenergic receptor blockade on lipid metabolism. Am J Med, 80 (Suppl 2a), 104

7. Krone, W, Betteridge, DJ and Galton, DJ (1979). Mechanism of regulation of 3-hydroxy-3-methylglutaryl coenzyme A reductase activity by low density lipoprotein in human lymphocytes. Eur J Clin Invest, 9,405

8. Krone, W and Greten, H (1984). Evidence for post-transcriptional regulation by insulin of 3-hydroxy-3-methylglutaryl coenzyme A reductase and sterol synthesis in human mononuclear leukocytes. Diabetologia, 26, 366

9. Betteridge, DJ, Krone, W, Reckless, JPD and Galton, DJ (1978). Compactin inhibits cholesterol synthesis in lymphocytes and intestinal mucosa from patients with familial hypercholesterolemia. Lancet, 11, 1342

10. Borda, ES, deBracco, MM, Cangiani, S et al. (1984). Alpha-adrenoceptor stimulated lymphocytes trigger the mechanical response of vas deferens: participation of arachidonic acid metabolites. Br J Pharmacol, 82, 863

11. Titinchi, S and Clark, B (1984). Alpha-2-adrenoceptors in human lymphocytes: direct characterization by ^{3}H-yohimbine binding. Biochem Biophys Res Comm, 121, 1

12. Brodde, DE, Engel, G, Hoyer, D et al. (1981). The beta-adrenergic receptor in human lymphocytes: subclassification by the use of a new radio-ligand, (+-)-^{125}iodopindolol. Life Sci, 29, 2189

13. Krone, W, Hildebrandt, F and Greten, H (1982). Effect of catecholamines on sterol synthesis in human mononuclear cells. Eur J Clin Invest, 12, 467

14. Krone, W, Müller-Wieland, D and Greten, H (1983). Regulation of cholesterol synthesis by catecholamines in human mononuclear leukocytes: roles of alpha-1-, alpha-2-, beta-1- and beta-2-adrenoceptors (abstract). Arteriosclerosis, 3, 492

15. Krone, W, Carl, U, Müller-Wieland, D and Greten, H (1984). Stimulation of beta-2-adrenergic receptors suppresses sterol synthesis in human mononuclear leukocytes. Biochim Biophys Acta, 804, 137

16. Krone, W, Müller-Wieland, D and Greten, H (1985). Effects of adrenergic antihypertensive drugs on sterol synthesis in freshly isolated human mononuclear leukocytes. J Cardiovasc Pharmacol, 7, 1134

17. Krone, W, Müller-Wieland, D and Greten, H. Regulation of cholesterol synthesis by alpha-adrenergic receptors in human mononuclear leukocytes. Biochem Biophys res Comm, in press
18. Krone, W, Nägele, B and Greten, H. Insulin and catecholamines regulate low density lipoprotein receptor activity in freshly isolated mononuclear leukocytes. Diabetes, in press
19. Nikkilä, EA, Tarskinen, MR, Rehnnen, S et al.(1978). Lipoprotein lipase activity in adipose tissue and skeletal muscle of runners: relation to serum lipoproteins. Metabolism, 27, 1661
20. Hooper, PL, Woo, W, Visconti, L and Pathak, DR (1981). Terbutaline raises high-density lipoprotein cholesterol levels. N Engl J Med, 305, 1455
21. Assmann, G and Schmitz, G (1986). Effect of antihypertensive drugs on cellular cholesterol metabolism: A challenge for further research. J Cardiovasc Res, 8, (suppl 2), 572

18
Blood platelets: their role in atherogenesis and arterial thrombosis and their inhibition, in particular by calcium antagonists

E.F. Lüscher

INTRODUCTION

Blood platelets play their major role in physiological and pathological processes by adhering to injured sites on the vascular wall, followed by the formation of aggregates , which when consolidated will form a "haemostatic plug" responsible for the spontaneous arrest of bleeding from smaller wounds or, particularly in arteries, a "white thrombus" which will interfere with normal blood circulation. An activation process is a prerequisite for aggregate formation and in its course platelets release a wide variety of substances, among them growth factors which have been implicated in atherogenesis.

This brief review will first deal with the basic phenomena of adhesion and activation, followed by a survey of the different hypotheses on platelet participation in atherogenesis. Finally, the interference with platelet activity and with atherogenesis will be touched upon with emphasis on the role of calcium antagonists.

It should be noted that the covered topics fill several books and that therefore only a superficial version of the state of the art can be given.

PLATELETS, THROMBOSIS AND ATHEROGENESIS

The adhesion of platelets to the vascular wall

The intact vascular wall is non-thrombogenic; however, platelets will immediately adhere to sites of endothelial injury, in particular to collagen fibers of the subendothelium. At higher flow rates, adhesion in order to be effective requires the presence of von Willebrand factor (vWF), a plasma protein which reinforces the linkage of the platelets to collagen.

Particularly in relation to atherognesis the question arises, whether visible damage is always a prerequisite for platelet deposition. This is not the case: there appear to exist sites of increased permeability in the vascular wall, to which platelets and leukocytes adhere before signs of the formation of an atherosclerotic lesion are discernible [1]. Tobacco smoke as well as the application of catecholamines leads in animals to platelet adhesion to the vascular endothelium [2]. This is of interest because smoking and stress are known risk factors for coronary thrombosis and atherosclerosis.

Platelet activation

Depending on the nature and the extent of the endothelial injury, adhesion will be followed by the more or less pronounced formation of aggregates. Only platelets which have undergone an activation process will aggregate and consequently aggregation is only one of many manifestations which result from activation. The more important of these manifestations, besides aggregation, are: pseudopod formation, synthesis and release of prostaglandins (PG), thromboxane A_2 (TXA_2) and of platelet activating factor (PAF), contractile activity, the rapid release from specific storage organelles of a large number of substances, and the acquirement of procoagulant properties.

Activation can be brought about by a wide variety of agonists, among them thrombin, ADP, adrenaline, serotonin, PGG_2, H_2, and E_2, TXA_2, PAF, and collagen. ADP, adrenaline and serotonin are released from storage organelles (termed dense bodies) and the PG's, TXA_2 and PAF are products of the activated cell. Thrombin forms by the intrinsic pathway on the surface of activated platelets. Thus, activation is characterized by a series of feedback mechanisms which propagate and potentiate the activation process.

The role of calcium ions in platelet activation

Many of the manifestations of the activated platelet are calcium-dependent. This is obvious for actomyosin-based contractile activity, for the cleavage of arachidonic acid from phospholipids by calmodulin-controlled phospholipase A_2, which is a prerequisite for PG and TX-formation, and for several other manifestations of activity as well. Calcium ionophores which transport Ca^{2+}-ions passively through the plasma membrane are indeed excellent activators of the platelet [3]. It is today established that the mobilization of Ca^{2+}-ions within the cell is the result of the activatition, as a consequence of the reaction of an agonist with the corresponding receptor, of the phosphatidylinositol metabolism in the course of which phosphatidylinositol-4,5-bisphosphate (PIP_2) is degraded to diacylglycerol (DAG) and inositoltrisphosphate (IP_3)[4]. IP_3 is a powerful releaser of calcium ions from an intracellular storage organ, the dense tubular system. Activation is also linked to the opening of calcium channels in the plasma membrane and this influx of the cation amplifies the activation process. Recent observations make it likely that PIP_2-degradation is initiated via the activation of phospholipase C by the action of G- (or N-) proteins [5], which appear to depress the calcium requirement of this enzyme to the intracellular level of the resting cell (10^{-7}M).

Platelets and atherosclerosis

As early as in 1844, von Rokitansky had postulated that arteriosclerosis was linked to a thrombotic event, a hypothesis which
more recently was taken up again by Duguid [6]. Modern methods allow
to detect quite often within plaques organized platelet- and fibrin
thrombi [cf.2]. The question remains, whether these are causative
or only a consequece of other pathogenetic processes.

For quite different reasons, platelets have again been discussed as a causative factor in atherogenesis, because they release
in the course of their activation mitogenic factors. The major
component is "platelet-derived growth factor" (PDGF)[7], which
is a powerful stimulator of the proliferation of smooth muscle
cells and fibroblasts (but not of endothelial cells). Platelet adhesion followed by activation and subsequent release of PDGF was
made responsible for the thickening of the vascular wall, which
would later develop into a typical atherosclerotic plaque.

More rcently the important role of the macrophage in atherogenesis has become more and more evident. These cells invade the
vascular endothelium in an early stage and persist underneath the
intima in the form of foam cells. Macrophages are also a source
of PDGF [8] and so are endothelial cells [9]. Accordingly, the
new hypothesis of atherogenesis [10] assigns the platelets no longer a dominant, but at best an auxiliary role. On the other hand,
it remains a fact that thrombocytopenic animals will not develop
atherosclerosis [11] and the same is true for pigs with severe
von Willebrand disease [12].

The inhibition of platelet activity

Whereas the importance of platelets for atherosclerosis remains
still controversial, their crucial role in the initiation of arterial thrombosis is undisputed. In view of the high incidence of
coronary thrombosis with subsequent myocardial infarction in industrialized countries, the last years have seen a remarkable effort in the development of agents capable of interfering with
platelet activity [cf. reviews 13, 14]. Several of these products
have undergone large-scale clinical trials [cf. 15], which have
established their effectiveness but have also shown the limits
of their effects. The points of attack of these agents are manyfold
[16]; quite often they interfere with one of the feedback mechanisms, whereby the PG-TX-pathway is particularly often the target.
Other agents appear to impair the platelet-fbrinogen interaction,
which is a prerequisit for aggregation, or they block receptors
for important agonists.

The DTS_2, the calcium storage organ of platelets not only makes
available Ca^{2+}-ions, but is also capable of accumulating them in
an energy-dependent process which is stimulated by cyclic AMP [17].
Agents which activate adenylate cyclase, the enzyme which synthe-
sizes cAMP, therefore would be expected to be inhibitors of platelet activity. This is indeed the case: prostacyclin (PGI_2), PGE_1

or adenosine are such cyclase activators and belong to the most powerful platelet inhibitors [18].

Calcium antagonists and platelet inhibition

In view of the important role of calcium ions in platelet activation it was to be expected that calcium antagonists should be particularly efficient inhibitors. In vitro an inhibitory effect is easily demonstrable for verapamil [19, 20] as well as for nifedipine and diltiazem [20, 21]. However, significant effects are only observed with concentrations which are 2 to 3 orders of magnitude higher than those used in patients [23]. On the other hand there is increasing experimental evidence that combinations of calcium antagonists with other drugs, such as e.g. aspirin, may be much more potent than each drug alone [24].

CALCIUM ANTAGONISTS AND THE PREVENTION OF ATHEROSCLEROSIS

Different from thrombosis, calcium antagonists alone appear to exert a significant effect on the initiation and progression of atheroscleosis. Numerous experiments [25, 26, 27]have demonstrated that atherogenesis is suppressed by their application in animals fed an atherogenic diet. Here again, a critical dose seems to exist and this may explain some negative results [28].

What is the mode of action of the calcium antagonists? First of all it must be pointed out that most available data have been obtained on animals fed with a diet rich in fat. In this context the observation that calcium antagonists stimulate the receptor-mediated endocytosis of LDL [29] is particularly relevant. It is of interest that Watanabe rabbits have no LDL-receptors and that in these animals calcium antagonists have no protective effect. [30].

It must be pointed out, however, that it is well established that atherogenesis is also observed in the absence of hyperlipidaemia and it would be of considerable interest to study the effect of blockers of calcium flux also under these conditions. One is also inclined to ask, whether calcium antagonists may not also exert an effect on macrophages, which as outlined above, appear to play a key role in atherogenesis. Experimental data on this important point are as yet missing. However, in this context it is noteworthy that nifedipine inhibits DNS synthesis in PDGF-stimulated smooth muscle cells [31]. Finally ist must also be recalled that there is little doubt that thrombotic events often accompany plaque formation andtherefore platelet inhibition appears worth discussing also in relation to atherogenesis. It is obvious that a solution of the problem on how and by what mechanisms atherosclerosis is influenced by drugs will only come from further studies which must take fully into account the complexity of this process.

1.   Rowsell, HC, Mustard, JF, and Downie, HG (1965). Experimental atherosclerosis in swine. Ann N Y Acad Sci, 127, 743
2.   Woolf, N (1982). Pathology of Atherosclerosis. (Boston, Durban, Singapore, Sydney, Toronto, Wellington: Butterworth)
3.   Massini, P and Lüscher, EF (1974). Somme effects of ionophores for divalent cations on blood platelets - comparison with the effects of thrombin. Biochim Biophys Acta, 372, 109
4.   Watson, SP, Ruggiero, M, Abrahams, SL, and Lapetina EG (1986). Inositol 1,4,5-triphosphate induces aggregation and release of 5-hydroxytryptamine from saponin-permeabilized human platelets. J Biol Chem, 261,5368
5.   Baldassare, JJ and Fisher, GJ (1986). GTP and cytosol stimulate phosphoinositide hydrolysis in isolated platelet membranes. Biochem Biophys Res Commun, 137, 801
6.   Duguid, JB (1948). Thrombosis as a factor in the pathogenesis of aortic atherosclerosis. J Pathol Bacteriol, 60, 57
7.   Deuel, TF and Huang, JS (1984). Platelet-derived growth factor. Structure, function, and roles in normal and transformed cells. J Clin Invest, 74.669
8.   Glenn, KC and Ross, R (1981). Human moncyte-drives growth factor(s) for mesenchymal cells: activation of secretion by endotoxin and concanavalin A (conA). Cell , 25, 603
9.   Gajdusek, C, DiCorletto, P, Ross, R and Schwartz, SM (1980). An endothelial cell-derived growth factor. J Cell Biol, 85, 467
10.   Ross, R (1986). The pathogenesis of atherosclerosis - an update. New Engld J Med, 314, 488
11.   Friedman, RJ, Stemerman MB, Wenz, B, Moore, S, Gauldie, J, Gent, M, Tiel, ML, and Spaet TH (1977). The effect of thrombocytopenia in experimental arteriosclerotic lesion formation in rabbits. J Clin Invest, 60, 1191
12.   Fuster, VD, Bowie, EJW, Lewis JC, Fass, DN, Owen, CA, Brown, AL (1978). Resistance to arteriosclerosis in pigs with von Willebrand's disease. J Clin Invest, 61, 722
13.   Verstraete, M, Dejana, E, Fuster, VD, Lapetina, E, Moncada, S, Mustard, JF, Tans, G, and Vargaftig, B (1985). An overview of antiplatelet and antithrombotic drugs. Haemostasis, 15, 89
14.   Bertelé, V, Salzman EW (1985). Antithrombotic therapy in coronary artery disease. Arteriosclerosis. 5, 119
15.   Boissel, JP (1986). Registry of multicenter clinical trials. Seventh report - 1985. Thromb Haemostas, 55, 282
16. Verstraete, M (1982). A pharmacological approach to the inhibition of platelet adhesion and platelet aggregation. Wright-Schulte Lecture. Haemostasis, 12, 317
17.   Käser-Glanzmann, R, Jakábová, M, George, JN, and Lüscher, EF (1977). Stimulation of calcium uptake in platelet membrane membrane vesicles by adenosine 3',5' cyclic monophosphate and protein kinase. Biochim Biophys Acta, 466, 429
18.   MacIntyre, DE, Shaw, AM, Bushfield, M, MacMillan, LJ, McNicol, A, and Pollock, WK (1985). Endogenous and pharmacological mechanisms of the regulation of human platelet cytosolic free Ca^{2+}.

Nouv Rev Fr Hématol, 27, 285

19.   Ikeda, Y, Kikuchi, M, Toyama, K, Watanabe, K, and Ando, Y (1981). Inhibition of human platelet function by verapamil. Thromb Haemostas,45, 158

20.   Han, P, Boatwright, C, Ardlie, NG (1983). Effect of the calcium-entry blocking agent nifedipine on activation of human platelets and comparison with verapamil. THromb Haemostas, 50, 513

21.   Coeffier, E, Cerrina, J, Jouvin-Marche, E, and Benveniste, J (1983). Inhibition of rabbit platelet aggregation by the Ca^{2+}-antagonists verapamil and diltiazem and by trifluoperazine. Thromb Res, 31, 565

22.   Kiyamoto, A, Sasaki, Y, Odawara, A, and Morita, T (1983). Inhibition of platelet aggregation by diltiazem. Comparison with verapamil and nifedipine and inhibitory potencies of diltiazem metabolites. Circ Res 52 (Suppl 1), 115

23.   Klaus, W, Latta, G, and Schroer, K (1985). The influence of nifedipine on platelet function. In: Lichtlen, PR (ed.) "Recent Aspects of Calcium Antagonism". p.139 (Stuttgart:Schattauer)

24.   Greer, IA, Walker, JJ, Calder, AA, and Forbes, CD (1985). Aspirin with an adrenergic or a calcium-channel blocking agent as a new combination therapy for arterial thrombosis. Lancet, I, 31.

25.   Rouleau, JL, Parmley, WW, Stevens, J, Wikman-Coffelt, J, Sievers, R, Mahley, RW, and Havel, RJ (1983) Verapamil suppresses atherosclerosis in cholesterol-fed rabbits. Am Coll Cardiol 1, 1453

26.   Willis, AL, Nagel, B, Churchill, V, Whyte, MA, Smith, DL, Mahmud, I, and Puppioni, DL (1985). Antiatherosclerotic effects of nicardipine and nifedipine in cholesterol-fed rabbits. Arteriosclerosis, 5, 250

27.   Sugano, M, Nakashima, Y, Matsushima, T, Takahama, K, Takasugi, M, Kuroiwa, A, and Koido, O (1986). Suppression of atherosclerosis in cholesterol-fed rabbits by diltiazem injection. Arteriosclerosis, 6, 237

28.   Overturf, ML and Smith, SA (1986). Failure of nifedipine to reduce atherogenesis in cholesterol-fed rabbits. Artery, 13, 267

29.   Stein, O, Leitersdorf, E, and Stein, Y (1985). Verapamil enhances receptor-mediated endocytosis of low ensity lipoproteins by aortic cells in culture. Arteriosclerosis, 5, 35

30.   Tilton, GD, Buja, LM, Bilheimer, DW, Apprill, P, Ashton, J, McNatt, J, Kita, T, and Willerson, JZ. Failure of a slow channel calcium antagonist, verapamil, to retard atherosclerosis in the Watanabe heritable hyperlipidemic rabbit: An animal model of familial cholesterolemia. J Am Coll Cardiol, 6, 141 (1985)

Nilsson, J, Sjölund, M, Palmberg, L, von Euler, AM, Jonzon, B, and Thyberg, J (1985). The calcium antagonist nifedipine inhibits arterial smooth muscle cell proliferation. Atherosclerosis, 58, 109

PRIMARY AND SECONDARY PREVENTION: DIFFERENT EXPERIENCES

19
Prevention of coronary heart disease - links with other chronic disorders
F.H. Epstein

The thesis is proposed that measures which, according to present knowledge, are likely to prevent premature coronary heart disease will, at the same time, diminish the toll and burden from other major chronic diseases. Thus, life might be further prolonged and disability amongst the elderly diminished. The scientific evidence for this view is still no more than suggestive but worth reviewing because, if true, the impact on the preventability of chronic disease as a whole would be profound. Supportive data come from a consideration of mortality rates, the influence of life styles, the sharing of risk factors and the clustering of disease in the same people.

MORTALITY RATES
Support for the thesis comes from correlations in terms of secular changes in mortality in different countries. Particular attention is given to the secular trends for "heart disease" (defined as non-rheumatic heart disease and hypertension) and "cancer other than lung". Lung cancer trends must be viewed separately because lung cancer mortality is rising in almost every country, so that its inclusion would obscure the trends for other types of cancer. The data for 26 countries summarized in the Table are part of a more comprehensive analysis [1] of which the secular trends for heart disease have already been reported, comprising the same countries listed in the publication [2]. For the purpose of this analysis, changes of less than 5 percent have been defined as "no change" because no reliance can be placed on trends of lesser magnitude. There are 2 approximately equal time periods between 1950 and 1978 and 2 age groups, subdivided by sex, forming 8 groups. Depending on the group, between 0 and 20 percent of the countries show divergent trends for the 2 conditions "heart disease" and "cancer other than lung". It can be concluded that secular trends for the 2 con-

ditions do not move in opposite directions in most of the comparisons; in fact, in 7 of the 8 groups the percentage is 15 % or less. It is true that the trends are not very often consonant either; e.g. in younger men during the second time period, the trends were fully consonant in only 10 of the 26 countries. Considering that the two conditions have only some but not all causes in common and taking into account the vagaries of death certification, especially across countries, a much higher degree of consonance could have hardly been expected. It is, however, gratifying and compatible with the proposed thesis that, in the majority of countries, a change in trend for one condition went along with no change for the other, remembering that most of the changes refer to heart disease since the secular trends for heart disease are more marked than those for cancer.

If, instead of changes over time, countries are compared at one point in time, it becomes more difficult to show that countries with a high cardiovascular mortality also have high mortalities from all other causes which would again suggest the existence of common causes. Such analyses are still in progress. However, there is a striking example of such a correlation within the United States, indicating that there is an almost linear relationship between cardiovascular and non-cardiovascular mortality in the different States of the Union so that, at one end of the scale, there is a high mortality from all causes while, at the other, mortality from all causes is low [3]. It would seem, therefore, that there are all-pervading influences, relating to life styles and the environment, which are conducive either to health or to disease in general. It would be worthwhile to look for similar regional differences within the same country elsewhere.

LIFE STYLES

For the present purpose, "life style" is used as a general term, including habits like eating, smoking, drinking, taking exercise and patterns of coping with the strains and stresses of daily existence. Some of the components of life style have specific biological effects, such as smoking or certain dietary constituents like the different fatty acids. Presumably, there are also non-specific components, relating to psychosocial interactions with biological processes like neuro-hormonal mechanisms and immunity [4].

The single, most persuasive piece of evidence for the importance of life styles in this connection comes from the Alameda County Study in which a very simple index of 7 daily habits, reflecting a scale from "healthy" to "unhealthy" life styles, was correlated not only with the risk of dying from heart disease but also cancer and other major causes of death [5]. Further data will come from other community studies, particularly intervention studies, supplementing information already available from the North Karelia project which indicate that the decline in coronary heart disease mortality was accompanied by a reduction in the mortality from cancer [6]. In the Rome trial, on the other hand, there was no change in cancer mortality to parallel the decline in coronary heart disease mortality [7].

COEXISTENT MORTALITY TREND PATTERNS FOR "HEART DISEASE" AND "CANCER OTHER THAN LUNG" FOR MEN AND WOMEN DURING TWO TIME PERIODS: 1950-1954 TO 1960-1964 (I) AND 1965-1969 TO 1975-1978 (II)

TREND PATTERN	NUMBER OR COUNTRIES IN EACH CATEGORY:							
	MEN				WOMEN			
	PERIOD I		PERIOD II		PERIOD I		PERIOD II	
	Age 45-64y.	Age 65-74y.	Age 45-64y.	Age 65-74y.	Age 45-64y.	Age 65-74y.	Age 45-64y.	Age 65-74y.
Consonant: up or down for both conditions	2	5	10	9	10	10	12	19
Up or down for one condition and no change for the other	13	11	7	13	10	9	8	5
No change for either condition	1	1	5	2	0	0	3	1
Divergent: trend for the two conditions in opposite directions	4	3	4	2	0	1	3	1
Total - all countries	20	20	26	26	20	20	26	26
Percent of "Total" divergent	20%	15%	15%	8%	0%	5%	12%	4%

N.B.: Period I includes only 20 countries since the data for 6 of the 26 countries included in Period II were incomplete

Definition of trends: a change of 5% or more in either direction is considered an "up" or "down" trend; changes of less than 5% are defined as "no change"

It is relevant in this context that the well-documented inverse social class gradient for coronary heart disease mortality is also present for other major causes of death, as shown impressively by data from the British Civil Servants Study [8]. There is further evidence from the Gothenburg Study that several social attributes and activities influence total mortality but the data are not presented in terms of specific causes of death [9].

Concerning nutrition, it was shown in the Zutphen Study that dietary fibre intake is inversely correlated with mortality from both coronary heart disease and cancer [10]. High intake of fat is associated not only with high mortality from coronary heart disease but also cancer of the colon and breast [11]. It may also be mentioned that low selenium intake shows a correlation with heart disease and cancer mortality, at least in Finland [12].

RISK FACTORS

The question whether coronary heart disease risk factors are predictive for other diseases as well has so far been systematically addressed only in analyses of the data from the Italian cohort of the 7-Country Study. However, such links were reported in terms of prevalence data from the Tecumseh Community Health Study some 25 years ago [13]. The prospective Italian data indicate that the multiple logistic function derived for coronary heart disease has predictive value also for stroke, cancer and total mortality though serum cholesterol is associated only with coronary heart disease risk [14]. Smoking is obviously a risk factor for both heart and lung disease, apart from some other disorders. The fact that the multiple logistic function carries a measure of universal predictive power deserves further attention.

CLUSTERING OF HEALTH AND DISEASE

It is common experience that human beings can be aligned along a spectrum of disease susceptibility so that there are those who hardly ever get sick at all while, at the opposite end, there are people who constantly have one or the other complaint. At the baseline examination of the Tecumseh Study, careful medical histories were obtained and it did, indeed, emerge that some two-thirds of all major illnesses tended to cluster amongst around a third of the population; unfortunately, this preliminary analysis was never pursued further. Clusters of mostly minor illnesses were also found in a study in New York [15]. A systematic analysis of this question was made as part of the Kiryat Yovel Study in a health district adjacent to the University Hospital in Jerusalem, detecting several clusters in which specific diseases occurred in the same persons significantly more often than expected by chance alone [16].

CONCLUDING REMARKS

Ultimately, every disease must be caused by a constellation of mechanisms which is specific for it. To use Sherrington's term, there is a "final common path" which leads to specific pathological changes. At the same time, there are likely to be distinct factors and influences which impinge simultaneously on a number of final common paths. This phenomenon would be responsible for a linkage between different disorders sharing common predisposing factors. If these factors are amenable to change through modifications in life styles or otherwise, the prevention of several diseases as the result of the same preventive measures would be the consequence. The plea is made to start thinking along these lines, in addition to searching for disease specific preventive measures [17, 18].

While, on the scientific front, there is still much room for research, there are overriding arguments in favour of comprehensive, rather than categorical community prevention programmes on the practical level. It is wasteful in terms of resources and unreasonably demanding on people's time to stage separate preventive activities for several different diseases, even if they do not share common links. For these reasons, the World Health Organization has launched integrated chronic disease prevention programme, based on W.H.O. headquarters in Geneva [19] and the so-called "CINDY" programme which is coordinated by the W.H.O. Regional Office for Euro in Copenhagen. If further research provides additional evidence that common links between these diseases do, indeed, exist, the justification for such integrated programmes will be greatly strengthened.

SUMMARY

Much evidence has accumulated to indicate that premature coronary heart disease can be prevented to a great extent by appropriate changes in life style. Several lines of evidence suggest that the same changes are likely to protect at the same time against a number of other chronic disorders. Thus, these preventive measures will have an impact which can be assumed to go far beyond their influence on heart disease alone, protecting health in the population on a broad front.

REFERENCES

1. Thom, TJ, Epstein, FH, Feldman, JJ and Leaverton, PE (in preparation). Total mortality and mortality from heart disease, cancer and stroke in men and women 35-74 years of age in 26 countries, 1950 to 1978.
2. Thom, TJ, Epstein, FH, Feldman, JJ and Leaverton, PE (1985). Trends in total mortality and mortality from heart disease in 26 countries from 1950 to 1978. Int. J. Epidemiol. 14, 510
3. Sauer, HI and Enterline, PE (1959). Are geographic variations in death rates for the cardiovascular diseases real? J. Chronic Dis. 10, 513
4. Anon (1985). Emotions and immunity. Lancet 2, 133
5. Wingard, DL, Berkman, LF and Brand, RJ (1982). A multivariate analysis of health-related practices. Am. J. Epidemiol. 116, 765
6. Puska, P, Pukkala, E, Teppo, L, Tuomilehto, J and Kuulasmaa, K (to be published). Changes in cancer incidence in North Karelia, an area with a comprehensive preventive cardiovascular program.
7. Research Group of the Rome Project of Coronary Heart Disease Prevention (1986). Eight-year follow-up results from the Rome Project of Coronary Heart Disease Prevention. Prevent. Med. 15, 176

8. Marmot, MG, Shipley, MJ and Rose, G (1984). Inequalities in death - specific explanations of a general pattern? Lancet 1, 1003

9. Welin, L, Tibblin, G, Svärdsudd, K, et al. (1985). Prospective study of social influences on mortality - the study of men born in 1913 and 1923. Lancet 1, 915

10.Kromhout, D, Bosschieter, EB, Coulander, C.deL (1982). Dietary fibre and 10-year mortality from coronary heart disease, cancer and all causes. Lancet 2, 518

11.Doll, R and Peto, J (1982). The causes of cancer. p.1205. Oxford, Oxford University Press.

12.Salonen, JT, et al. (1985). Risk of cancer in relation to serum concentrations of selenium and vitamins A and E: matched case-control analysis of prospective data. Brit. med. J. 1, 417

13.Epstein, FH, Francis Jr, T, Hayner, NS, et al. (1965). Prevalence of chronic diseases and distribution of selected physiologic variables in a total community, Tecumseh, Michigan. Am. J. Epidemiol. 81, 307

14.Menotti, A, Conti, S, Dima, F, et al. (1983). Prediction of all causes of death as a function of some factors commonly measured in cardiovascular population surveys. Prevent. Med. 12, 318

15.Hinkle Jr, LE and Wolff, HG (1958). Ecologic investigations of the relationship between illness, life experiences and the social enrivonment. Ann. Int. Med. 49, 1973

16.Abramson, JH, Gofin, J, Peritz, E, et al. (1982). Clustering of chronic disorders - a community study of coprevalence in Jerusalem. J. Chronic Dis. 35, 221

17.Epstein, FH and Holland, WW (1983). Prevention of chronic diseases in the community - one-disease versus multiple-disease strategies. Int. J. Epidemiol. 12, 94

18.Epstein, FH (1983). Preventing coronary heart disease and prevention of other chronic disorders - are there common links? Heartbeat 3,2.

19.Glasunov, IS, Grabauskas, V, Holland, WW and Epstein, FH (1983). An integrated programme for the prevention and control of non-communicable diseases. J. Chronic Dis. 36, 419

20
Therapy versus prevention of coronary heart disease

P. Puddu and M. Muscari

The prevention of coronary heart disease (CHD) is usually
classified as Pre-primary, Primary or Secondary according
to the subjects to whom it is addressed and according to
its purposes, and it includes various types of
intervention : from hygienic-dietetic measures, to the
use of anti-hypertensive, anti-dislipidemic, anti-anginal
and anti-platelet drugs, up to coronary surgery.
According to this type of classification Therapy,
strictly defined as treatment of coronary events IN
PROGRESS, is limited to Nitroglycerin administration and
to Coronary Intensive Care, including within the latter
also emergency invasive techniques, such as coronary
thrombolysis, angioplasty or surgery performed during
acute or threatening infarction.

The fields of application for Prevention or Therapy
may be approximately quantified taking into account that:
a) nearly 1/5 of coronary events are sudden and
unexpected deaths, on which the only possible
intervention is of preventive type; b) more than 2/3 of
CHD deaths occur before hospital admission, and also in
this case it is necessary to refer to prevention, unless
intensive care will become quickly available where the
patient is, which is more theoretical than practical; c)
only the rest of CHD deaths may be affected by therapy,
as well as by prevention.

Therefore, as everybody knows, "preventing is always
better than treating". On the other hand, since often
intention does not coincide with the actual ability of
acting, according to present knowledge and means, do more
significant results have to be expected from prevention
or from therapy ? And which is the most useful kind of
prevention (pre-primary, primary or secondary) ?

Taking as reference the United States, in the period
1968-1981 mortality from CHD decreased by 31.8 % [1] :
answers to the previous questions could arise from an
analysis of the possible explanations of this trend. The
interventions of preventive and therapeutic type that
were available and mostly diffuse in the United States in

the years 1968-81 will be shortly discussed here. Of course, the possibility also exists that the observed decrease in mortality has not been caused by human intervention, but that it represents a phase of a cyclic event,controlled by unknown factors.

CORONARY CARE UNITS (CCU)

The contribution of CCU to decreased mortality from CHD has been assessed only in retrospective studies, or in prospective but non-randomized studies (in which patient destination to CCU or general ward was usually defined according to age or bed availability), or in randomized studies concerning only low-risk patients.

Taking into account the above mentioned limitations, the studies performed at the end of the sixties and at the beginning of the seventies showed a significant favourable effect of CCU, since case fatality rates fell on an average from 35 to 15-20 % [2-4]. On the contrary, the studies performed from 1974 onwards did not show any further decrease in mortality [5-7]. In this respect Goldman et al. [8] showed that in 63 acute care hospitals in the Boston area the mortality rate from myocardial infarction did not change between 1973-74 and 1978-79, while during the same period the general mortality from myocardial infarction was still decreasing.

It seems therefore that CCU may have contributed to decreasing mortality trends from their introduction up to about 1973. The subsequent further decline has not been paralleled by the diffusion of significant major innovations in coronary care, and therefore it must be explained by other factors.

BETA-BLOCKERS

In a study by Hampton [9] the results of the main trials concerning beta-blocker administration after a suspected myocardial infarction have been pooled and evaluated as 95 % confidence intervals. The trials have been grouped into two categories: a) those in which treatment began more than three days after the onset of symptoms and b) those in which treatment began within three days. While the trials with "late" treatment showed an overall trend towards a mortality reduction, the results of many trials with "early" treatment suggested the possibility of an increase in mortality.

The Beta-blocker Heart Attack Trial (BHAT) is one of the main studies concerning this subject [10]. It is one of the trials with "late" beginning of treatment, and the effect of propranolol on mortality resulted significantly favourable. It should be noted that the percent cumulative mortality curves relative to placebo and propranolol diverged during the first twelve months of follow-up, and thereafter were substantially parallel.

In a trial concerning oxprenolol [11] it has been shown that the drug yielded an evident advantage in terms of mortality compared to placebo when treatment began within four months of infarction, and the survival curves for placebo and oxprenolol were still diverging at six years. On the other hand, an apparent harmful effect of the drug was demonstrated when tratment started more than twelve months after infarction, deaths being concentrated among the patients who discontinued oxprenolol a year or more before.

The main practical implications of these trials are the following : 1) Mortality may be reduced by about 25 % when beta-blockers are given "late". 2) Too early or too late interventions with beta-bolckers may be useless (if not harmful). The beginning of treatment may be advisable between 5 and 28 days after infarction. 3) Beta-blockers should be maintained for at least one year. 4) The possibility of deleterious effects arising early or late after withdrawal of beta-blockers should be always kept in mind. 5) In the absence of other specific indications, it seems prudent to reserve treatment with beta-blockers to patients less than 65-70 years old.

In conclusion, the wide diffusion of beta-blockers may have contributed to reduce mortality from CHD by an action of secondary prevention, although an exact assessment of its role is not possible.

ANTI-PLATELET DRUGS

AMIS (Aspirin Myocardial Infarction Study, 1980) was the first large trial concerning the effects of anti-platelet drugs [12]. Aspirin was administered at high doses (500 mg twice a day), beginning treatment 8 weeks-5 years after myocardial infarction. Both men and women were admitted to the trial. No difference in cumulative rates for coronary events was found, after a three year follow-up, between the group treated with Aspirin and the one treated with placebo.

PARIS (Persantine Aspirin Reinfarction Study, 1980) was the second large trial concerning anti-platelet drugs [13]. This study shared many features with AMIS, but it tested, besides high-dose Aspirin, Aspirin associated with Dipyridamole. Also in this trial the cumulative event rates (total, CHD and sudden deaths) did not show any significant difference between placebo and treated groups, considering all the patients participating to the trial. On the other hand, when the patients entered within six months of a previous myocardial infarction were considered separately, it was shown that the curves relative to placebo and treated groups diverged, and the advantage of a treatment with antiplatelet drugs became significant for coronary deaths.

The Veterans Administration Cooperative Study [14] was performed in 1983 with different criteria : 1) Low-dose aspirin (324 mg once a day); 2)Beginning of randomization within 51 hours of hospital admission for unstable angina; 3) Inclusion of men only. The study showed a decrease in the end points by about 50 % in the aspirin-treated group. This value was highly significant for myocardial infarction, and close to significance for death.

Therefore it is possible to conclude that low-dose aspirin, possibly associated with another antiplatelet drug with different mechanism of action, given early in unstable angina and perhaps after myocardial infarction, may reduce mortality up to 50% (acting as secondary prevention), especially in men. The impact of this kind of treatment on decreasing mortality trends is recent and difficult to be quantified.

CORONARY BY-PASS SURGERY

CASS (Coronary Artery Surgery Study) [15] is the largest and most recent comparative study concerning the effects on CHD mortality of medical vs surgical therapy. The randomized study created a great sensation since it did not show any significant difference in survival between the patients who underwent coronary artery by-pass surgery and those assigned to medical therapy. On the other hand it must be emphasized that among the patients in the CASS Registry screened for participation to randomization, 33.2 % were assigned directly to medical therapy since they had normal coronary arteries or minimal vessel disease or no operable vessels, 38 % were excluded because the severity of angina or of coronary lesions did not allow randomization, and only a 4.7 % of patients actually participated to the trial, representing those (28.8 %) in whom the choice of treatment was uncertain. The true impact of coronary artery by-pass surgery on mortality trends should be estimated from the results obtained in the most severe patients, who electively undergo surgery. Since these patients are not randomizable for ethical reasons, the only possible analysis is retrospective. The analysis of the five-year survival data for all the patients in the CASS Registry (left main diseases excluded) shows an advantage arising from surgical therapy, significant in patients with three vessel disease and severe angina or ejection fraction less than 50 % [16]. The elective indication of surgical therapy for patients with severe left main coronary stenosis is widely accepted [17, 18].

The conclusion is that coronary by-pass surgery : a) does reduce mortality in severe cases; b) often relieves symptoms in patients not taking advantage from medical

therapy, thus improving their quality of life; c) may
have in part contributed to the general decrease in
mortality from CHD, but it does not appear to have played
a major role.

PRE-PRIMARY AND PRIMARY PREVENTION

With the exception of the studies on hypertension control
[19-21], none of the main trials on pre-primary and
primary prevention could demonstrate a significant
decrease in CHD mortality [22-28]. For some trials this
could be expected, since they were designed to evaluate
different or combined end-points; on the other hand, the
goal of reaching a statistical significance for a
decrease in CHD mortality would probably need too large
samples of "normal" population. Therefore, it may be more
useful to consider which changes in prevalence rates of
main risk factors occurred between the first and the
second half of the seventies [29]. Among white americans,
35 to 74 years of age, the percentage of hypertensive
subjects did decrease, and to a greater extent in women
(from 22.2 to 19 % in men and from 19 to 14.5 % in
women). No significant change occurred, instead, in the
prevalence rates of hypercholesterolemic subjects and of
heavy smokers, with even a trend to an increase in
hypercholesterolemic men and in woman smokers. On the
other hand, the overall change of risk factors may
explain less than half of the observed decrease in CHD
mortality [30].

CONCLUSIONS

The decrease in CHD mortality observed in the U.S.A. in
the years 1968-1981 seems to be attributable to the
cumulative action of multiple factors : mainly
interventions of secondary prevention, primary prevention
due to hypertension control and coronary intensive care
(the latter at least in the first half of the seventies).
The role of life-style and dietetic changes in pre-
primary and primary prevention is difficult to ascertain,
and objective proofs in favor of it are scanty.
      All the previous discussion has been centred on the
decrease in CHD mortality observed in the United States.
However, it should be kept in mind that, although in the
presence of similar advances in therapy and prevention,
in some nations of eastern and western Europe CHD
mortality rates are actually increasing [31]. Clearly,
some important factors in the pathogenesis and
progression of CHD are still unknown. Before we
understand them, it is tempting to believe in
"spontaneous epidemic fluctuations" of the disease.

REFERENCES

1. National Heart, Lung, and Blood Institute (1983). Fact Book for Fiscal Year 1982. U.S. Department of Health and Human Services. Public Health Service. National Institutes of Health. NIH Publication.

2. Langhorne, WH (1967). The Coronary Care Unit. A year's experience in a community hospital. JAMA, 201, 662.

3. Christiansen, I, Iversen, K and Skouby, AP (1971). Benefits obtained by the introduction of a coronary care unit. A comparative study. Acta Med Scand, 189, 285.

4. Hofvendahl, S (1971). Influence of treatment in a coronary care unit on prognosis in acute myocardial infarction. Acta Med Scand, 519 (suppl), 1.

5. Astvad, K, Fabricius-Bierre, N, Kjaerulff, J and Lindholm, J (1974). Mortality from acute myocardial infarction before and after establishment of a coronary care unit. Br Med J, 1, 567.

6. Mather, HG, Morgan, DC, Pearson, NG, Read, KLQ, Shaw, DB, Steed, GR, Thorne, MG, Lawrence, CJ and Riley, IS (1976). Myocardial infarction: a comparison between home and hospital care for patients. Br Med J, 1, 925.

7. Hill, JD, Hampton, JR and Mitchell, JRA (1978). A randomized trial of home-versus-hospital management for patients with suspected myocardial infarction. Lancet, i, 837.

8. Goldman, L, Cook, F, Hashimoto, B, Stone, P, Muller, J and Loscalzo, A (1982). Evidence that hospital care for acute myocardial infarction has not contributed to the decline in coronary mortality between 1973-74 and 1978-1979. Circulation, 65, 936.

9. Hampton, JR (1983). The use of beta blockers following myocardial infarction - doubts. Eur Heart J, 4 (suppl. D), 151.

10. Beta-Blocker Heart Attack Trial Research Group (1982). A randomised trial of propranolol in patients with acute myocardial infarction. I. Mortality results. JAMA, 247, 1707.

11. Taylor, SH, Silke, B, Ebbutt, A, Sutton, GC, Prout, BJ and Burley, DM (1982). A long-term prevention study with oxprenolol in coronary heart disease. N Engl J Med, 307, 1293.

12. Aspirin Myocardial Infarction Study Research Group (1980). A randomized, controlled trial of aspirin in persons recovered from myocardial infarction. JAMA, 243, 661.

13. The Persantine-Aspirin Reinfarction Study Research Group (1980). Persantine and aspirin in coronary heart disease. Circulation, 62, 449.

14. Lewis, HD, Davis, JW, Archibald, DG, Steinke, WE, Smitherman, TC, Doherty, JE, Schnaper, HW, LeWinter, MM, Linares, E, Pouget, JM, Sabharwal, SC, Chesler, E and De Mots, H (1983). Protective effects of aspirin against

acute myocardial infarction and death in men with unstable angina. Results of a Veterans Administration Cooperative Study. N Engl J Med, 309, 396.

15. CASS Principal Investigators and Their Associates (1983). Coronary Artery Surgery Study (CASS): a randomized trial of coronary artery bypass surgery. Survival data. Circulation, 68, 939.

16. Loop, D (1985). CASS continued. Circulation, 72 (suppl. II), 1.

17. Takaro, T, Hultgren, H, Lipton, M, Detre, K and participants in the Veterans Administration Cooperative Study Group (1976). VA Cooperative Randomized Study for Coronary Arterial Occlusive Disease. II. Left main disease. Circulation, 54 (suppl. III), 107.

18. European Coronary Surgery Study Group (1979). Coronary bypass surgery in stable angina pectoris: survival at two years. Lancet, i, 889.

19. Hypertension Detection and Follow-up Program Cooperative Group (1979). Five year findings of the Hypertension Detection and Follow-up Program: 1. Reduction in mortality of persons with high blood pressure, including mild hypertension. JAMA, 242, 2562.

20. Report of the Management Committee (1980). The Australian therapeutic trial in mild hypertension. Lancet, i, 1261.

21. Helgeland, A (1980). Treatment of mild hypertension: a five year controlled drug trial. The Oslo Study. Am J Med, 69, 725.

22. National Public Health Laboratory of Finland (1981). Community control of cardiovascular disease: the North Karelia Project. WHO Regional Office for Europe, Copenhagen.

23. Hjermann, I, Velve Byre, K, Holma, I and Leren, P (1981). Effect of diet and smoking intervention on the incidence of coronary heart disease. Report from the Oslo Study Group of a randomized trial in healthy men. Lancet, ii, 1303.

24. WHO Collaborative Group (1983). Multifactorial trial in the prevention of coronary heart disease. 3. Incidence and mortality results. Europ Heart J, 4, 141.

25. MRFIT Research Group (1982). Multiple risk factor intervention trial. Risk factor changes and mortality results. JAMA, 248, 1465.

26. Cooperative Trial in the Primary Prevention of Ischemic Heart Disease Using Clofibrate (1978). Report from the Committee of Principal Investigators. Br Heart J, 40, 1069.

27. Lipid Research Clinics Program (1984). The lipid research clinics coronary primary prevention trial results. JAMA, 251, 351.

28. Miettinen, TA, Huttunen, JK, Naukkarinen, V, Strandberg, T and Vanhanen, H (1986). Long-term use of Probucol in the multifactorial primary prevention of vascular disease. Am J Cardiol, 57, 49H.

29. Health - United States and Prevention Profile 1983:
Report of the National Center for Health Statistics
(1984). US Dept of Health and Human Statistics.
Publication 84, 1232.
30. Borhani, NO (1985). Prevention of coronary heart
disease in practice. Implications of the results of
recent clinical trials. JAMA, 254, 257.
31. Pisa, Z and Uemura, K (1984). CVD mortality trends
in 27 industrial countries in 1970-1980. WHO internal
communication 84.21.

21
Prevention in Europe - facts, fallacies and future
G. Lamm

FACTS

Almost 20 years passed since the first decline in CHD mortality in the USA was observed. Since then we constantly hear that not only is the decline continuing, but it is spreading to other countries as well. If CHD is a waning phenomenon, why are we still debating whether and how best prevention should be instituted?

Table 1 answers this question by showing that in 1981-84 the countries leading the rank-list of CHD mortality were practically the same as twenty years ago. (We shall return to the notable exceptions later.)

Table 1. Age-standardized mortality from CHD in 1981-84
Rates per 100,000 population aged 40-69 years

Males			
UK-N.I.	567.4	PL	290.9
UK-Sc.	564.7	FRG	289.0
SF	538.0	NL	287.7
IRL	479.9	BLG	284.3
CS	471.8	A	282.4
UK-E.W.	455.0	RO	239.9
H	441.0	B	225.5
N	363.8	I	206.4
DK	353.1	CH	199.4
S	331.1	YU	189.6
		F	128.8

Pisa-Uemura

The impressive changes in the last decade shown in Fig. 1 (1) could not completely reverse the picture in Europe - yet. Thus prevention is still an issue in Western Europe in spite of declining mortality, as the rates are still too high. For the Eastern Countries prevention seems to become a crucial problem. Hungary for instance is not only the country with the third greatest increase in CHD mortality in ten years - over 30% - but it has taken already the 7th place in the level of CHD mortality; in the youngest male age group it has already "beaten" Finland. The first fact is thus, that prevention of CHD is as actual as ever.

171

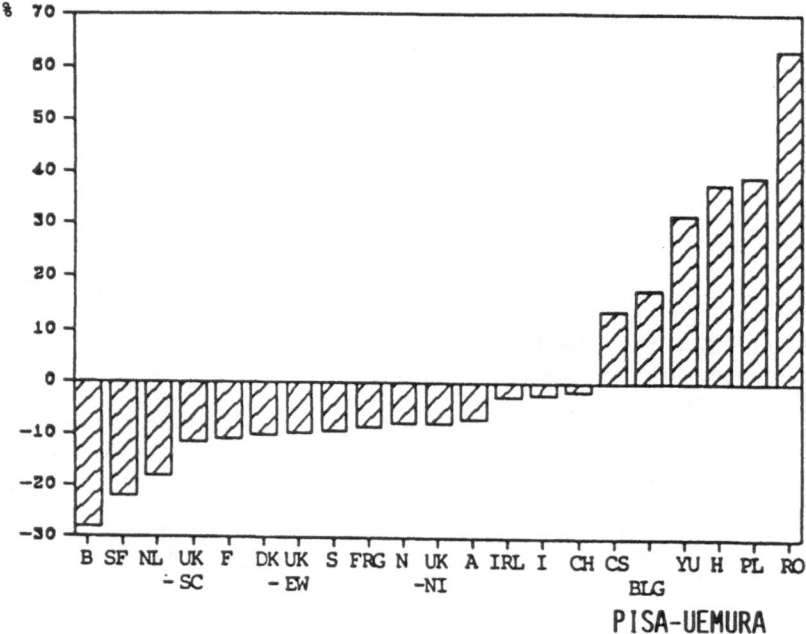

PERCENTAGE CHANGE IN AGE-STANDARDIZED RATES - CHD

1971-4/1981-4

MALES; Age 40-69 years; EUROPE

PISA-UEMURA

Figure 1

Fact number two is, that changes in CHD mortality are more conspicuous and pronounced in the young, than in the old. Table 2 shows this fact clearly, irrespective whether one looks at the increase (by adding up the % increase in these countries) or the decrease (proceeding in the same manner).

Table 2. 10 year percentual change in IHD mortality according to age, males, % Sum of individual countries

		Increase	Decrease
	40-44 years	378	290
"Young"	45-49 "	354	261
	50-54 "	380	137
	55-59 "	301	98
"Old"	60-64 "	175	105
	65-69 "	145	103

Young people catch on more quickly and easily with the new life-style, whether it is in the direction of more moderation and health consciousness, like in the West. In Eastern Europe where quick but still insufficient improvements in economy allowed in the last fifteen years to catch-up with earlier western gluttony and intoxication with alcohol and tobacco, it was again the young who adopted as firsts the new life-style.

Fact 3 is that changes in CHD mortality mirror changes in life-style. Two examples from the many should stress this point.

In Hungary the per capita consumption of cigarettes per day rose by 13% in 10 years. In Finland - with the largest decrease in CHD mortality -it fell by 17% in the same period. Going beyond a single pair comparison, in all other western countries cigarette use declined by 3%, while in the East it rose by 11% (2).

In 1980 the Hungarians were eating 6% more calories a day than twenty years earlier. The contribution of fat to total calories increased by 21%.

Though simple correlations can never be proof of causality it is instructive to look on the graph (Figure 2) of Szostak et al. (3) demonstrating the excellent correlation between changes in CHD mortality and animal fat consumption between 1968 and 1977 in 23 countries.

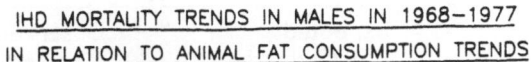

IHD MORTALITY TRENDS IN MALES IN 1968–1977
IN RELATION TO ANIMAL FAT CONSUMPTION TRENDS

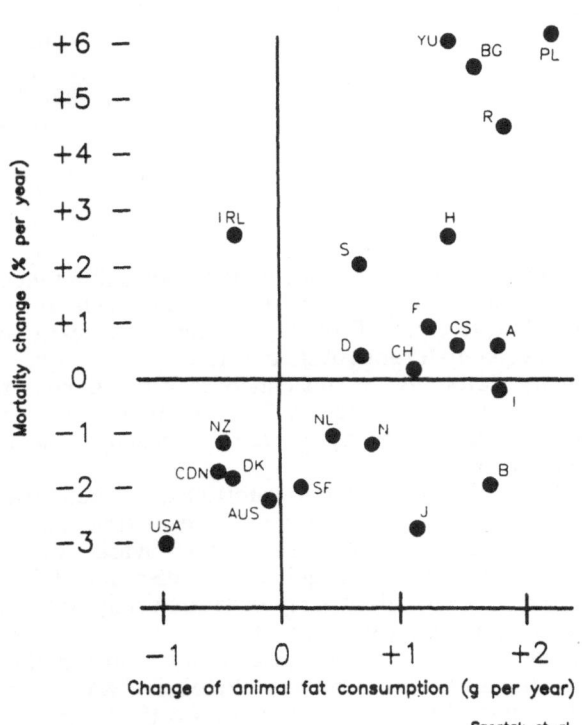

Change of animal fat consumption (g per year)

Szostak et al

Figure 2

The fact that behaviour and life-style-defined risk factors exert major impact on the level of CHD in a population and similarly on its changes is now recognized by practically everybody in Europe. One more example is quoted here therefore, mainly because it is new. At the 10th World Congress of Cardiology last month, the WHO-ERICA Research Group presented a remarkable table (Table 3). In this centralized analysis of 36 epidemiological studies from 18 countries in Europe between 1970 und 1980 it was shown that applying risk coefficients from another study to our own risk-factor data, we could predict pretty well the CHD mortality in the next five years. The fairly good fit between expected (predicted) and observed deaths is even more remarkable, if one considers the two factors speaking against a good fit. First, that "outside" coefficients were used (provided by A. Menotti from the European part of the 7 Country Study). Second that the expected deaths were calculated from large studies, but still with limited number of subjects - around 25.000 altogether - while the observed deaths came from national mortality statistics as reported to WHO (4).

Table 3. Risk prediction from WHO/ERICA-Study and observed national IHD mortality data, males

Age groups	Expected	Observed
	IHD deaths / 10,000 in 5 years	
40 - 44 years	46,5	46,6
45 - 49 "	83,9	76,8
50 - 54 "	123,0	132,9
55 - 59 "	270,0	227,8

FALLACIES

In view of these facts and their increasingly broad acceptance by many populations one may wonder, why the debate among medical scientists is still flaring up from time to time. Probably because it is difficult to find a common language between different subspecialities.

There are many fallacies or misconcepts that pave the way of population wide prevention with pot holes, whether they are natural depressions or digged deliberately by vested interests. I should like to review the most common ones.

The first is the belief based on our traditional medical training, that prevention is simply early cure. We need from time to time sobering lessons like AIDS, where unfortunately no cure is yet available, to consider measures reducing the probability of acquiring the disease. The experience with some cancers also teaches, that early detection may - by definition - prolong survival, but do not offer real prevention.

The next mistake is mixing up risk assessment with individual prediction. Let us consider the following example. Professor XY the outstanding representative of his specialty applies the best available set of screening tests to all his patients in order to detect risk for CHD. His battery of tests makes very few mistakes: out of hundred tests it says only once, that disease is likely to come, when it is not, and similarly only once in hundred,

174

that it is unlikely, when in fact CHD will occure in the not too far distance. In other words his test has only 1 false positive and 1 false negative with 98% correct predictions.

Now let us consider the case of patient N.N. coming to see this famous, Academy Award winning professor.

He is impressed by professor Oscar's good record, that is why he is coming to see him. But his question before entering the surgery is: "Am I or not the one false positive?" (Most patients would like to learn that they are healthy.) And the answer - or the probability - to this question even in the excellent setting of professor Oscar's office is 50 to 50. One could of course argue, that by improving the diagnostic accuracy to 100% instead of 98% one could reach a "true" prediction, but in that ideal case one should term prediction as predestination and call professor Oscar simply God.

There are still many doctors, who equate screening with prevention. Forgetting what was said about early detection and prevention, there is another fallacy in this belief. Even if one could - but unfortunately we can't - deal with complete success with all those at the highest risk, the bulk of the cases would still remain untouched as shown by the simple graph (Figure 3) of population attributable risk. This in essence says, that the majority of new CHD cases comes not from the relatively small proportion

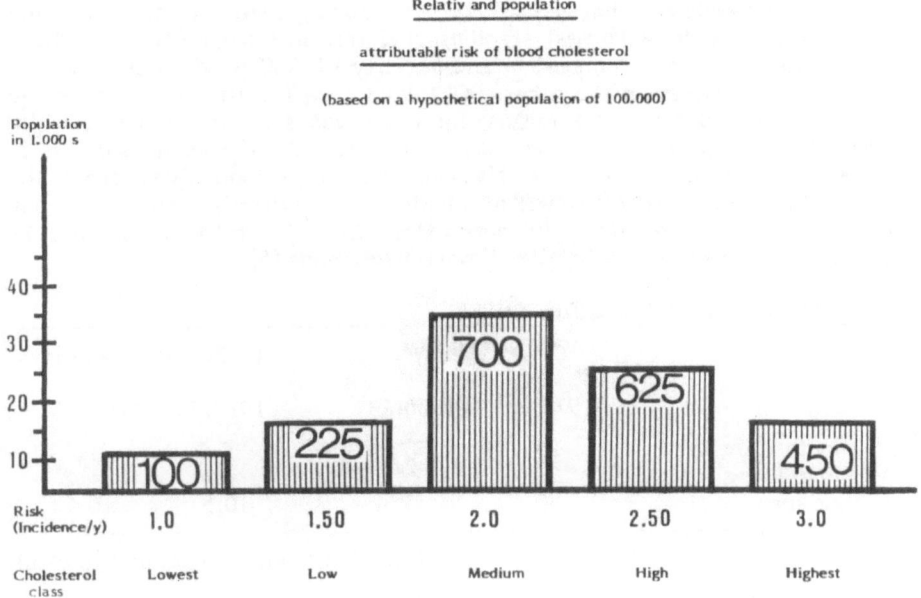

Figure 3

175

of the population with very high risk, but from the large number of those with moderate to medium risk. Thus screening and successful "treatment" of high risk subjects, would take care only of a fraction of the problem.

It is claimed frequently, as the major hindrance to prevention, that we are in lack of appropriate treatment. This of course is to a large extent true, but only with limitations. Table 4 shows on 3 selected examples that the link between pathogenesis, treatment and prevention is very weak. Successful prevention of cholera in London by closing the Broad-street pump was achieved well prior the knowledge of pathogenesis and therapy of cholera. The elucidation of pathogenesis and treatment of diabetes by Best and Banting contributed very little to the prevention of diabetes. Finally therapy was still nowhere, when decline of TBC started due to improvements in socioeconomic conditions.

Table 4.   Better Treatment = Prevention?

	Pathogenesis	Treatment	Prevention
Cholera	no	no	yes
Diabetes	yes	yes	no
TBC	yes	no	yes

Better treatment alone is not a guarentee for reduction of mortality. There can be little doubt, that the treatment of acute myocardial infarction improved tremendously between 1970 and now. Still as shown by the experience of the three longest standing registers in Europe (Table 5) there is no relation between changes in case fatality of AMI on the one hand and CHD mortality trends on the other. In Finland case fatality increased while mortality came down - a smaller increase was seen in Hungary, while mortality went up sharply. One may argue that there was no success in dealing with sudden death and thus one should exclude these from the comparison. The situation however remains essentially the same when one excludes deaths in the first 24 hours after onset. Mortality between 1-28 days does not reflect either national mortality trends (5).

Table 5.   3 AMI Register Study

	Case fatality %		1 - 28 day mortality %	
	1970/71	1980/81	1970/71	1980/81
North Karelia	25	37	6,5	5,8
Heidelberg	26	27	6,4	4,2
Budapest	40	47	10,5	10,5

Östör - Gyarfas - Tuomilehto et al.

Finally let us consider one of the most frequently used fallacy. According to this claims for changes of our present way of life, especially of our eating, drinking and idling habits are unwarranted. What I should like to stress here, is not whether these suggested changes are or not based on sound evidence or whether they will confer this or that much benefit. The misleading character of this statement is, that it tacitly assumes, that lifestyle is something stable, firmly established, unchanging. There is really no need to prove this, only remind people that ٦ur eating and drinking habits are exposed to substantial changes in relatively short periods. The first reminder comes from the EEC study reported by DeGennes and Epstein (6) - Table 6 showing tremendous changes in four decades, especially in the second part of that period. As to drinking, it is worthwhile to quote the experience of our host land from a recent paper of La Vecchia et al. As it is shown in Figure 4 per capita alcohol consumption is on a steady and steep increase, with a dip only during the years of World War 2. Why should one endure changes which are definitely not health-conducive and at the same time tolerate to be admonished to abstain from alterations which could - and many of us are convinced they will - promote health?

Table 6.   Changes in eating in the EEC Nine

	Level 1934/38	Increase % until 1955/56	Increase % 1973
Meat, kg/year	46	18	72
Cheese, kg/year		5,9	79
Calories/day	2,875	2	13
Fat calories %	31	6,4	35

after De Gennes, Epstein et al.

TRENDS IN PER CAPITA TOTAL
ALCOHOL CONSUMPTION IN ITALY
(averaged to unity over the whole period)

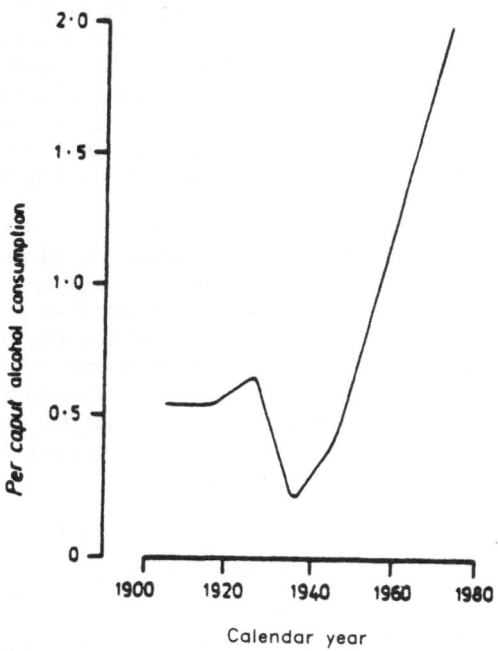

La Vecchia et al

Figure 4

FUTURE

In spite of such non negligible problems progress is encouraging. Clinical medicine and public health are coming closer together day by day. It is now mutually recognized that the high risk strategy is unseparable from medical thinking and ethics. It is admitted at the same time that its effectivity will be low if it goes isolated from the population strategy (8). Among the many indications for hope in this field is the Consensus Statement of the European Atherosclerosis Society signed a few months ago in Neaples by 26 experts from 15 European countries.

But beyond the boundaries of our own profession, governments and their specialized institutions are increasingly ready to promote prevention. On behalf of the Regional Office for Europe of WHO we collected last year the official statements on CVD prevention from Europe (Table 7). There is little doubt that we missed some countries and that others will follow the example of the 9 sooner or later.

Table 7. Policy statements on prevention of CVD in Europe after 1980

FRG	2	Netherland	5
Finland	3	Norway	1
Hungary	1	Sweden	1
Italy	2	U.K.	6
Irland	1		

The problems of air pollution, dying forests, atomic waste are sensitizing people not only toward the health of their environment, but also for their own. If doctors use this favorable atmosphere to invite and lead people to a more sound life-style already from childhood on, we can hope for a continuing decline of CHD, but also of other chronic diseases.

There is hope even for the countries in Eastern Europe, where CHD is still increasing. With the further improvement of economy and growing freedom of choice to spend money on homes, culture and travel instead of eating, smoking and drinking only, the turning point might be reached soon even there.

New knowledge about the pathogenesis and treatment of CHD is accumulating day by day. It is enough to remember of the new insights in lipid-metabolism and of the recent findings in coagulation and platelets. It may bring better undestanding of the effect of diet on atherosclerosis, although it is unlikely that it will basically change the firm link between life-style and disease. We need more research whether it is basic, clinical or public health. Beyond that we need to stress repeatedly that health has many more facets than a single medical one and for its promotion not only the medical profession must join its ranks. Health is a problem for the whole society.

LITERATURE

1. Uemura, K and Pisa, Z (1986). Recent trends in cardiovascular disease mortality in 27 industrialized countries. World Health Statistics Quarterly, in print

2.   Editorial note (1984). JAMA 252/1, 23

3.   Szostak, WB, Cybulska, B and Sekula, W (1985).   Nutrition and ischaemic heart disease mortality, II. Nutritional and mortality trends in 1968-1977 in 23 countries.   Polish Journal of Human Nutrition and Metabolism, 12/2, 73

4.   WHO ERICA Research Group (1986). The US pooling project revisited. 10th World Congress of Cardiology, Washington 1986

5.   Östör-Lamm, E, Gyarfas, I, Tuomilehto, J, et al. (1986).   Acute myocardial Infarction: trends in Europe reflected by the three oldest registers: Heidelberg - Budapest - North Karelia.   10th World Congress of Cardiology, Washington 1986

6.   De Gennes, JH, Epstein, FH, et al (1977).   Influence on health of different fats in food. Commission of the European Communities, Information on Agriculture No. 40

7.   La Vecchia, C, Decarli, A, Mezzanotte, G, Cislaghi, C (1986). Mortality from alcohol related disease in Italy. J. Epid. Comm. Health 40, 257

8.   Rose, GA (1985). Sick individuals and sick populations. Int. J. Epid. 14, 32

9.   European Artherosclerosis Society (1986). A policy statement on the strategy for the prevention of CHD. European Heart Journal, in press

22
Low linoleic acid - a new risk factor for coronary heart disease
M.F. Oliver, D.A. Wood, R.A. Riemersma, R.A. Elton and M. Thomson

INTRODUCTION

While there is a vast literature indicating how saturated fatty
acids differ from polyunsaturated fatty acids in their effects on
plasma lipoproteins, interest in the specific effects of individual
fatty acids on the pathogenesis of coronary heart disease (CHD) has
been small in comparison. There are a number of reasons for this.
They include the facts that (1) the whole field of CHD has been
dominated for years by cholesterol metabolism (2) cross-cultural
surveys of food habits have indicated that there are strong
relationships between dietary saturated fatty acids and serum
cholesterol, on the one hand, and age-standardised five-year CHD
rates on the other and (3) effect of polyunsaturated fatty acids
in lowering plasma cholesterol and low density lipoprotein
cholesterol (LDL) has come to be regarded as an adequate end in
itself, because of the presumed but unproven benefit which
populations and individuals may obtain from reduction of raised
serum cholesterol and LDL cholesterol.

The possibility that coronary-prone populations and patients
with CHD might be relatively deficient in some fatty acids,
particularly linoleic acid, has only recently been considered
seriously, although with increase public health awareness of the
advisability of increasing the P/S ratio, the consumption of
linoleic acid has increased.

The main essential fatty acid for the maintenance of normal
biology in men is linoleic acid (C18:2n6); it is the principal
precursor of archidonic acid (C20:4n6), which is itself an
essential fatty acid in some species, and the main precursor fatty
acid for many prostaglandins.

POPULATION STUDIES

Over the last 10 years, we have demonstrated that there is an
inverse relationship between adipose linoleic acid and CHD in
different populations. The Edinburgh-Stockholm Study[1] showed
that healthy men in a coronary-prone population (Edinburgh) had

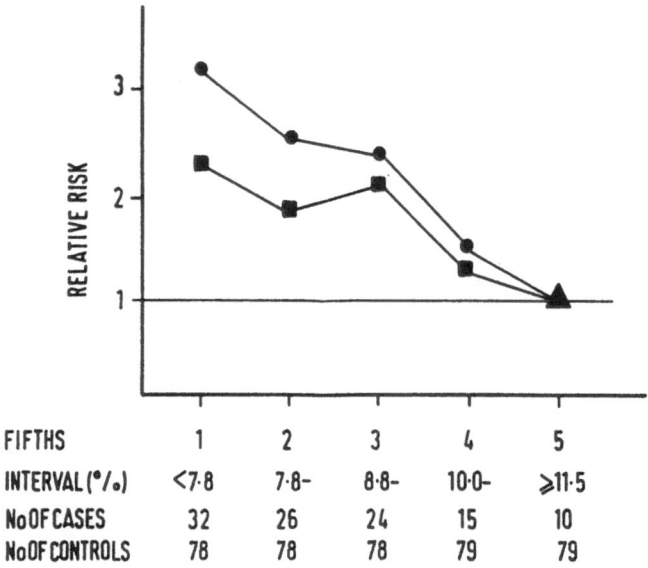

Figure 1 Relative risks of angina pectoris by quintiles of adipose linoleic acid (%) in controls. Circles = adjusted risk; squares = risk adjusted for other risk factors.

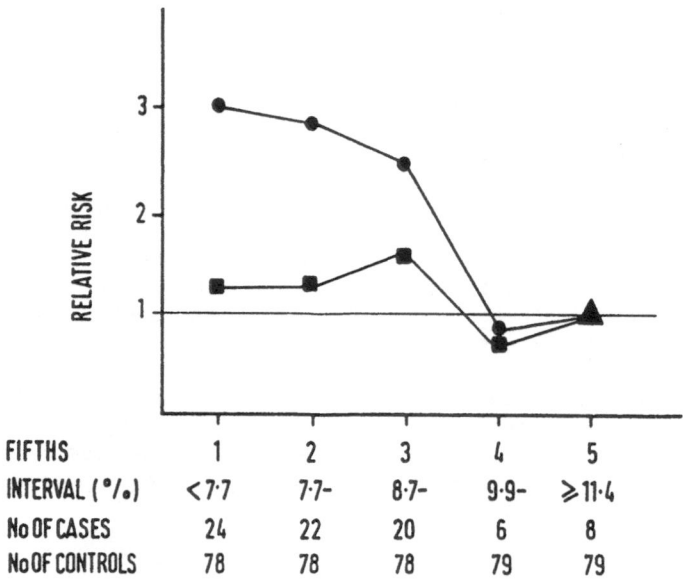

Figure 2 Relative risks of acute myocardial infarction by quintiles of adipose linoleic acid (%) in controls. Circles = adjusted risk; squares = risk adjusted for other risk factors.

significantly lower adipose linoleic acid than comparable men aged
40 in Stockholm, where the incidence of coronary heart disease was
one-third.   This inter-population difference in the concentration
of adipose linoleic acid has recently been confirmed by us with
the demonstration of low adipose linoleic acid concentrations in
North Karelia and Scotland, in contrast to relatively high levels
in South Italy where CHD is far less common[2].

We have also demonstrated that, within a random population of
400 men in Scotland, apparently healthy individuals who were found
to have occult CHD had lower adipose linoleic acid concentrations
than comparable healthy men with CHD[3].   These data were obtained
from 28 men who answered an angina questionnaire positively or who
were found to have electrocardiographic evidence of Q wave
infarction.   The men were unaware that they had coronary heart
disease and, since they had not reported this to anyone, there can
be no question of them being advised to change their diet.

Thus, it has been possible to demonstrate between populations
and within populations that CHD is associated with low concentrations of adipose linoleic acid.

CASE-CONTROL STUDY

Confirmation of these findings is now available from our
recently completed formal case-control study[4].   This shows that
there is an inverse relative risk of angina pectoris and
myocardial infarction of more than 3 to 1 according to the proportions of adipose linoleic acid: thus, there were more than
three times the number of cases in the lowest quintile of adipose
linoleic acid compared with a large control population (Figs 1
and 2).   The data for patients with angina were obtained from
those who had angina for the first time during the preceding one
month: in these subjects a multivariate analysis indicated that
the inverse relative risk of low adipose linoleic acid and CHD was
independent of all other risk factors.   The data from patients
with myocardial infarction were obtained from those arriving
acutely without previous myocardial infarction or angina in an
Intensive Care Unit.   The reason for emphasising the recent onset
of symptoms is that neither the angina patients nor the patients
with myocardial infarction were aware of impending CHD and therefore we assume that the adipose linoleic acid concentrations truly
reflect their long-term dietary habits.   Multivariate analysis
for the myocardial infarct patients showed that the low adipose
linoleic acid content was independent of all other risk factors,
with the exception of cigarette smoking.

We have also identified that cigarette smokers, independently
of the presence of CHD, have lower concentrations of adipose
linoleic acid than non-smokers[3].   More important, perhaps,
cigarette smokers consume linoleic acid[4].   Why this should be is
not clear, although it is possible that non-smokers are more
health conscious and therefore take more edible oils.   This is
one of the first indications that cigarette smoking might lead to

to CHD by influencing food consumption adversely.

Low adipose linoleic acid must result from a low dietary intake of linoleic acid and, from a 7-day prospective weighed record in 140 normal men[5], the correlation coefficient with dietary linoleic acid was +0.58.

The turnover of adipose linoleic acid is in the region of 10-12 months[6]. Thus, the lower concentrations of linoleic acid in adipose tissue found in these cross-sectional surveys reflect long-term eating habits and not recent intake. It is difficult to believe that coronary-prone people select a diet low in linoleic acid months before they develop any symptoms and the possibility therefore arises that there are also major metabolic differences either in absorption, catabolism, storage or mobilisation of fatty acids; and these are under study.

It is not clear what the biological significance is of low tissue levels of the essential fatty acid, linoleic acid, and it has yet to be shown whether the increased relative risk for CHD applies equally in populations with a high intake of edible oils. But the importance of the finding is emphasised further by the identification of low serum phospholipid linoleic acid as a prospective marker for subsequent CHD[7].   There is evidence to suggest that, at least in the short term, linoleic acid is capable of reducing blood pressure[8].

CONCLUSION

Far more needs to be learned about the influences of long chain polyunsaturated fatty acids on the pathogenic processes which lead to CHD.   Meanwhile, there appears to be a strong case for increasing the proportion of linoleic acid in those living in communities where the intake is low.

REFERENCES

1. Logan RL, Thomson M, Riemersma RA et al (1978). Risk factors for ischaemic heart disease in normal men aged 40. Lancet, i,949.
2. Riemersma RA, Wood DA, Butler S et al (1986). Linoleic acid in adipose tissue and coronary heart disease. Brit Med J. 292, 1423
3. Wood DA, Butler S, Riemersma RA et al (1984). Adipose tissue and platelet fatty acids and coronary heart disease in Scottish men. Lancet, ii, 117.
4. Wood DA, Riemersma RA, Butler S et al (1987). Linoleic and eicosapentaenoic acids in adipose tissue and platelets and risk of coronary heart disease. Lancet, In Press.
5. Thomson M, Fulton M, Wood DA et al (1985). A comparison of the nutrient intake of some Scotsmen with dietary recommendations. Human Nutrition: Applied Nutrition 39A, 443
6. Van Staveren WA, Deurenberg P, Katan MB et al. (1986). Validity of the fatty acid composition of subcutaneous fat tissue micro-biopsies as an estimate of the long term average fatty acid com-position of the diet of separate individuals. Am J Epid. 123,455.

7. Miettinen TA, Naukkarinen V, Huttunen JK et al (1982). Fatty-acid composition of serum lipids predicts myocardial infarction. Brit Med J. 285, 993.
8. Puska P, Iacono JM, Nissinen A et al (1983). Controlled randomised trial of the effect of dietary fat on blood pressure. Lancet i, 1.

23
The US National Cholesterol Education Program
B.M. Rifkind

Considerable changes are currently taking place in the attitudes of U. S. physicians, other health professionals and the public to cholesterol and coronary heart disease (CHD). An increasing awareness of the role of dietary fat and blood cholesterol in CHD can be traced to gradual advances in our understanding over the past two decades. However, it has been markedly stimulated by 3 recent events, namely the report of the Lipid Research Clinics Coronary Primary Prevention Trial (LRC-CPPT), the recommendations of the U.S. National Institutes of Health Consensus Development Conference on Lowering Blood Cholesterol and the recent initiation of the National Cholesterol Education Program (NCEP). I will deal briefly with each of these.

LIPID RESEARCH CLINICS CORONARY PRIMARY PREVENTION TRIAL[1,2]

The Lipid Research Clinics Program Coronary Primary Prevention Trial was designed to test the hypothesis that reducing elevated cholesterol levels would prevent CHD. By the time it was initiated in 1973 there was already a considerable spectrum of evidence relating cholesterol to CHD derived from animal studies, observations on the composition and natural history of the atherosclerotic plaque, detailed studies of various genetic hypercholesterolemias especially familial hypercholesterolemia, metabolic studies of the plasma lipids and lipoproteins and many different epidemiological approaches. Many clinical trials of cholesterol-lowering had also been previously conducted using diet or drug for the primary or secondary prevention of CHD. Most of them had yielded encouraging results but none of them had been held to be conclusive on account of problems such as inadequate numbers of participants, inadequate periods of follow-up, failure to apply randomization and to use a double-blind design, statistical problems in analysis and inadequate cholesterol-lowering.

The design of the LRC-CPPT attempted to address these problems. The trial was a multi-centered, randomized, double-blind study which tested the efficacy of cholesterol-lowering in reducing risk of CHD in 3,806 asymptomatic middle-aged men with primary hypercholesterolemia (Type II hyperlipoprotemia). Men were required to have a plasma cholesterol level of 265 mg/dl or greater (the 95th percentile based on population studies) and an LDL cholesterol level of 190 mg/dl or greater. Individuals whose LDL cholesterol level fell below 175 mg/dl after treatment with the special LRC-CPPT diet were excluded. Individuals were free of clinical manifestations of CHD, so that the study was a primary prevention trial.

After a series of visits eligible participants were randomized into two groups, each of which received the LRC-CPPT diet which was designed to reduce plasma cholesterol levels by 3-5%. In addition, one of the groups also received cholestyramine resin at a prescribed dose of 6 packets (24G) a day. The other group received a placebo. Comparison of the two treatment groups with respect to 83 variables compared at baseline showed that the randomization process had resulted in 2 almost identical groups. All men were followed for a minimum of 7 and up to 10 years with the average period of follow-up being 7.4 years.

The cholestyramine group experienced average plasma total and low density lipoprotein cholesterol reductions of 13.4% and 20.3% respectively which were 8.5% and 12.6% greater reductions than those obtained in the placebo group. The cholestyramine group experienced a 19% reduction in risk ($p < 0.05$) of the primary endpoint - definite CHD death and/or definite nonfatal myocardial infarction - reflecting a 24% reduction in definite CHD death and a 19% reduction in nonfatal myocardial infarction. (Figure)

Several other indices of CHD were monitored and corresponding reductions in CHD were found for those in which a sufficient number of events occurred to allow for a meaningful comparison. Thus, the incidence rates for new positive exercise test, angina and coronary bypass surgery were significantly reduced by 25, 20, and 21% respectively in the cholestyramine group.

When the cholestyramine treatment group was analyzed separately, a 19% reduction in CHD risk was also associated with each decrement of 8% in total cholesterol or 11% in LDL cholesterol levels ($p < 0.001$). Furthermore, the CHD incidence in men sustaining a fall of 25% in total plasma cholesterol or 35% in LDL cholesterol levels, typical responses to the prescribed dosage of cholestyramine resin, was half that of men who remained at pretreatment levels.

No conclusive evidence of serious toxicity was observed in the LRC-CPPT. An equal number of malignancies occurred in each group. More gastrointestinal cancers were found in the cholestyramine group, mainly in the buccal cavity and pharynx. No increase in colon-rectal cancers was seen. A follow-up of the participants in the CPPT is being conducted for a further 5 years with particular emphasis on monitoring cancer experience.

The LRC-CPPT findings show that reducing total plasma cholesterol levels by lowering LDL cholesterol diminishes the incidence of CHD morbidity and mortality in men at high risk for CHD because of raised LDL cholesterol levels.

NIH CONSENSUS DEVELOPMENT CONFERENCE[3]

A year after the LRC-CPPT was reported a Consensus Development Conference on Lowering Blood Cholesterol to Prevent Heart Disease was convened at the National Institutes of Health. The Consensus Panel of lipoprotein experts, cardiologists, primary care physicians, epidemiologists, bio-medical scientists, bio-statisticians, experts in prevent medicine, and lay representatives heard a series of expert presentations on various aspects of cholesterol and CHD research. The panel concluded that elevated blood cholesterol level is a major cause of coronary artery disease. They believe that it had been established, beyond a reasonable doubt, that lowering definitely elevated blood cholesterol levels (specifically blood levels of LDL-C) will reduce the risk of heart attacks due to coronary heart disease. After careful review of genetic, experimental, epidemiologic, and clinical trial evidence they recommended treatment of individuals with blood cholesterol levels above the 75th percentile (upper 25% of values). Further they were persuaded that the blood cholesterol levels of most Americans was undesirably high, in large part because of the high dietary intake of calories, saturated fat and cholesterol.

Specifically it was recommended that:
1. Individuals with high risk blood cholesterol levels (Table I) be treated intensively by dietary means under the guidance of a physician, dietitian, or other health professional; if response to diet is inadequate, appropriate drugs should be added to the regimen.
2. Adults with moderate risk blood cholesterol levels (Table I) should be treated intensively by dietary means especially it additional risk factors are present. Only a small proportion should require drug treatment.
3. The panel also recommended that all Americans (except children under two years of age) be advised to adopt a diet that reduces total dietary fat from the current level of about 40% of total calories to 30% total calories, reduces saturated fat intake to less than 10% of total calories, increases polyunsaturated fat intake but to no more than 10% of total calories, and reduces daily cholesterol intake to 250-300 mg or less. (Table 2)

To implement these and related recommendations it was further recommended that new and expanded programs be planned and initiated to educate physicians, other health professionals, and the public to the significance of elevated blood cholesterol and the importance of treating it.

THE NATIONAL CHOLESTEROL EDUCATION PROGRAM[4]

The National Cholesterol Education Program (NCEP) was initiated in October 1985 by the National Heart, Lung, and Blood Institute. The overall objective of the NCEP will be to reduce

CHD morbidity and mortality related to elevated blood cholesterol by developing a national education effort and by stimulating extensive cooperation and coordination among responsible government agencies and interested public organizations. As in the case of the highly successful predecessor program the National High Blood Pressure Education Program, the NCEP will operate as a partnership. A Coordinating Committee has been established for the NCEP to ensure effective mobilization of the resources and energies of all interested organizations. Membership of this committee comprises representatives from over 20 participating organizations representing most of the major medical organizations in the United States with a a current or potential role in the area of cholesterol education. These include the American Medical Association, the American Heart Association, the American College of Cardiology, the American Dietetic Association and public interest groups such as the American Red Cross.

The NCEP is designing programs for health professionals, patients with elevated cholesterol, and the American public that are not only increasing their awareness of the importance of lowering elevated blood cholesterol levels but which are providing them with the information and skills necessary to achieve lowering through dietary change and appropriate drug treatment. Cholesterol-lowering research programs will be developed for implementation in the workplace and from cooperation in existing workplace wellness and disease prevention programs. An additional focus will be made on encouraging curriculum changes in primary and secondary schools that will alert students to the role of blood cholesterol as a risk factor for heart disease and the benefits of lowering elevated levels by diet and other means. A special emphasis will be placed on reaching minority groups and other special audiences by developing materials and programs responsive to their particular needs.

A substantial decline in mortality from CHD has been observed in the U.S. over the past 15-20 years. Although it is not possible to pinpoint the precise factors responsible for this, there is little doubt that increasing emphasis on control of risk factors has made a significant contribution. It is believed that the new NCEP offers great promise for furthering the decline in cardiovascular mortality.

Table I. Cholesterol Values for Selecting Adults at Moderate and High Risk Requiring Treatment

Age	Moderate Risk	High Risk
20-29	200 mg/dl (5.17 mM)	220 mg/dl (5.69 mM)
30-39	220 (5.69)	240 (6.21)
40+	240 (6.21)	260 (6.72)

Table II. Recommended Diet for General Population Aged 2 Years and Older

	% Total Calories
Total fat	30%
Saturated fat	10% or less
Polyunsaturated fat	increase to no more than 10%
Cholesterol	250-300 mg/day

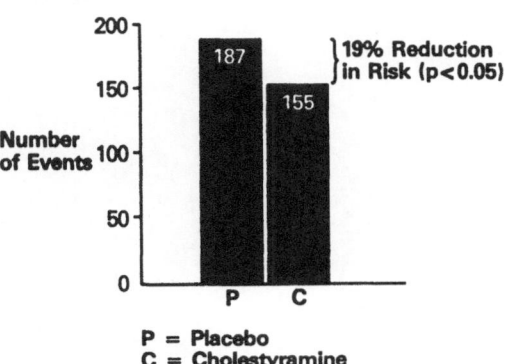

LRC-CPPT

PRIMARY ENDPOINT (DEFINITE CORONARY HEART DISEASE DEATH AND/OR NONFATAL MYOCARDIAL INFARCTION)

19% Reduction in Risk (p<0.05)

187 — P
155 — C

Number of Events

P = Placebo
C = Cholestyramine

Figure 1

191

References

1. Lipid Research Clinics Program. The Lipid Research Clinics Coronary Primary Prevention Trial Results I. Reduction in incidence of coronary heart disease. JAMA 251:351-364, 1984
2. Lipid Research Clinics Program. The Lipid Research Clinics Coronary Primary Prevention Trial Results II. The relationship of reduction in incidence of coronary heart disease to cholesterol lowering. JAMA 251:365-374, 1984
3. Consensus Conference Statement on Lowering Cholesterol to Prevent Heart Disease. JAMA 253:2080-2086, 1985.
4. Lenfant C. A new challenge for America: The National Cholesterol Education Program. Circulation 73:855-856, 1986

24
The WHO European Multifactor Preventive Trial of CHD

A. Menotti, on behalf of the WHO European
Collaborative Group

The WHO European Multifactor Preventive Trial of Coronary Heart
Disease (CHD), also known as WHO Collaborative Trial, represents
one of the major attempts, started in the early seventhies, aimed
at answering two crucial questions concerning the primary prevention of the disease, i.e.: (1) whether the major risk factor could
be modified in a substancial and permanent way; (2) whether such
changes, if any, were accompanied by a reduction of CHD incidence
and mortality over a period of 6 years. The main characteristics of
this study was that to adopt, as statistical units, pairs of
occupational groups called "factories" made of men aged 40-59 and
to allocate at random one member of each pair to intervention and
the other to control. This approach, which is different from those
of all other similar studies, has needed a peculiar procedure for
the conduction of the study and for the final analysis of data.

MATERIAL AND METHODS
    The study was conducted in five European countries, i.e. Great
Britain, Belgium, Italy, Poland and Spain. The latter country
contributed only to study the risk factor changes and not incidence
and mortality data. Excluding the Spanish section, 40 pairs of
factories have been enrolled for a total of 60,881 men; out of them

Members of the Group; Belgium: Dr G. De Backer, Dr M. Kornitzer,
Mrs M. Dramaix, Prof C. Thilly (data co-coordinator); Italy: Prof A.
Menotti, Prof G. Ricci, Prof G.C. Urbinati, Prof G. Farchi; Poland:
Prof S.I. Rywik, Prof J. Sznajd, Prof W.B. Szostak, Dr M. Magdon,
Dr J. Charzewska; Spain: Prof I. Balaguer-Vintro, Dr L. Tomas-Abadal
Dr S. Sans; GB: Prof G. Rose (chairman), Prof H.D. Tunstall Pedoe,
Dr R.F. Heller, Mr M.J. Shiphey; World Health Organisation (European
Office): Dr G. Lamm.

30,486 were assigned to intervention and 30,392 to control. An entry screening for the measurement of some classical coronary risk factors was offered to all men in the intervention factories and to about 10% of men in control factories.

The factors considered for this analysis are age, systolic blood pressure, serum cholesterol, cigarettes smoked per day and body mass index. All measurements were taken following standardized procedures. Subsequently the following operations have been performed: (a) intensive preventive action on an individual basis in order to modify risk factor levels in men belonging to the upper 15% (a little more in Italy) of an entry risk score based on five factors and in hypertensives, in the intervention factories; (b) general health education for all men belonging to intervention factories; (c) annual re-screening for risk factors of high risk men and of a random 10% in intervention factories; (d) biennal rescreening at 2nd and 4th anniversary of the same original 10% random sample of men in control factories; (e) continuous monitoring for 6 years of non fatal cardiovascular events, based on absenteism from work and subsequent check of each suspect diagnosis; (f) continuous monitoring of all deaths and their causes for 6 years; (g) final screening for risk factors at the end of 6 years offered to all men in both intervention and control factories.

More details on methodology and diagnostic criteria can be found elsewhere (1-5).

The 90% of the control men not examined at entry   screening and 2 and 4 years later formed the at risk popolation for incidence measurement.

The core of the analysis was based on the independent estimate for each pair of factories of risk factor changes and coronary incidence and mortaltiy. Risk factor changes were obtained by calculating for each man the estimate of the multiple logistic function (MLF) theorical risk from entry, 2-year, 4-year and 6-year examination. The coefficients were computed ad hoc from the experience of the European cohorts of the Seven Countries Study (2) in 5 years. Individual changes were then averaged for the estimation of the overall net change of each intervention and control factory. The final effect of intervention was expressed in each factory pair, by the log e of the ratio of the intervention to the control rate. The relation of outcome to the risk factor changes was estimated by means of a modification of the maximum likelihood regression method of Pocock et al. (6) which is expressed by log e $(p_i/p_c) = a + b(\text{delta MLF}) + E$; where p_i is the rate of events in intervention factory; p_c is the rate of events in control factories; a is a constant; delta MLF is the net change of risk factors as summarized by the multiple logistic function; b is the slope of the regression; E is an error term.

Table 1. Participating centres and study population

Centers		Intervention	Control
Great Britain	(GB)	9734	8476
Belgium	(B)	8509	10900
Italy	(I)	3131	2896
Poland	(P)	9115	8120
All Centers		30486	30392

RESULTS

The number of men enrolled in the four countries are given in Table 1. The overall participation rate to the first examination was of 86%. The entry levels of major risk factors were similar in the overall intervention and control groups, although differences were found when comparing different countries.

The impact of intervention on risk factors (Table 2) suggests that in Great Britain and in Poland the preventive procedure was poor or poorly accepted, whereas in Belgium and in Italy the changes of the mean levels of risk factors and of the combined MLF estimate were much more satisfactory. The net result on the lumped national groups reflects a balance between good and poor results, which are also influenced by the different size of the national groups themselves.

The six year outcome, in terms of CHD incidence and mortality, (Table 3) is a kind of replica of the results obtained on risk factor levels. The treatment has apparently produced an adverse effect in Great Britain, a limited and contraddictory effect in

Table 2. Net percent change in risk factors for all men in trial, averaged over all examinations.

Factors	GB	B	I	P	ALL
cholesterol	−0.4	−0.9	−4.8	+1.2	−1.2
cigarettes/day	−15.6	−3.7	−5.5	−9.0	−8.9
weight	−0.4	+0.2	−1.9	−1.0	−0.4
systolic BP	−1.6	−2.3	−4.1	−1.2	−2.0
combined MLF	−3.9	−15.8	−28.2	−5.4	−11.1

Poland and a much better effect in Belgium and Italy with a substancial decrease of CHD incidence and mortality (statistically significant in Belgium). Overall a reduction of 7% of fatal CHD, of 15% of non fatal CHD, of 10% total CHD and of 5% of all death are outcomes not far from what could be expected on the basis of risk factor changes.

The results of the computation of the regression method of Pocock et al. do correspond to a weighted regression where the incidence differences are weighted according to the inverse of variance of each factory pair. (Table 4). The slopes for fatal CHD and total CHD are significant (p less than 0.05; 2 tails). This simply means that risk factor changes, as described by the summary MLF, explain in a significant way the observed differences in CHD incidence. The intercept, or constant a which anyhow is not significant, represents any effect of the intervention for zero net change in risk factors, whereas the slopes measure the strenght of the relation between risk factor change and outcome. The value of the intercept, which is small and negative, suggests that there might have been a slight extra reduction in CHD in intervention groups not accounted for by the MLF summary of measured risk factor changes.

When the regression of the difference in the intervention/control rates have been calculated, (instead of the log e of their ratio), against the measured risk factor changes, it appeared that for each reduction in risk factors corresponding to a predicted decline in total CHD of 10 cases per 1000 in 6 years, there was an observed decline of 6.2 per 1000. In the regression quoted above it is possible to recognize four quadrants corresponding to the presence of factory pairs which could be classified as true positives (decrease of factors and of incidence), and true negatives (increase of factors and of incidence) which behaved according with the theory of risk reversibility. On the other hand

Table 3. Net percent difference in 6-year CHD incidence and mortality between intervention and control, by centre.

Event	GB	B	I	P	All (*)
Fatal CHD	+8	−21	−30	+3	−7 (p=0.8)
Total CHD	+5	−24	−14	−16	−10 (p=0.07)
All Deaths	−14	−17	−6	−5	−5 (p=0.4)

(*) Adjusted for effect of allocating groups, not individuals.

a few factories pairs could be classified as false positive (decrease of factors and increase of incidence) or false negatives (increase of factors and decrease of incidence).

DISCUSSION
This study has to be viewed in comparison with the three other major multifactor trials recently completed. The Oslo study

Table 4. Slopes and intercepts values for the regression of differences in incidence of CHD ($\log e$ Pi/Pc) on difference in risk factor changes for the trial as a whole.

Events	Slope	SE	Intercept	SE
Fatal CHD	+0.310(*)	0.138	−0.028	0.069
Total CHD	+0.246(*)	0.118	−0.064	0.057
All Deaths	+0.151	0.133	−0.027	0.060

(*) p less than 0.05 (2 tails)

provided positive results, but it was confined to high risk men (7). The MRFIT ended up with moderate decrease in both risk factors and CHD mortality (8). The Goteborg trial did not show any net difference between intervention and controls, neither for factors nor for incidence (9).

In this trial, which is the largest of the four, we found that the intervention effort was followed by a reduction of 7% in fatal CHD, 15% in non fatal CHD, 10% in total CHD and 5% in total mortality. These benefits, although small, are of great public health interest. They were obtained by a realitively cheap effort but, more important, the regression analysis on factory pairs has demonstrated that there is a kind of proportionality between the intervention effort and the final outcome, like in a dose-effect response. The fact that only 62% of the expected reduction was really achieved can be explained by measurements defects, delay in risk reversal and perhaps adverse effects of the anti-hypertensive drugs.

Some problems have been met in the interpretation of the Polish results which in part were of the false negative type.

The overall experimental evidence shows that advice on risk factors control is effective to the extent of its acceptance.

REFERENCES

1. WHO European Collaborative Group (1974). An international controlled trial in the multifactorial prevention of coronary heart disease. Int J Epidem 3, 219.

2. WHO European Collaborative Group (1980). Multifactorial trial in the prevention of coronary heart disease. 1 Recruitment and initial findings. Euro Heart J, 1, 73.

3. WHO European Collaborative Group (1982). Multifactorial trial in the prevention of coronary heart disease. 2. Risk factor changes at two and four years. Euro Heart J, 3, 184.

4. WHO European Collaborative Group (1983). Multifactorial trial in the prevention of coronary heart disease. 3 Incidence and mortality results. Euro Heart J, 4, 141.

5. WHO European Collaborative Group (1986). European Collaborative Trial of Multifactorial prevention of coronary heart disease: final report on the 6-year results. Lancet, 8486, 869.

6. Pocock SJ, Cook DG and Beresford, SAA (1981). Regression of area mortality on explanatory variables: what weighting is appropriate ? Appl Statistics, 30, 286.

7. Hjermann, I, Velve Byre, K, Holme, I, and Leren, P (1981). Effects of diet and smoking intervention on the incidence of coronary heart disease. Lancet, ii, 1303.

8. Multiple Risk Factor Intervention Trial Research Group (1982). Multiple risk factor intervention trial. Risk factor changes and mortality results. JAMA, 248, 1465.

9. Wilhelmsen, L, Berglund, G, and Elmfeld, D, Tibblin G, Wedel H, Pennert K, Vedin A, Wilhelnesson C, Werkö L, (1986) The multifactor primary prevention trial in Göteborg, Sweden. Euro Heart J, 7, 279.

25
Epidemiology and clinical features of hypertension in the elderly
G. Abate and M. Zito

AGE TRENDS IN BLOOD PRESSURE - PREVALENCE OF HYPERTENSION IN THE EL-
DERLY.

It has long been recognized that basal resting systolic and diastolic
blood pressure values increase with advancing adult age.
In particular, the longitudinal observations of the Framingham Study
indicate that diastolic pressure values rise with age until the mid-
50s and then plateau until about age 65, after which they decline in
subsequent decades.
The values in the two sexes are parallel over time, and persistently
lower in women in respect to men.
Systolic pressure presents a distinctly different age trend. Its rise
continues unabated at least until age 75; the values in women are ini
tially lower than those of men, but after age 60, they are higher in
the same sex, depending on a steeper increase over time.
According to these epidemiological data, hypertension, however
defined, is very common in the elderly.
The prevalence values in different studies range from 35% to 65%, depending on sex, race, the definition of the upper limits of "normali-
ty" and the methods by which the pressures were obtained.
This general trend, which is typical for Western and affluent so
cieties, cannot be considered as a "normal" phenomenon.
Even in these populations, not all persons exhibit a rise in pressure
in adult life; moreover in some isolated, primitive ethnical groups
the pressure values are sensibly lower and stable over time.
These observations draw to the conclusion that the rise of pressure values age-related isn't only caused by aging per se, but that
it in some way reflects the intrusion of a disease process.
Between them, the increased rigidity of the aorta and peripheral arte
ries is worthy of note, because of loss of elastic fibers in the arte
rial media, accompanied by increased collagen and calcium deposits.
The aorta is no longer able to dampen the peaks of the arterial pres-

sure generated by the left ventricle and so the systolic pressure inclines to increase.

Besides that, a reduced sensitivity of the baroceptors area must be acknowledged; subsequently the reactive baroreflex function, following hypertensive or hypotensive situations is impaired and the blood pressure values reset on higher levels.

HAZARD OF HYPERTENSION

Hypertension is a prominent contributor to overall mortality, doubling the risk of death, and to cardiovascular mortality in particular, where the risk in the elderly is tripled compared to normotensive persons of the same age.

Moreover, the risk of every major cardiovascular sequela of hypertension is increased in the elderly hypertensive subjects.

The impact of hypertension is greater for the risk of stroke and cardiac failure and least for occlusive peripheral arterial disease.

The attributable risk, which takes into account the high prevalence of hypertension and the relative risk, is also as great in the elderly as in the young.

Thus, there is nothing to suggest a lesser hazard of hypertension in the elderly.

Also the isolated systolic hypertension, too often considered an innocuous, normal accompaniment of advanced age, cannot be considered at all well tolerated.

In fact, the analysis of every component of blood pressure, including pulse pressure, suggest that nothing is clearly superior to the systolic pressure in predicting cardiovascular events, in general, and stroke in particular.

Moreover the relative impact of other associated risk factors must be considered.

Despite the fact that the impact of cholesterol, glucose tolerance and cigarette smoking diminishes with advancing age, multivariate risk profiles made up of these variables, blood pressure and ECG-LVH, have been found to be a predictor of risk both in the elderly and in the young.

So, in assessing the gravity of hypertension in the elderly, several factors must be taken into account, among them the height of the systolic pressure, the number of associated cardiovascular risk factors and whether or not there is target organ involvement.

CLINICAL AND PHYSIOPATHOLOGICAL FEATURES

On the basis of the epidemiological data just reported, and of the re sults of recent therapeutical trials, it is generally accepted that the hypertensive status in the elderly must be correctly treated, in order to reduce the cardiovascular mortality and the incidence of car diovascular events.

Such therapeutical intervention however cannot be indiscriminately di rected to all the elderly hypertensives, but it is necessary to take into account some particular clinical and physiopathological features.

1) Complications and other unrelated diseases.

While in young patients hypertension is frequently asymptomatic, and usually detected in the course of a common medical screening in other wise healthy subjects, in the elderly, on the contrary, the prevalence of cardiovascular complications is higher and hypertension is asso ciated with many other unrelated diseases.

In such a way, the expectancy of life may be highly reduced, and hypertension plays a minor role as a risk factor for overall mortality. In this respect the paper of Rajala e Co., who, in a recent longitudi nal study in the population over 85 in Tampere, Finland, found the striking evidence of reduced mortality rates in hypertensive compared to normotensive subjects, is worthy of note.

These results have been confirmed by personal observation on elderly people (mean age 73), living in istitutions: hypertension was associa ted with an higher incidence rate of stroke and cardiac failure, and with an higher mortality rate for cardiovascular events; despite that the overall mortality rate was lower in hypertensive compared to nor- motensives.

It is possible to draw the conclusion that the treatment of hyperten- sion cannot be considered mandatory, whenever the expectancy of life is reduced in the elderly by other unrelated diseases or poor general conditions.

2) Pseudohypertension.

It is well known that in clinical conditions the evaluation of blood pressure, by means of the cuff sphigmomanometer, is based on an outer compression, which acts indirectly against the homeral artery.

Therefore the thickness of tissued interposed between the cuff and the vessel, and the compliance of the artery "in se", may influence the validity of the measure.

In the elderly the vessel walls may be less compliant; so a greater outer compression may be necessary in order to balance the intravascu lar pressure, and the values clinically observed can overrate the re- al ones inside the artery.

The existence of pseudohypertension must be suspected:

a) in patients with arterial rigidity (Osler's manuever positivity);
b) when there is a discrepancy between the high values and long cour- se of hypertension and relative mild impairment of target organs;
c) when there is the onset of symptoms of "hypotension" after treat- ment, which "normalises" the blood pressure values.

3) Variability of blood pressure.

The tecnniques of blood pressure continuous intra-arterial monitoring have clearly demonstrated wide fluctuations in the same subjects during the day and in the course of different stressing events.
In the elderly such a variability is greater than in the young, because of different physiopatologic conditions (reduced baroceptor responsiveness, aortic compliance, intravascular volume, iuxta-glomerular apparatus responsiveness, imbalance between beta and alpha adrenoceptors), which impairs the short and long term homeostatic control.
The consequences of such a greater variability can be of some value in the elderly, who are prone to cerebral ischemic lesions as a consequence of even limited falls in arterial blood pressure.

CONCLUSIONS

Hypertension in the elderly must be regarded as a major cardiovascular risk factor.
Treatment is advisable as general philosophy.
However several factors must be taken into account on the clinical ground: among them the age, the specific complications, other unrelated diseases, the physiopathological background, the possible side effects of treatment, the psychological and socio-economic conditions.
The therapy must be undertaken only after an extensive individual evaluation, with the aim not only of reducing the cardiovascular mortality and morbidity, but, overall, of improving the quality of life.

BIBLIOGRAPHY

1) Amery A., Brixko P., Clement D., e al.: "Mortality and morbidity results from the European Working Party on High Blood Pressure in the Elderly trial".
Lancet 1, 1349, 1985.

2) Bulpitt C.J.: "The prognosis of essential hypertension". In Hand Book of Hypertension, Vol. 6, Epidemiology of Hypertension Elsever Oxford, 1985.

3) Corneli M., Zito M., Santicchia S., D'Aviero M., Cervone C., Amatetti M., Fici F., Abate G.: "Ipertensione arteriosa nell'anziano: studio retrospettivo su soggetti istituzionalizzati (Nota 1)".
La riforma medica, 115, 122, 1986.

4) Kannel W.: "Hypertension and aging" Human Biology and Pathology - Van Nostrand Reinhold Company - N.Y. 1985.

5) Mancia G., Zanchetti A.: "Arterial Blood pressure recording in human hypertension". Atherosclerotic Rev., 7, 325, 1980.

6) Messerly F.H., Ventura H.O., Amodeo C.: "Osler's maneuver and pseu̱ dohypertension". New. Engl. J. Medicine, 24, 1548, 1985.

7) Rȧjala S., Haevisto M., Heikiheimo R.: "Blood pressure and mortali̱ ty in the very old". Lancet 1, 520, 1983.

8) Zito M., Corneli M., Santicchia S., D'Aviero M., Cervone C., Amatetti M., Fici F., Abate G.: "Ipertensione arteriosa nell'anziano: studio retrospettivo su soggetti istituzionalizzati (Nota 2)".
La riforma Medica, 101, 123, 1986.

26
Atherosclerosis precursors in children. The Bologna study. Preliminary data

G.P. Salvioli, G. Faldella, R. Alessandroni,
R. Rossini, M. Lanari, S. Alati and C. De Marchis

INTRODUCTION

Atherosclerosis lesions start considerably earlier than the onset of clinical disease. It is now generally agreed that atherosclerosis may start as early as in childhood and adolescence. Studies of arterial pathology have shown that fatty streaks are present in the aortas of children as young as three years of age. By the age of 20 years, raised lesions significant to the development of clinical disease begin to appear in coronary arteries (1,2,3).

For primary prevention it is therefore essential to study the occurrence and development of cardiovascular risk factors and their determinants in childhood and adolescence. Serum cholesterol, cigarette smoking, arterial blood pressure, consumption of alcohol, physical inactivity, family history of death from cardiovascular diseases and evidence of diseases such as diabetes mellitus, are the main risk factors currently recognised (4,5,6,7).

A prospective study, to be carried out from 1986 to 1988, was designed to obtain data on the risk factors of atherosclerosis and its determinants in Bologna school age children and to plan educational programmes in school that enable children to make informed choices concerning their health and lifestyle.

The study plan consists of three successive stages. In the first stage, participants are enrolled and the cardiovascular risk factors prevalent among them are assessed. The second stage is an educational programme in which the results of initial boold tests and assessment of diet and lifestyle are discussed with the children, who will then be informed about existing cultural and social trends and correct eating and lifestyle habits. At the end of the study the efficacy of the programme will be evaluated by reassessing all the parameters considered at the ontset.

SUBJECTS AND METHODS

The study is underway in three secondary schools of Bologna, a large wealthy Italian town, traditionally famous for its learning and rich food.

In January 1986, all first year students (aged about 12) were invited to participate in the project and were informed about the study design. Two or three weeks before the medical examination, each family received a general questionnaire on the socioeconomic background of the family, the environment where the children were living, the childrens'general health and development and the parents' and grand-parents' state of health.

Physical activity of the children was estimated by a multiple choice questionnaire. Each student was asked to choose his physical activity pattern out of the following:

1. Usually reads, watches television, goes to the cinema or spends leisure-time in sedentary activities (sedentary);
2. Walks, rides a bicycle or spends at least four hours a week moving outdoors (moderately active);
3. Spends leisure-time playing sports such as swimming, tennis, jogging, athletics (active);
4. Regulary participates in some type of sport, several times a week (very active).

Girls were asked whether they menstruated and if so, whether their cycles were regular.

Medical examination of the subjects took place in school; height (H) and weight (W) were measured and body mass index (BMI = Kg/m2) calculated. The triceps skinfold (TS) thickness was measured over the left arm with a Holtain caliper to 0.2 mm readings. The caliper provided a pressure of 10 gms/sq.mm over its entire operating range.Measurements were taken twice and averaged for analysis.

Blood pressure (BP) was measured with a standard mercury gravity sphygmomanometer, using a cuff that covered at least 2/3 of the left arm surface. Systolic pressure (SBP) was recorded for Korotkoff's first phase and diastolic pressure (DBP) for Korotkoff's fourth phase. Measurements were taken in a sitting position and repeated three times, taking the lowest value as final. The readings were taken to the nearest five millimetres of mercury. Heart rate (HR) corresponding to the lowest BP was also recorded (for more details see our communication "Blood pressure in children. Does body position affect measurement?", in this book).

At the medical examination each student was asked about smoking. The following questions were asked : Have you ever smoked?, Do you smoke now?, If so, how many cigarettes do you smoke a day?. Each student was given a seven day diary, previously explained, in which he had to record everything he ate and drank during the week.

After the diary was completed, venous blood samples were taken, after a 12 hours fast, for evaluation of serum total cholesterol (TC), high-density lipoproteins cholesterol (HDL-C), triglycerides (TG), glucose (G), and uric acid (U) concentrations. The blood was allowed to clot for three hours, and thereafter the serum was separated by centrifugation and sent for biochemical analysis in the Atherosclerosis Laboratory of I Clinica Medica of Bologna University.

TC, HDL-C and TG were carried out in duplicate by methods advised by the Italian Lipid Clinic Group (8,9,10). Serum TC concentrations were measured using a fully enzymatic Boehringer CHOD-PAP kit serum; HDL-C concentrations were measured from the serum supernatant after precipitation of VLDL- and LDL-lipoproteins with dextran sulphate. Serum TG concentrations were determined using Boehringer's fully enzymatic CPD-PAP system. Lipid quality control was checked with the WHO laboratory in Prague.

The data were processed using specific programmes developed for this study on an IBM computer linked to the Central University Computer (CINECA).

Statistical methods included Student's t test and correlation analysis.

RESULTS

The total number of invited students was 481 and 447 (92.9%) entered the study. 33 of them were excluded as they were $\geq$ 13 years or $\leq$ 11 years old or had not had

207

blood tests. Thus the results refer to 414 students, 207 males, mean age = 11.80 years (SD=0.3), and 207 females, mean age = 11.74 years (SD=0.3).

To date, nutritional data have not yet been processed and thus cannot be discussed in this paper.

Morbidity from cardiovascular disease among the parents and grandparents.

Family history of 122 students (29.5%) was positive for myocardial infarction (MI) or cerebrovascular disease. MI had occurred in the fathers of 6 students and in both the father and a grandparent of another three. MI alone had occurred in one or more grandparents of 55 students. Cerebrovascular disease alone had occurred in one or more grandparents of 39 students. Finally, both MI and cerebrovascular disease had occurred in a grandparent of 19 students.

Hypertension was referred by 5.3% of the fathers and 4.2% of the mothers; 15.8% of the students had one or more grandparents affected with hypertension.

Cigarette smoking

9 students, 7 males (3.5%) and 2 female (1%), admitted to having smoked. None of them was a regular smoker. Among the parents, 199 fathers (50.6%) and 157 mothers (38.3%) were regular smokers. In the homes of 247 students (60.2%) there was at least one regular smoker. This was true for all 9 students who had smoked.

Physical activity

Sedentary pattern of physical activity was chosen by 11 (5.4%) males and 22 (10.7%) females; moderately active pattern by 86 (41.9%) males and 85 (41.4%) females; active pattern by 51 (24.9%) males and 87 (42.5%) females; very active pattern by 57 (27.8%) males and 11 (5.4%) females.

Height, weight, body mass index, skinfold

Mean and standard deviation of height, weight, BMI and triceps skinfold thickness, by sex, are summarized in table 1.

Table 1.　　　　Heigt, weight, body　mass index　and
triceps skinfold in secondary school
students aged about 12.

	Sex	N	Mean	SD	Min	Max
H	M	199	149.2	7.9	131.0	174.0
(cm)	F	204	149.3	7.3	128.0	170.0
W	M	199	44.4	10.3	25.0	73.0
(Kg)	F	204	44.0	9.3	28.0	69.0
BMI	M	199	19.8	3.3	14.0	30.2
(Kg/sq.m)	F	204	19.5	3.3	10.9	31.9
TS	M	200	14.8	6.7	4.3	34.5
(mm)	F	206	15.6	5.7	5.6	31.0

55　　of　　206　females　(26.7%)　had　　menarche.
Menstruations were regular in 69% of them.

Blood pressure

Mean　systolic　pressure　and　standard　deviation　(in
brackets) was 120.8 (14.3) mmHg in males and 122.3 (15.9)
mmhg in females.　Mean diastolic pressure was 75.1　(9.5)
mmHg　in males and 74.6 (9.9) mmHg in females.　Suggested
upper limits of normal BP in children aged 10-14 are　124
mmHg　for SBP and 84 mmHg for DBP (11).　　40.8% males and
44.4 % females had SBP equal to or greater than 125　mmHg
and　19.4%　males and 18.6% females had DBP equal　to　or
greater　than　85 mmHg.　After excluding subjects with　a
heart　rate　equal to or greater than 85/min to　cut　off
those　subjects whose high blood pressure could have been
caused by anxiety,　these figures were respectively 35.2%
and 33% for SBP and 15.2% and 13.9% for DBP.

Serum lipids

Mean　and standard deviation of serum total　cholesterol,
high-density lipoproteins cholesterol and　triglycerides,
by sex, are summarized in table 2.
Serum TC concentrations ranging from 180 to 199 mg/dl
were found in 26.1% males and 26.6% females. Values equal
to　or　greater than 200 mg/dl of serum TC were found　in
17.4%　males　and 18.8 %　females.　HDL-C　concentrations
lower　than 40 mg/dl were found in　1.5% males and　4.4%

females; TG concentrations equal to or greater than 150 mg/dl were found in 2.9% males and 3.8% females (12).

Table 2. Total cholesterol, high-density lipoproteins cholesterol and triglycerides concentrations in secondary school students aged about 12.

	Sex	N	Mean	SD	Min	Max
TC	M	207	175.2	26.8	101.0	276.0
(mg/dl)	F	207	178.1	27.1	127.0	257.0
HDL-C	M	206	55.2	8.0	30.2	85.0
(mg/dl)	F	206	53.8	8.2	29.0	75.5
TG	M	207	65.2	24.2	30.0	170.0
(mg/dl)	F	207	69.5	26.7	26.0	220.0

CORRELATIONS

In order to study interrelationships between physical measurements of the human body and between physical variables and serum lipids, correlation coefficients were calculated and are listed in table 3.

Height, weight and BMI were highly correlated with each other, both in males and in females. Triceps skinfold thickness was more correlated with weight and BMI ($P < 0.001$) than with height ($P < 0.05$). Blood pressure values significantly correlated with anthropometric measurements. Serum lipids were significantly correlated with each other. Serum triglycerides showed a direct correlation with blood pressure and with physical parameters: Total cholesterol was positively correlated with triceps skinfold thickness in males but not in females: In males, a low correlation was also present between total cholesterol and systolic blood pressure. HDL-cholesterol correlated negatively with weight alone.

All variables in the 122 students with a family history positive for myocardial infarction and/or cerebrovascular disease were compared with those of the other 292 with a negative family history. No significant difference was found in either mean values or correlation coefficients.

Table 3. Correlation coefficients between studied
variables

	Sex	W	BMI	TS	SBP	DBP	TC	HDL-C	TG
W	M	-	.89	.65	.58	.41	-.06	-.18	.27
	F	-	.85	.69	.50	.42	-.14	-.18	.13
BMI	M	.89	-	.81	.56	.39	.07	-.13	.38
	F	.85	-	.77	.46	.38	-.03	-.15	.20
TS	M	.65	.81	-	.45	.33	.21	-.07	.37
	F	.69	.77	-	.36	.27	.04	-.09	.16
SBP	M	.58	.56	.45	-	.65	.14	-.04	.32
	F	.50	.46	.36	-	.68	-.08	-.11	.14
DBP	M	.41	.39	.33	.65	-	.10	-.06	.26
	F	.42	.38	.27	.68	-	-.13	-.12	.18
TC	M	-.06	.07	.21	.14	.10	-	.24	.24
	F	-.14	-.03	.04	-.08	-.13	-	.30	.23
HDL-C	M	-.18	-.13	-.07	-.04	-.06	.24	-	-.22
	F	-.18	-.15	-.09	-.11	-.12	.30	-	-.18
TG	M	.27	.38	.37	.32	.26	.24	-.22	-
	F	.13	.20	.16	.14	.18	.23	-.18	-

if r>0.23 P<0.001;   if r>0.18 P<0.01;   if r>0.14 P<0.05

CONCLUSIONS

The first stage of our study on atherosclerosis precursors in childhood has shown quite a high prevalence of risk factors in an Italian 12 year old population, particularly high serum total cholesterol concentrations. Although at this age serum cholesterol concentration of each subject may be influenced by his/her degree of sexual maturation, intraindividual correlation of serum cholesterol concentrations over time has been demonstrated in children aged 12 (13,14). This age is also a critical period for adopting lifestyle habits which will be maintained throughout adulthood. Hence, this year's educational programme aims to develop childrens' awareness of primary health care and preventive medicine. Emphasis will be placed on regular physical activity, maintenance of ideal body weight, discouraging smoking, and teaching the basic elements of a healthy diet (15).

ACKNOWLEDGEMENTS

We are grateful to Prof.G.C.Descovich for his helpful advice and suggestions and for analyzing the blood samples.
This study is supported by the Emilia Romagna Region, Programma di ricerca sanitaria finalizzata per il triennio 1985-87.

References

1. Holman, RL, McGill, HC, Strong, JP and Geer, JC (1958).The natural hystory of atherosclerosis: the early aortic lesions as seen in New Orleans in the middle of the 20th century. Am J Pathol, 34, 209

2. Strong, JP and McGill, HC (1969). The pediatric aspects of atherosclerosis. J Atheroscler Res, 9, 251

3. McNamara, JJ, Molot, MA, Stremple, JF and Cutting, RT (1971). Coronary artery disease in combat casualties in Vietnam. JAMA, 216, 1185

4. Frerichs, RR, Srivivasen, SR, Webber, LS and Berenson, GS (1976). Serum cholesterol and trigliceride levels in 3446 children from a biracial community: The Bogalusa heart study. Circulation, 54, 302

5. Morrison, JA, deGroot, I, Edwards, BK, Kelly, RA, Rauh, JL, Mellies, M and Glueck, CJ (1977). Plasma cholesterol and triglyceride levels in 6775 school children, aged 6-17. Metabolism, 26, 1199

6. Viikari, J, Akerblom, HK and Uhari, M (1985). Atherosclerosis precursors in children. Acta Paediatr Scand, Suppl 318

7. Pagnan, A, Ambrosio, GB, Vincenzi, M, Mormino, P, Maiolimo, P, Gerin, L, Barbieri, E, Cappelletti, F and Dal Palù, C (1982). Precursors of atherosclerosis in children. The Cittadella study. Follow-up and traking of total serum cholesterol, triglycerides and blood glucose. Prev Med, 11, 381

8. Manual of laboratory operations (1974). Lipid Research Clinic Program. Lipid and Lipoprotein Analysis. p.628. DHEW pubblication No. (NIH) 75. (Washington, D.C.: US Department of Health, Education and Welfare)

9.   Block, WD (1966). An improved automated determination of serum total cholesterol with a single reagent. Clin Chem, 12, 681

10. Kessler, G and Lederer, H (1966). Fluorimetric measurements of triglycerides. In: Automation in Analytical Chemistry. p.341.(New York Medical)

11. The Joint National Committee on Detection, Evaluation, and Treatment of High Blood Pressure (1984). The 1984 Report of the Joint National Committee on Detection, Evaluation, and Treatment of High Blood Pressure. Arch Intern Med, 144

12. Berenson, GS and Epstein, FH (1983). Conference on blood lipids in children: optimal levels for early prevention of coronary artery disease. Workshop Report: Epidemiological section. April 18 and 19, 1983. American Health Foundation. Prev Med, 12, 741

13. Orchard, TJ, Donahue, RP, Kuller, LH, Hodge, PN and Drash, AL (1983). Cholesterol screening in childhood: Does it predict adult hypercholesterolemia? The Beaver County experience. J Pediatr, 103, 687

14. Clarke, WR, Schrott, HG, Leaverton, PE, Connor, WE and Lauer, RM (1978). Traking of blood lipids and blood pressures in school age children: The Muscatine study. Circulation, 58, 626

15. Lamm, G (1985). Risk factors and their prevention in infancy and childhood. In: Nutrition and atherosclerosis risk factors. pag.54. 3rd Congresso Nazionale della Società Italiana di Pediatria Preventiva e Sociale - Nipiologia. Bologna, May 6-8, 1985. (Torino: Minerva Medica).

27
From observational to intervention programmes.
The Brisighella study

G.C. Descovich, A. Dormi, A. Gaddi, G.L. Magri,
G. Mannino, S. Rimondi, Z. Sangiorgi and S. Lenzi

INTRODUCTION

The past target of epidemiology concerned the study of
chronic degenerative/proliferative diseases, with the aim
of detecting and evaluating some suspected etiological
and/or risk factors (RF).
The second step was to confirm the influence of these RF,
follow the RF level modification during a long-term
period of observation, formulate suggestions concerning
their spontaneous trend (related to the environment
influence), and (the interpretative epidemiology) assess
the association or correlation among RF and diseases,
predicting fatal and/or non fatal new events, to best
identify main real RF.
This approach will make it possible to reach the third
step: a statement for intervention programmes against
"sure" RF in terms of prevention of ATS and CHD.
From both the theoretical and experimental points of
view, several nutritional parameters may be "related" (as
"etiological" and/or "risk" factors) to plasma total
cholesterol levels, to atherosclerosis itself and to
ATS-dependent vascular damage.
Unfortunately, a lot of dietary consituents are
responsible for several aspects, and on the other hand,
all the diet constituents are usually pooled in the food
consumed from day to day.
However, it may be useful to discriminate only a few
"major" dangerous factors (i.e. cholesterol and
saturated fats in the diet), thus decreasing the
difficulties in data analysis and increasing the power of
preventive indications. Alternatively, an integrated
approach may be advanced in which several major diet
constituents are focused and none, a priori, regarded as
"the major one".
The USA, Italy and Europe Consensus Conferences [1-3]
indicate the first solution (target: diet cholesterol and
saturated fat reduction) as better.

Taking into account: a) the relevance and priority of nutritional habit modification (NHM) in preventive intervention planning, and b) the concurrent urgency in defining the NHM type, it is doubtless that if a preventive intervention is to be applied to the whole national population, only an easy, few target-intervention can be adopted.

On the contrary, in smaller population samples, an integrated approach may be more useful and, perhaps, more effective.

This paper briefly reports part of the results obtained from the Brisighella Epidemiological Study, concerning nutritional habit changes during the observational phase and the relationships between these changes and new even incidence of disease. The purpose of this study is to identify the nutritional parameters which it is necessary to modify in order to perform a Community Medicine Multi Intervention Study (CMMIS), against several RF common for different diseases.

MATERIALS AND METHODS

The Brisighella Study started in 1972, on the rural population of this little village near Ravenna, in the Emilia Romagna Region. For this purpose 2939 subjects aged from 14 to 84 were enlisted (1491 males and 1448 females). Personal history, clinical, behavioural and laboratory parameters were recorded for each subjects according to the protocol described elsewhere [4]. All the methods (clinical, instrumental, biochemical, nutritional and behavioural records, etc) adopted were the same advised by CNR, US-NHI and Italian Lipid Clinics. Every 4 years, a control of the whole population was performed, without any intervention or influence on the population untill 1984. Nutritional habits were studied at each control by means of both questionnaire and dietary daily record (seven day questionnaire). Nutrition components analysis was performed by Virgo and Mizar biomedical statistical programmes [5].

To detect possible relationships between diet spontaneous changes and disease and/or death incidence several mathematical models were adopted, particularly multifactorial models following the method suggested by Walker and Duncan [6].

Up to 1984, more than 1000 disease new cases were recorded [7], 214 persons died (all causes) and among them 104 from coronary heart disease.

With the collaboration of the Health Dept. and

Agricultural Dept. of the Emilia Romagna Region, in 1985-1986 a Community Medicine Multi Intervention Study was planned, and it is now starting on the ˙Brisighella population.
The preventive protocol to be applied is based both on mass media (local radio and/or TV Companies; newspaper), population-oriented messages (public meetings, posters, booklets), and on individual messages (by hospital physicians and general practitioners and by specialized personnel, such as school teachers, dietitians, nurses and other experts).

RESULTS

Tables I (males) and II (females) illustrate the nutritional habit "spontaneous" changes during the 12 years of follow-up. In the Tables, only the foods (in g/day) are reported: variations of food constituents described elsewere [4,7], are consistent for a marked decrease, in both sexes, of P/S ratio (from 0.31 in 1972 to 0.19 in 1984) and for an increase in absolute animal saturated fat amount and a reduction of fish intake. Some potentially favourable variations were also recorded, such as the increase in vegetable proteins and the decrease in total cholesterol intake.

TABLE I: BRISIGHELLA STUDY LONGITUDINAL SURVEY (1972-1984)
DAILY FOOD INTAKE (g/day) IN MALES

	1972	1984	DIFFERENCE (%)
MILK - DAIRY PRODUCTS	220.9	184.6	- 16.4
EGGS	34.9	24.3	- 30.3
SALAMI - HAM	52.1	40.7	- 21.9
BUTTER - LARD	14.7	20.7	+ 20.4
OLIVE OIL	19.7	22.1	+ 12.2
OTHER VEGETABLE OILS	10.8	7.5	- 30.5
FISH	34.0	29.9	- 12.1
MEATS	179.8	152.4	- 15.2
VEGETABLES	123.2	156.2	+ 26.8
FRUITS	225.6	183.7	- 18.5
BREAD - PASTA	496.0	417.9	- 15.9
SUGARS	83.2	62.9	- 24.4
WINE - BEER	728.0	537.0	- 26.2

Unfortunately, the absolute value of these variations
is very low if compared to the baseline (1972) values.
From these data, it may be stated that a slight and
progressive deterioration of nutritional patterns of
the whole Brisighella population occurred from 1972 to
1984.
Variations of some biochemical parameters during the
twelve year follow-up are reported in Table III.
As shown in Table III, total plasma cholesterol, the
major RF for atherosclerosis, progressively increased
from 1972 to 1984 both in males and females.
Triglycerides and BMI also rise during the follow-up.
On the contrary, diastolic and systolic blood pressure
showed only minimal changes. The absence of an expected
increase (age related) in blood pressure can be
explained by good hypertensive pharmacological control
carried out by Brisighella general practitioners.
In fact, at the 1980 control, about 5% of Brisighella
population was receiving proper chronic hypotensive
treatment (by diuretics and beta-blockers) and another
5% was on other hypotensive drugs (particularly
reserpine).

TABLE II: BRISIGHELLA STUDY LONGITUDINAL SURVEY
(1972-1984)
DAILY FOOD INTAKE (g/day) IN FEMALES

	1972	1984	DIFFERENCE (%)
MILK - DAIRY PRODUCTS	220.9	188.0	- 14.9
EGGS	24.6	18.9	- 23.1
SALAMI - HAM	40.5	30.2	- 25.4
BUTTER - LARD	13.4	16.8	+ 25.4
OLIVE OIL	17.3	21.8	+ 26.0
OTHER VEGETABLE OILS	11.8	8.7	- 26.2
FISH	27.9	26.7	- 4.3
MEATS	136.0	115.9	- 14.8
VEGETABLES	125.8	155.1	+ 10.3
FRUITS	233.3	199.5	- 14.5
BREAD - PASTA	328.1	288.7	- 12.0
SUGAR	78.7	58.7	- 25.4
WINE - BEER	268.3	207.6	- 22.6

On the contrary, at the same control, only very few
patients (< 1%) were (discontinuously !) treated by
major hypolipidemic drugs (such as cholestyramine or

fibrates).

A first step of nutritional and metabolic RF analysis
was carried out by Multiple Logistic Function (MLF),
analysing firstly the relative influence of 23
variables (Table IV).
The solution of the Multiple Logistic Function obtained
in the Brisighella male citizens who underwent to a
fatal acute myocardial infarction demonstrates a high
predictive power of the classic "main" risk factors.
In fact, age, physical activity (protective), smoking
habits, SBP and total plasma cholesterol have very high
coefficients.
On the other hand, animal protein, lipid and
carbohydrate intakes contribute to the prediction of
the AMI fatal new events.
A protective, but not statistically significant effect
might be attributed to the P/S ratio; on the contrary,
cholesterol intake appears to be slightly predictive
for AMI.
Surprisingly, a very high predictive power was found
for some anthropometric parameters, namely for
skinfolds sum and width/height index (WHI).

TABLE III: BRISIGHELLA STUDY LONGITUDINAL SURVEY
(1972-1984)
SPONTANEOUS TREND OF MAJOR ATS RISK FACTORS

		MALES		FEMALES	
		1972	1984	1972	1984
S.B.P.	(mmHg)	143.4	144.0	143.1	142.3
D.B.P.	(mmHg)	87.8	88.6	87.2	84.6
TC	(mg/dl)	222.6	247.2	226.2	259.6
TG	(mg/dl)	152.9	174.1	129.1	155.8
FBS	(mg/dl)	84.9	90.1	83.3	87.6
SUA	(mg/dl)	5.4	5.3	4.7	3.4
BMI	- -	24.7	26.2	25.1	25.8

Obviously not all the variables listed in the MLF
solution can be modified, but it is possible to draw a
very impressive suggestions for the intervention
programmes planned for the Brisighella population,
according to Finalized Research Programmes of the
Emilia Romagna Region.

TABLE IV: BRISIGHELLA STUDY LONGITUDINAL SURVEY (1972-1984)
MYOCARDIAL INFARCTION: 23 PARAMETERS MLF SOLUTION

Parameter	Coefficient	SE	t	p
Constant	- 29.9376	4.1086	-	-
Age (yr)	0.0225	0.0096	2.343	< 0.02
Physical Act. (code)	- 0.1657	0.0398	4.163	< 0.001
Smoking (cig/day)	0.2204	0.0477	4.620	< 0.001
Height (cm)	0.1038	0.0219	4.739	< 0.001
Weight (Kg)	- 0.0454	0.0140	3.892	< 0.001
Biacromial Diam. (cm)	- 0.2472	0.0339	7.292	< 0.001
Bicrestal Diam. (cm)	- 0.1789	0.0516	3.467	< 0.001
Wrist circumf. (cm)	0.1266	0.0648	1.953	n.s.
Arm circumf. (cm)	0.0273	0.0411	0.664	n.s.
Skinfoold sum (mm)	0.0229	0.0064	3.578	< 0.001
SBP (mmHg)	0.0209	0.0034	6.147	< 0.001
TC (mg/dl)	0.0096	0.0017	5.647	< 0.001
FBS (mg/dl)	0.0066	0.0046	1.434	n.s.
SUA (mg/dl)	0.0114	0.0049	2.326	< 0.02
Food Calories (Cal/day)	- 0.1221	0.0277	4.573	< 0.001
Alcohol (g/day)	- 0.0010	0.0003	3.333	< 0.01
Animal protein (g/day)	0.5112	0.1097	4.659	< 0.001
Lipids (g/day)	1.1043	0.2427	4.550	< 0.001
P/S ratio	- 0.0046	0.0084	0.534	n.s.
Food cholest. (mg/day)	0.0005	0.0005	1.000	n.s.
Carbohydrates (g/day)	0.4995	0.1093	4.569	< 0.001
Fibers (g/day)	0.0115	0.0042	2.738	< 0.01
WHI (*)	0.3989	0.0730	5.464	< 0.001

(*) (Biacromial diameter + bicrestal diameter)/height.

Our aims are the following: decrease the cholesterol level in the whole population by means of a reduction in meat, dairy products and saturated fats intake; reduce salt and alcohol intakes with to reduce BP without pharmacological treatment; promote physical activity and all hygienic measures to increase the efficacy of all targets.

This means a new cultural trend for a permanent and safe life-style, avoiding the dangerous risk of a psychological negative involvement.

Another type of strategy should be devoted to the high risk individuals for which together with the Brisighella medical hosptal staff and the general Practitioners, a lot of special protocols will be planned.

Special attention will be paid to the smoking habits
and an education programme for school children is under
study to stop children starting smoking rather than
stopping heavy smokers.

This Study, included in the WHO ERICA Project was
partially supported by a grant of Health Dept. of
Emilia Romagna Region and by the Bologna University.

REFERENCES

1) Consensus Conference (1985). Lowering blood cholesterol to prevent heart disease. JAMA,
   253, 280.
2) Consensus Conference (1986). Abbassare la colesterolemia per ridurre la cardiopatia
   ischemica. CNR, Roma, May 1986.
3) European Atherosclerosis Group (1986). A strategy for the prevention of coronary heart
   disease, a policy statement of the European Atherosclerosis Group. Naples, 19th 20th June.
4) Descovich GC, Lenzi S (1982): "The Brisighella Study", MTP Press, Lancaster- Boston- The
   Hague- Dordrecth, 367.
5) Mannino G, Guidi S (1978): "Mizar: un programma interattivo guidato di statistica
   sanitaria", Informatica- Ed. Dedalo, Roma.
6) Walker S, Duncan DB (1967): "Estimation of the possibility of an event as a function of
   several indipendent variables", Biometrika, 54, 167.
7) Dormi A, Perini P, Magri GL, Mannino G, Descovich GC, Lenzi S (1984). La funzione
   logistica multipla. Applicazioni in una popolazione in studio. In: Lenzi S, Descovich GC
   (eds) "Atherosclerosis and Cardiovascular Diseases", Editrice Compositori, Bologna, 317.

APPENDIX

All Researchers listed in the appendix must be considered "Authors" of the present paper. Authors of previous papers will also be considered Author of the present one and are listed elsewhere [4].

BRISIGHELLA STUDY MEMBERS
Present Composition

Chairman: Prof. S. Lenzi.

Principal Investigator: Prof. G.C. Descovich.
Coordinators of Medical Staff: Gaddi A, Rimondi S.
Coordinator of Biological Staff: Sangiorgi Z.

Bologna Medical Researchers: Barozzi G, Ceredi C, D' Addato S, Dalmonte G, Finazzo L, Greci M, Gualandi A, Knottner M, Magri F, Magri GL, Manganaro G, Matteucci A, Mezzetti M, Minardi A, Vigna M.
Bologna Biochemical Laboratory Staff: Copparoni G, Forni M, La Regina G.
Bologna Dietitian Staff: Rocca P, Faggioli E, Borlotti ML, Vici D.
Bologna Biometrics Laboratory Staff: Dormi A, Braiato A.
Mathematic consultant: Prof. G. Mannino, Numerical Analysis FP, Mathematics Institute, Modena University.

Brisighella Hospital Staff: Santarella M, Sarti A, Zambon A, Pagano G, Ramponi R, Quercia O, Zucchini R, Montanari FM, Casadei-Giunchi D, Folco-Zambelli E.
Brisighella Medical Staff: Savorani L, Trere' G, Gamberi I, Drei I, Valpondi FM.
Brisighella Coordination Staff: Bandini R, Alboreti B, Silvestrini F.
Brisighella Anagraphic Staff: Sbarzaglia L.

We gratefully acknowledge all the Brisighella Mayors and Administrators who from 1972 continuosly supported this Study: Pelliconi E (Mayor, 1972-1979), Piancastelli A (Mayor, 1979-1981), Galassini V (Mayor, 1981-1983 and 1987-), Bartoli G (Mayor, 1983-1987), and Laghi A, Savorani R, Morini T, Montevecchi A, Liverani F, Patuelli G, Marchetti A, Bandini A, Cardini E, Rondinini C, Tassi D, Baldi V, Gagliani D, Cavina L, Tredozzi P, Punti PD, Sangiorgi C, Neri R, Samore' T.

LIPID REGULATION IN THE PREVENTION OF CORONARY HEART DISEASE

28
Relationship of glucose intolerance and elevated triglyceride: implications for gemfibrozil

G. Steiner

BACKGROUND: HYPERINSULINEMIA AND HYPERTRIGLYCERIDEMIA

Recent studies have suggested that the smaller triglyceride-rich lipoproteins may be atherogenic [1-3]. This, plus the observations that 70% of the population of triglyceride-rich lipoprotein particles in the plasma are those in the smaller (i.e. Sf 12-60, 250-350A) subpopulation [4], makes it particularly relevant to understand the factors regulating the metabolism of this family of lipoproteins. Our studies have focused on the role of insulin in the regulation of the metabolism of the triglyceride-rich lipoproteins. This is because of the close association of both insulin deficiency [5] and of hyperinsulinemia with hypertriglyceridemia [6-8].

This review will concentrate on hyperinsulinemia because, not only is it seen in hypertriglyceridemics without diabetes [6-8], but also it is seen very often in diabetics [9] and may be responsible for some of the abnormalities seen in their triglyceride-rich lipoprotein metabolism. In those with insulin-treated diabetes the hyperinsulinemia may be partly because of an inability to supply just the appropriate amount of insulin at all times of day. More importantly, in those receiving insulin subcutaneously the peripheral insulin concentration is supraphysiologic even though the hepatic portal venous insulin concentration may be physiologic. This contrasts with the normal situation in which the heparin/portal insulin concentration may be 3 to 4 times greater than that in the periphery. This reflects the fact that insulin, when released from the pancreas, first passes through the liver and that organ extracts a significant proportion of the insulin before it reaches the periphery. Obviously this same situation does not apply when insulin is administered peripherally. In those with type II diabetes who are treated without exogenous insulin, a number of factors may contribute to hyperinsulinemia. These include insulin resistance due to the frequently associated obesity and even insulin-resistance in the absence of obesity [10]. These considerations become all the more interesting in view of the epidemiologic [11-13] and pathophysiologic [14] studies that show a link between hyperinsulinemia and early atherosclerosis.

HYPERINSULINEMIA AND TRIGLYCERIDE TURNOVER

VLDL triglyceride production rates have been observed to be positively correlated with serum insulin levels in humans. These studies were conducted in people who had chronic changes in their levels of endogenous insulin in association with obesity and a variety of nutritional states [15] or in association with steroid treatment [16]. Obviously, although triglyceride production rates and insulin levels were positively related to each other, in these two models there could have been many factors other than insulin to explain this.

To examine further the relationship between chronic hyperinsulinemia and the metabolism of the triglyceride-rich lipoproteins, it was necessary to turn to models in which factors such as obesity would not play a role. This was done by studying rats made hyperinsulinemic by giving them 6 units of insulin per day over two weeks. To avoid hypoglycemia, the rats were also given a 10% sugar solution in place of their drinking water. These hyperinsulinemic rats were compared to controls that did not receive exogenous insulin, but were still given the same amount of sugar solution (sugar-supplemented controls) and to normal rats receiving chow ad lib and water to drink (chow controls). Somewhat surprisingly, neither the hyperinsulinemic rats nor the sugar-supplemented controls became any more obese than the chow fed controls [17]. Hyperinsulinemia was found to be associated with an increase in triglyceride production, even over that seen in the control rats receiving the sugar supplement alone [18]. However, this effect of insulin was only seen when the sugar solution contained fructose (i.e. fructose itself or sucrose) but not when it contained only glucose [19]. Although the reason for this is not yet clear, it may relate to the observations that most of an orally administered fructose load is taken up by the liver, whereas most of a similar glucose load is taken up by extrahepatic tissues.

In spite of the insulin-induced increase in triglyceride production, the rats' plasma triglyceride concentrations did not always increase. In those rats receiving their exogenous insulin subcutaneously the plasma triglyceride concentration actually fell, suggesting that insulin had increased triglyceride removal even more than it increased triglyceride production. This was probably attributable to the increased activity of lipoprotein lipase observed in their adipose tissue [18-20].

No such increase in lipoprotein lipase or decrease in triglyceride concentration was seen when the insulin entered the body via the hepatic portal vein. In rats receiving insulin by that route there still was a similar increase in triglyceride production. The differences in the effects of insulin on the balance between production and removal were paralleled by differences in the relative concentrations of insulin in the hepatic portal vs peripheral circulation [20]. Such observations may clearly have relevance to the route by which insulin reaches the body. This, together with its timing and the dose of insulin may then influence the triglyceride concentration seen in association with hyperinsulinemia.

TRIGLYCERIDE TURNOVER, IDL AND ATHEROSCLEROSIS

If the turnover of triglyceride-rich lipoproteins is accelerated, it is reasonable to expect that there would be an increase in the generation of their catabolic remnants. We and others [20,21] have shown that the Sf 12-60 lipoproteins conform to the kinetic characteristics of VLDL-remnants and, as a consequence, have used this ultracentrifugal range to define the intermediate density lipoproteins (IDL). In recent studies [1] we have extended the work of others [2,23] demonstrating an association between elevated levels of IDL and early coronary artery disease.

HYPERTRIGLYCERIDEMIA AND INSULIN RESISTANCE

As noted above, hyperinsulinemia is often seen in hypertriglyceridemic individuals. In order to explore the basis for this we undertook to determine whether hypertriglyceridemics might be resistant to insulin. To avoid the confounding influence of obesity which is frequently associated with hypertriglyceridemia, we selected only lean individuals for this study. Glucose turnover was measured at a variety of insulin concentrations in lean hypertriglyceridemic and in normolipidemic individuals. Those with hypertriglyceridemia were found to be resistant to insulin [24].

The basis for this insulin resistance has not yet been fully defined. However, Bieger et al showed that monocytes and erythrocytes of hypertriglyceridemic individuals bound less insulin than did those of normolipidemic individuals [25]. This was consistent with our earlier findings that VLDL could down-regulate insulin receptors on IM-9 lymphocytes and on adipocytes in vitro [7]. Recently Cordera et al found a similar decrease in insulin binding by the erythrocytes of hypertriglyceridemics [26]. However, this was not restored to normal when the hypertriglyceridemia was treated. These findings suggested that the insulin resistance was either not secondary to the hypertriglyceridemia, or it was due to a post-binding rather than a binding problem.

To examine whether insulin resistance is secondary to the hypertriglyceridemia, we have conducted some preliminary studies in hypertriglyceridemics. They were treated with Gemfibrozil alternating with placebo. Oral glucose tolerance tests were conducted in the same individuals on each treatment regimen. Insulin resistance, as judged by insulin/glucose ratios, increased or decreased in parallel with the alterations in plasma triglyceride levels. This was independent of any weight changes, dietary changes or non-lipid related drug effects. Hence, it appears hypertriglyceridemia and insulin resistance may be associated in a cause and effect manner. The mechanism responsible for this remains to be clarified.

IMPLICATIONS

Clearly any measures which can break the cycle of hypertriglyceridemia, hyperinsulinemia, increased VLDL turnover and increased IDL generation might reduce the risk of atherosclerosis. In addition to these considerations, hyperinsulinemia itself appears to increase the risk of atherosclerosis. As reducing plasma triglyceride levels will reduce insulin resistance and thereby reduce plasma insulin levels, one might anticipate that this too might diminish the risk of atherosclerosis.

REFERENCES

1. Steiner, G, Schwartz, L, Shumak, S and Poapst, M (1987). The association of increased levels of intermediate density lipoproteins with smoking and with coronary artery disease. Circulation, 75, (in press)
2. Reardon, MF, Nestel, PJ, Craig IH and Harper, RW (1985). Lipoprotein predictors of the severity of coronary artery disease in men and women. Circulation, 71, 881
3. Zilversmit, DB (1979). Atherogenesis, a post-prandial phenomenon. Circulation, 60, 473
4. Poapst, M, Reardon, M and Steiner, G (1985). The relative contribution of triglyceride-rich lipoprotein particle size and number to plasma triglyceride concentration. Arteriosclerosis, 5, 381
5. Steiner, G, Poapst, ME and Davidson, JK (1975). Production of chylomicron-like lipoproteins from endogenous lipid by intestine and liver of diabetic dogs. Diabetes, 24, 263
6. Steiner, G (1986). Hypertriglyceridemia and carbohydrate intolerance: Interrelationship and therapeutic implications. Am J Cardiol, 57, 27G
7. Steiner, G and Vranic, M (1982). Insulin and hypertriglyceridemia: A vicious cycle with atherogenic potential. Int J Obesity, 6(suppl 1), 117
8. Olefsky, JM, Farquhar and JW, Reaven, GM (1974). Reappraisal of the role of insulin in hypertriglyceridemia. Am J Med, 57, 551
9. Nikkila, EA (1981). High density lipoproteins in diabetes. Diabetes, 30(suppl 2), 82
10. Reaven, GM and Olefsky JM (1978). Role of insulin resistance in the pathogenesis of hyperglycemia. In: Katz, HM and Mahler, RJ (eds.) "Diabetes, Obesity and Vascular Disease". p.229. (New York: John Wiley and Sons)
11. Pyorala, K (1979). Relationship of glucose tolerance and plasma insulin levels to the incidence of coronary heart disease: results from two population studies in Finland. Diabetes Care, 2, 131
12. Ducimitiere, P, Eschwege, L, Papoz, PL, Claude RJR and Rosselin, G (1980). Relationship of plasma insulin levels to the incidence of myocardial infarction and coronary heart disease mortality in a middle-aged population. Diabetologia, 19, 205

13. Welborn, TA and Wearne, K (1979). Coronary heart disease incidence and cardiovascular mortality in Busselton with reference to glucose and insulin concentrations. Diabetes Care 2, 131

14. Stout, RW (1979). Diabetes and atherosclerosis - the role of insulin. Diabetologia, 16, 141

15. Streja, DA, Marliss, EB and Steiner, G (1977). The effects of prolonged fasting on plasma triglyceride kinetics in man. Metabolism, 26, 505

16. Cattran, DC, Steiner, G, Wilson, DR and Fenton, SSA (1979). Hyperlipidemia after renal transplantation: natural history and pathophysiology. Ann Int Med, 91, 554

17. Martin, C, Desai, KS and Steiner, G (1983). Receptor and postreceptor insulin resistance induced by in vivo hyperinsulinemia. Can J Physiol Pharmacol, 61, 802

18. Steiner, G, Haynes, F, Yoshino, G and Vranic, M (1984). Hyperinsulinemia and in vivo very-low-density lipoprotein triglyceride kinetics. Am J Physiol, 246, E187

19. Kazumi, T, Vranic, M and Steiner, G (1986). Triglyceride kinetics: Effects of dietary glucose, sucrose or fructose alone or with hyperinsulinemia. Am J Physiol, 246, E197

20. Kazumi, T, Vranic, M and Steiner, G (1986). Portal vs peripheral hyperinsulinemia and very low density lipoprotein kinetics. Metabolism, 35, (in press)

21. Reardon, MF and Steiner, G (1982). The use of kinetics in investigating the metabolism of very low and intermediate density lipoproteins. In: Berman, M, Grundy, SM and Howard, B (eds.) "Lipoprotein Kinetics and Modeling". (New York: Academic Press)

22. Reardon, MF, Fidge, NH and Nestel, PJ (1978). Catabolism of very low density lipoprotein B apoprotein in man. J Clin Invest, 61, 850

23. Jones, HB, Gofman, JW, Lindgr, FT, Lyon, TP, Graham, DM, Strisower, B and Michols AV (1951). Lipoproteins in atherosclerosis. Am J Med, 11, 358.

24. Steiner, G, Morita, S and Vranic, M (1980). Resistance to insulin but not to glucagon in lean human hypertriglyceridemics. Diabetes 29, 899

25. Bieger, WP, Michel, G, Borwich, D, Biehl, K and Wirth, A (1984). Diminished insulin receptors in monocytes and erythrocytes in hypertriglyceridemia. Metabolism, 33, 982

26. Cordera, R, Bertolini, S, Andraghetti, G, Pistocchi, G, de Alessi, M and Gherzi, R (1985). Insulin receptor binding on red cells of hypertriglyceridemic patients. Effect of a low fat, low carbohydrate diet. Diabete Metab, 11, 137

29
A comparison of different formulations and dosage administrations of gemfibrozil in types IIA and IIB hyperlipidemia

P. Kovanen, P. Koskinen and V. Manninen

SUMMARY

To assess the lipid-regulating effects of two new gemfibrozil formulations, a non-blind parallel group comparison was performed using Finnish industrial workers with types IIA and IIB primary hyperlipoproteinaemia. In all, 670 subjects were evaluated. After an initial dietary treatment period of 2 months, 321 subjects had serum total low density lipoprotein (T-LDL) cholesterol [serum total cholesterol minus high density lipoprotein (HDL) cholesterol] levels equal or above 5.2 mM (200 mg/dl) and thus qualified for the active 12-month drug phase of the trial. The patients were randomly allocated to one of three treatment groups. Groups 1 and 2 received a total daily dosage of gemfibrozil equal to 1200 mg, group 1 receiving the standard gemfibrozil dosage of two 300 mg capsules twice daily, and group 2 receiving a 600 mg tablet twice daily. Group 3 received a reduced total daily dose of 900 mg, given as a once-a-day dose of two 450 mg tablets in the evening.

The results show that the new gemfibrozil formulations are equal to the standard gemfibrozil dosage in their effects on blood lipoproteins. Substantial decreases were noted in serum triglycerides, serum cholesterol, LDL cholesterol and serum apolipoprotein B. The three formulations also produced similar increases in HDL cholesterol and its subfractions HDL2 and HDl3, as well as in serum apolipoproteins AI and AII. Furthermore, the types of side-effects, as well as the numbers of side-effects and of treatment failures (due to lack of efficacy and lack of patient compliance) were similar in the three treatment groups.

INTRODUCTION

The extensive clinical investigation of gemfibrozil has been undertaken with gemfibrozil dispensed in capsules. The usual dosage has been 1200 mg daily, given as two 300 mg capsules twice daily (see Ref. 1). Tablet formulations and the effects of an once-daily dosage are now being considered as alternatives. Therefore, a study was designed to compare the effect on serum lipoproteins and apolipoproteins of three formulations of gemfibrozil, the 300 mg capsules and, alternatively, tablets containing either 450 or 600 mg of the drug. In addition, the study was designed to compare once daily and twice daily dosing of gemfibrozil.

STUDY DESIGN AND PATIENT SELECTION

The study was designed as a non-blind, parallel treatment group evaluation of subjects with types IIA and IIB primary hyperlipidaemia. Candidates had to have serum "total low density lipoprotein (T-LDL) cholesterol (=serum total cholesterol minum HDL cholesterol) of 5.2 mM (200 mg/dl) or greater" to qualify. The 12-month active drug treatment phase of the study was preceded by a 2-month screening period, during which time the patients were prescribed an optimal diet for their diagnosed phenotype. If the T-LDL cholesterol remained at the 5.2 mM level or greater after 2 months of diet therapy, patients were entered into the active drug phase of the evaluation and randomized to one of three treatment groups (Table 1). Patients in group 1 received the standard gemfibrozil regimen. i.e. two 300 mg capsules two times a day. Those in group 2 also received a total daily dosage of 1200 mg, but given as one 600 mg tablet two times a day. Those in group 3 received a lower total daily dosage (900 mg) of gemfibrozil: two 450 mg tablets taken once daily in the evening. The patients were instructed to continue diet therapy during the active drug phase of the trial. Clinic visits were made after 1, 3, 6, 9 and 12 months of active drug treatment. In addition to a physical examination and history, a fasting serum sample was taken for a lipid profile at each clinic visit. As a safety precaution, clinical laboratory tests including haemotological tests and biochemical multichannel analyses were performed.

Initially, a total of 670 subjects were evaluated. The group consisted of industrial workers from southern and south-eastern Finland, as well as of subjects selected from the free-living population in the county of North Karelia in eastern Finland. Of the evaluated subjects, 416 qualified for, and were randomly assigned to, the screening phase of the study. After screening, 322 subjects fulfilled the criteria and were admitted to the active drug treatment phase. All of the admitted candidates exhibited either type IIA or IIB primary hyperlipoproteinaemia. Demographic characteristics of these patients were similar (Table 2).

Table 1 Different formulations and dosage administrations of gemfibrozil

Group	Total daily dose	Regimen
1	1200 mg	Two 300 mg capsules two times a day
2	1200 mg	One 600 mg tablet two times a day
3	900 mg	Two 450 mg tablets once daily in the evening

Table 2 Patient characteristics

	Group		
	1	2	3
No.	109	107	106
Mean age (years SD)	49 9	50 10	51 10
Sex (male/female)	75/34	74/32	69/37

RESULTS

Table 3 shows the initial values of serum lipids and apolipoproteins in the three treatment groups as well as the percent changes in these values observed after 1 month of active drug treatment. During the remaining 11 months of active drug treatment, the serum concentrations of all studied parameters remained at the same altered levels. In the three treatment groups, the observed changes were equal, and no significant differences were observed among the groups.

In accordance with previous studies, this study demonstrated that treatment with gemfibrozil effectively lowers the levels of serum triglycerides and serum total cholesterol. The decrease in serum total cholesterol resulted from a pronounced decrease in LDL cholesterol and from a less pronounced increase in HDL cholesterol. The increase in HDL cholesterol, again, resulted from an increase in both subfractions of HDL, HDL2 and HDL3. As expected from the observed decrease in the LDL cholesterol, the level of the protein component of LDL, the apolipoprotein B also decreased. Similarly, the apolipoproteins of the HDL fraction, apo AI and AII, increased in parallel with the observed changes found in HDL cholesterol.

Table 3 Mean serum lipid apolipoprotein concentrations in various treatment groups at entrance to trial and after 1 month of active drug treatment

Parameter	Group 1		Group 2		Group 3	
	Start	Change	Start	Change	Start	Change
Triglycerides	2.38	-42%	2.10	-39%	2.24	-34%
Total cholesterol	7.62	-14%	7.48	-13%	7.69	-13%
LDL cholesterol	5.59	-21%	5.52	-21%	5.70	-19%
Apolipoprotein B	180	-14%	176	-15%	181	-13%
HDH cholesterol	1.25	+14%	1.29	+13%	1.29	+12%
HDL2 cholesterol	0.70	+ 6%	0.70	+11%	0.69	+ 9%
HDL3 cholesterol	0.54	+29%	0.57	+26%	0.57	+24%
Apolipoprotein AI	115	+ 6%	120	+ 4%	115	+ 7%
Apolipoprotein AII	33	+14%	34	+15%	33	+15%

* The units of the values for triglycerides, total cholesterol and cholesterol in the various lipoprotein fractions are mmol/L, and those for the apolipoproteins are mg/100 ml.

Adverse effects

In each group the overall drop-out rate was the same; of those entering about 20% had dropped out at the end of the trial. In each group the major cause for discontinuing the treatment were either lack of efficacy, non-compliance and side-effects. In common with other studies with gemfibrozil, the major side-effects requiring withdrawal from the trial included gastrointestinal disturbances and various skin reactions.

DISCUSSION

The results of this study show that the efficacies of the capsule and tablet formulations are equal. Furthermore, even once-daily dosage appears to have the same effects on blood lipids and apolipoproteins as the conventional twice-daily dosage regimen. Finally, the study demonstrates that reducing the daily dosage by 300 mg, i.e. from 1200 mg to 900 mg, does not diminish the efficacy of the drug.

Low levels of serum LDL cholesterol and high levels of serum HDL cholesterol are associated with a low incidence of coronary heart disease [2,3]. Thus, decreasing of serum LDL cholesterol and, perhaps, increasing of serum HDL cholesterol may reduce the incidence of coronary artery disease [4]. Accordingly, the effects of the three formulations of gemfibrozil on blood lipoprotein metabolism should be considered beneficial in patients with type IIA and type IIB primary hyperlipidaemia.

In moderate hyperlipidaemia, the development of coronary heart disease is slow, thus requiring preventive measures to last for decades. A long lasting treatment, be it dietary, pharmacological or a combination of both, requires good patient compliance. Efficient new dosage regimens, such as once-daily administration of gemfibrozil, may help to achieve better results in the long term drug treatment of lipid disorders and, hence, be of value in the prevention of the development of coronary heart disease.

REFERENCES

1. Kovanen, PT, Koskinen, P and Manninen, V (1986). A comparison of different formulations and dosage administrations of gemfibrozil. *Am J Cardiol*, **57**, 31G
2. Kannel, WB, Castelli, WP and Gordon, T (1971). Serum cholesterol, lipoproteins and the risk of coronary heart disease: the Framingham study. *Ann Intern Med*, **74**, 1
3. Miller, GJ and Miller, NE (1975). Plasma high-density-lipoprotein concentrations and development of ischaemic heart disease. *Lancet*, **1**, 16
4. The Lipid Research Clinic's Program. Lipid clinic's coronary primary prevention trial results. II. The relationship of reduction in incidence of coronary heart disease to cholesterol lowering. *J Am Med Assoc*, **251**, 365

30
Coronary heart disease in Italy
M. Mancini, P. Rubba and G. Riccardi

CORONARY HEART DISEASE MORTALITY IN ITALY

It is known since long time that Coronary Heart Disease
(CHD) morbidities and mortalities show large variations in
different countries of the world (1).
There is a group of countries with exceedingly high CHD
mortality which includes Scotland, Ireland and Finland,
with the region North Karelia ranking first among all the
areas of the world. Other countries with intermediate
mortality are USA, Germany and the Scandinavian ones.
Lower mortality is found in Southern Europe (Italy,
France, Jugoslavia, Greece) and in the far East (Japan).
This picture is thought to reflect the different levels
of risk factors for CHD in each population. However even
in the group of low mortality areas, including Italy, CHD
represents the leading cause of death in the population.
Prospective data which have became available in recent
years confirm, also for Italy, the direct relationship
between incidence of CHD and major risk factors for
atherosclerotic cardiovascular disease such as
hyperlipidemia, cigarette smoking and hypertension (2).
In order to define priorities for the implementation of
preventive actions against CHD in Italy, the results of
two cross-sectional studies, performed in middle aged men
from different populations in Europe will be considered
(3,4).

COOPERATIVE STUDY ON ADIPOSE TISSUE FATTY ACIDS AND CORONARY HEART DISEASE

Males in the age range 40-49 years from four populations in Europe (North Karelia, South West Finland, Scotland, South Italy) were invited to undergo serum lipids and adipose tissue fatty acids analysis. Table I describes adipose tissue composition in the four areas with different incidence of CHD. Mortality (deaths/100.000) in this age range is 212 for North Karelia, 146 for South West Finland, 140 for Scotland and only 43 for South Italy. Adipose tissue analysis (5) suggests that these differences might be related to a relatively higher consumption of mono- and poly-unsaturated fatty acids in South Italy as compared to Northern Europe.

TABLE I

ADIPOSE TISSUE FATTY ACIDS				(Men 40–49 years)
	SAT. (%)	MONO. (%)	POLY. (%)	P/S ___	CHD DEATHS x 100.000
ITALY	26	59	15	0.58	43
SCOTLAND	36*	54*	10*	0.30*	140
SW FINLAND	38*	52*	10*	0.26*	146
N KARELIA	39*	53*	9*	0.23*	212

Significance versus Italy; *)p < 0.01

Table II shows mean serum lipid concentrations in the four areas: total serum cholesterol goes in parallel with the mortality gradient.

TABLE II

S E R U M L I P I D S (Men 40–49 yrs)				
COUNTRY	n	CHOL tot (mg/dl)	HDL	TG (mg/dl)
ITALY	74	208	46	179
SCOTLAND	131	224	51	150
SW FINLAND	83	248*	51	138
N KARELIA	102	257*	54	158

Significance versus Italy: *)p < 0.01

No difference is detected in triglycerides; HDL cholesterol is highest in North Karelia and lowest in Italy. The different blood pressure levels might also contribute to explain the differences in CHD mortality (table III). There are data suggesting that the lower systolíc and diastolic blood pressure levels in South Italy might be related, at least to some extent, to the regular consumption of olive oil in this area (6). However dietary habits in Italy are changing and tending to become, especially in the towns of North Italy, more and more similar to those in Northern Europe (7). Therefore also in this country much attention should be given to the dietary approach for the population strategy of CHD prevention.

Among other things even if there is no evidence that alcohol affects the coronary risk in Italy, it seems advisable for a healthy behavior to encourage some reduction in the daily wine consumption (table III).

NON LIPIDIC RISK FACTORS FOR CHD (Men 40–49 years)						
COUNTRY	N	SBP (mmHg)	DBP	SMOKE (%)	BMI (kg/m^2)	ALCOHOL (g/week)
ITALY	74	128	84	55	26	454
SCOTLAND	131	135*	83	47	26	292*
SW FINLAND	83	146**	90**	35	27	78**
N KARELIA	102	143**	88**	44	28	78**

Significance versus ITALY:*)$p < 0.05$;**)$p < 0.01$

TABLE III

THE STOCKHOLM - NAPLES STUDY

This cross sectional survey on 50 year old men, randomly selected from people living in Stockholm and Naples gives further support to the idea that serum cholesterol and blood pressure are relatively lower in Italy as compared to countries of Northern Europe (table IV and V). It has also been found that in Sweden there is a high frequency of late pre-beta lipoproteins (8), which are thought to be highly atherogenic. They have been detected in 34% of Stockholm men as compared to 19% among those living in Naples (table VI).

TOTAL SERUM, LDL,HDL CHOLESTEROL-TRIGLYCERIDES (mg/dl) IN NAPLES AND STOCKHOLM (Men, 50 yrs)				
	CHOLESTEROL			TG
	SERUM	LDL	HDL	SERUM
Naples n=73	211	138	48	134
Stockholm n=77	241**	158**	54*	136

TABLE IV

(Mean values) *)p < 0.05; **)p < 0.01

The data of low HDL cholesterol already found in the Cooperative Study (Table II) have been confirmed in the Stockholm-Naples Study (TABLE IV).

Despite the overall risk of CHD is relatively smaller in Italy, nevertheless a substantial number of coronary deaths occur and low HDL cholesterol might be helpful to identify people at risk. There is much debate on the question whether HDL cholesterol is merely a predictor of CHD or definitely a causal factor (9). This question is still unsolved.

It is very likely that low HDL cholesterol in Italy is at least to some extent due to heavy cigarette consumption. In both the Cooperative and Stockholm-Naples studies (table III and V) the Italian population samples show the highest cigarette consumption, in parallel with the lowest HDL cholesterol concentration (table II and IV).

NON LIPIDIC RISK FACTORS FOR CHD					
	SBP (mmHg)	DBP	SMOKE (%)	BMI (Kg/m^2)	ALCOHOL (g/week)
Naples n=73	125	77	64	27	239
Stockholm n=77	134**	88**	43*	26	157**

TABLE V

(Mean values);*)p < 0.05;**)p < 0.01

SINKING (SpB) AND LATE (LpB) PRE–BETA LIPOPROTEINS		
		Mean VLDL
SpB	LpB	Chol/Tg
Naples n=64	14 (22%)	12 (19%)	.27
Stockholm n=68	16 (24%)	23 (34%)*	.30**

*)p < 0.05; **)p < 0.01

TABLE VI

In the second of the two surveys the amount of physical
activity has been investigated by using a widely accepted
questionnaire (10). It has been found that the percentage
of sedentery people is much higher in Naples as compared
to Stockholm (80% versus 20%, p < 0.01).
Lower physical activity in Naples is associated with a
higher fasting glucose concentration as compared to
Stockholm (table VII). However the glucose and insulin
response to a glucose load (100g orally) are nearly the
same in the two towns.
Sedentarism might also contribute to the lower HDL
cholesterol seen in Naples.
While an independent role of low HDL on CHD risk cannot
be excluded so far, there is no clear-cut evidence that
it is useful to raise HDL chlesterol by pharmacological
means.
Nevertheless it seems wise to modify those factors that
contribute to keep HDL low.

OGTT AND PHYSICAL ACTIVITY					
SERUM GLUCOSE		SERUM INSULIN		SEDENTARY	
0'	120'	0'	120'	work	leisure
mg/dl		mU/l		%	
Naples n = 73	91+2	90+4	8+1	40+4	51	79
Stockholm n = 77	84+2*	92+4	7+1	35+3	40	23*

*)p < 0.01   X+SEM

TABLE VII

In particular a preventive strategy in Italy should aim
to persuade to smoking cessation and to encourage a less
sedentary life style.

In summary a comprehensive approach to the correction of
all the known risk factors for CHD is advisable also in
Italy. Some priorities can be defined for the preventive
strategy in this country.
The number of cigarette smokers is exceedingly high and a
sedentary life style is almost the rule: this probably
contributes to a large extent to the low HDL cholesterol
concentrations.
Major emphasis should therefore be put on a widespread
anti-smoking advice, actively involving all health
operators. Encouragement of physical exercise during
leisure time should go together with the provision of
more facilities for sport or other recreational
activities requiring some energy expenditure.

REFERENCES

1) Keys A. (1970) Coronary heart disease in seven
countries. Circulation, 41(suppl. 1), 1-211

2) Menotti A., Conti S., Giampaoli S., Mariotti S., Rumi
A., Signoretti P. (1980) Prediction of coronary and other
causes of death by some coronary risk factors in fifteen
years. ISTISAN 1980/14, 1-19

3) Riemersma R.A., Wood D.A., Butler S., Elton R.A.,
Oliver M., Salo M, Nikkari T., Vartiainen E., Puska P.,
Gey F., Rubba P., Mancini M., Fidanza F. (1986) Linoleic
acid content in adipose tissue and coronary heart
disease. Br. Med. J., 292, 1423-1427

4) Olsson A.G., Holmquist L., Walldius G., Hadell K.,
Carlson L.A., Riccardi G., Rubba P., Pauciullo P.,
Mancini M. (1987) Metabolic differences in Northern and
Southern European males : Study of dietary habits, serum
apolipoprotein and lipid concentrations and glucose
metabolism (in preparation)

5) Beynen A.C., Hermus R.J.J., Hautvast J.G.A.J. (1980) A mathematical relationship between the fatty acid composition of the diet and that of adipose tissue in man. Am.J.Clin.Nutr., 33, 81-5

6) Rubba P., Mancini M., Fidanza F., Gautiero G., Nikkari T., Salo M., Elton R., Oliver M.F. (1987) Adipose tissue fatty acids and blood pressure in middle aged men from South Italy. Int.J.Epidem. (in press)

7) The Research Group ATS-RF2 of the Italian National Research Council (1981) Distribution of some risk factors for atherosclerosis in nine Italian population samples. Am.J.Epidem., 113, 338-46

8) Carlson K., Carlson L.A. (1975) Comparison of the behaviour of very low density lipoproteins of type III hyperlipoproteinemia on electrophoresis on paper and on agarose gel with a note on a late (slow) pre-beta VLDL lipoprotein. Scand.J.clin.Lab.Invest., 35, 655-60

9) Pocock S.J., Shaper A.G., Phillips A.N., Walker M., Whitehead T.P. (1986) High density lipoprotein cholesterol is not a major risk factor for ischaemic heart disease in British men. Br.Med.J., 292, 515-8

10)Saltin B., Grimby G. (1968) Physiological analysis of middle-aged and old former athletes. Comparison with still active athletes of the same ages. Circulation, 38, 1104-15

DIET: A RISK FACTOR AND A MEANS OF PREVENTION OF ATHEROSCLEROSIS AND CORONARY HEART DISEASE

31
Dietary fiber and lipid metabolism
D. Kritchevsky

Among the earliest experiments with dietary fiber were those carried out by Ershoff, whose lipid experiments consisted of comparing, in rats, the effects of a fiber-free diet, the same diet plus 1% cholesterol and the fiber-free cholesterol diet augmented with 5-10% of a dietary fiber.

Wells and Ershoff [1] found that 5% pectin reduced plasma cholesterol levels in rats by 17% and liver cholesterol by 41% [compared to rats fed the fiber-free regimen plus 1% cholesterol. Other vegetable gums such as guar gum, locust bean gum or carrageenan exerted a similar effect [2] but agar, cellulose and pectic acid did not [1]. In fact, cellulose and agar raised liver cholesterol levels. These different effects of pectin and cellulose have been confirmed by others. Pectin has been shown by other investigators to be hypocholesterolemic in rabbits fed cholesterol [3] or cholesterol-free diets [4], but cellulose appears to raise cholesterol levels in this species.

Judd and Truswell [5] have compared hypocholesterolemic effects of different types of pectins in rats and found high methoxyl pectins to be more effective than low methoxyl pectins; low molecular weight pectins were without effect.

In experiments in which rats were meal-fed diets containing 10% fiber liver cholesterol levels were reduced by guar gum, pectin and mannan; raised by cellulose, and unaffected by alginic acid [6]. When fed at the 15% level, cellulose increased liver cholesterol and total body cholesterol of rats while pectin, hemicellulose and lignin did not [7].

Schneeman et al. [8] fed rats a fiber-free, cholesterol-free diet or a fiber-free diet containing cellulose, wheat bran, oat bran, pectin or guar gum. The HDL-cholesterol levels were similar in all groups but analysis of the plasma apoproteins showed the wheat bran group to have significantly higher levels of apoE. The apoCII/CIII ratio was highest in the guar gum-fed rats and lowest in those fed wheat bran or cellulose.

The effects of dietary fiber on experimental atherosclerosis or aortic sudanophilia have been tested in rabbits, chickens and primates. Lambert et al. [9] reported in 1958 that a cholesterol-free, semipurified diet containing saturated fat was atherogenic for rabbits. Since saturated fat had no effect when added to stock ration [10] it was hypothesized that the fiber present in the commercial ratio had inhibited the atherogenic effect of the fat [11]. An alternate explanation for Lambert's findings was that the commercial diet contained enough polyunsaturated fat to counteract the effects of the added saturated fat. To test both possibilities rabbits were fed the semipurified diet, the same diet augmented with fat extracted from stock diet, a diet in which the residue was the lipid-extracted stock diet, and stock diet diluted with a high level of saturated fat. The fiber present in the stock diet was indeed shown to be protective [12] (Table 1). Moore [13] fed rabbits semipurified diets containing 20% butter with different types of fiber and found that diets containing wheat straw were significantly less hypercholesterolemic and atherogenic than diets containing cellulose or cellophane.

In general, the animal data suggest that gelling fibers are hypolipidemic whereas particulate fibers are not. The influence of various fiber additions on cholesterol levels in man was reviewed by Kay and Truswell in 1980 [14], there are more data today but the trend of the findings has not changed. Soft white wheat bran is without effect, but bran from hard red spring wheat is hypocholesterolemic [15]. Oat bran is hypocholesterolemic [16] probably because of its oat gum content. Generally, pectin is also hypocholesterolemic, the range of cholesterol reduction being about 10-15%. Other soluble fibers have also been shown to lower plasma cholesterol levels, among them, guar gum, locust bean gum and gum arabic. Gum tragacanth has no effect and results with karaya gum are inconsistent. Most of the substances tested were fed at levels of 10-20 g/day.

A group of subjects subsisting on a vegetarian diet had significantly lower plasma lipid levels than age and sex matched controls [17]. Studies among various groups of Seventh Day Adventists have shown that the vegans have significantly lower cholesterol levels than the lacto-ovo vegetarians or omnivores [18]. The vegans ingested significantly more pectin than the other groups, intake of other fibers was the same (Table 2).

Most of the substances which lower plasma cholesterol lower not only LDL-cholesterol but lower HDL-cholesterol as well. While these may appear to be opposite effects, if the ratio of HDL to LDL cholesterol is increased over control levels the result can still be considered beneficial. Soy hulls, corn bran and locust bean gum do not affect the ratio of HDL to LDL cholesterol; carboxymethylcellulose, oat bran, guar gum, beans and other legumes raise the ratio by at least 10%; and wheat bran and cellulose lower it by 7%. Vegetarians have lower levels of apoAI and apoB, than omnivores, both apoproteins being positively related to coronary risk. These data have been reviewed by Schneeman and Lefevre [19].

Dietary fiber is a generic term covering a number of substances of different structure and unique physiological effects. The precise mechanism of the hypolipidemic effect of fiber is not yet clear. Substances such as wheat bran which have laxative properties do not influence lipemia whereas the soluble, gelling fibers such as pectin or guar are hypocholesterolemic but do not affect intestinal transit time or fecal bulk. The effects of fibers on assembly of lipoproteins and on apolipoprotein spectra and metabolism require elucidation. The role of fiber metabolites, particularly short chain fatty acids on lipid metabolism remains to be clarified. As analytical methods become more precise we may expect to learn more about structure-function relationships which, in turn, could lead to design of fibers or concoction of fiber mixtures to do specific metabolic tasks.

ACKNOWLEDGEMENT

Supported, in part, by a grant (HL-03299) and a Research Career Award (HL-00734) from the National Institutes of Health (USA) and by funds from the Commonwealth of Pennsylvania.

REFERENCES

1.   Wells, AF and Ershoff, BH (1961). Beneficial effects of pectin in prevention of hypercholesterolemia and increase in liver cholesterol in cholesterol-fed rats. J Nutr, 74, 87
2.   Ershoff, BH and Wells, AF (1962). Effects of guar gum, locust bean gum and carrageenan on liver cholesterol of cholesterol-fed rats. Proc Soc Exp Biol Med, 110, 580
3.   Berenson, LM, Bhandaru, RR, Radhakrishnamurthy, B, Srinivasan, SR and Berenson, GS (1975). The effect of dietary pectin on serum lipoprotein cholesterol in rabbits. Life Sci, 16, 1533
4.   Hamilton, RMG and Carroll, KK (1976). Plasma cholesterol levels in rabbits fed low fat, low cholesterol diets: effects of dietary proteins, carbohydrates and fiber from different sources. Atherosclerosis, 24, 47
5.   Judd, PA and Truwell, AS (1985). The hypocholesterolaemic effects of pectins in rats. Br J Nutr, 53, 409
6.   Kritchevsky, D, Ryder, E, Fishman, A, Kaplan, M and DeHoff, JL (1982). Influence of dietary fiber on food intake, feed efficiency and lipids in rats. Nutr Rep Int, 25, 783
7.   Mueller, MA, Cleary, MP and Kritchevsky, D (1983). Influence of dietary fiber on lipid metabolism in meal fed rats. J Nutr 113, 2229
8.   Schneeman, BO, Cimmarusti, J, Cohen, W, Downes, L and Lefevre, M (1984). Composition of high density lipoproteins in rats. J Nutr, 114, 1320
9.   Lambert, GF, Miller, JP, Olsen, RT and Frost, DV (1958). Hypercholesteremia and atherosclerosis induced in rabbits by purified high fat rations devoid of cholesterol. Proc Soc Exp Biol Med, 97, 544
10. Kritchevsky, D and Tepper, SA (1964). Cholesterol vehicle in experimental atherosclerosis. 6. Long term effects of fats and fatty acids in a cholesterol-free diet. J Atheroscler Res, 4, 113

11. Kritchevsky, D (1964). Experimental atherosclerosis in rabbits fed cholesterol-free diets. J Atheroscler Res, 4, 103
12. Kritchevsky, D and Tepper, SA (1965). Factors affecting atherosclerosis in rabbits fed cholesterol-free diets. Life Sci, 4, 1468
13. Moore, JH (1967). The effect of the type of roughage in the diet on plasma cholesterol levels and aortic atherosis in rabbits. Br J Nutr, 21, 207
14. Kay, RM and Truswell, AS (1980). Dietary fiber: effects on plasma and biliary lipids in man. In: Spiller, GA and Kay, RM (eds.) "Medical Aspects of Dietary Fiber". p. 153. (New York: Plenum Medical Book Co.)
15. Munoz, JM, Sandstead, HH, Jacob, RA, Logan, GM, Reck, SJ, Klevay, LM, Dintzis, FR, Inglett, GF and Shuey, WC (1979). Effects of some cereals and textured vegetable protein on plasma lipids. Am J Clin Nutr 32, 580
16. Anderson, JW, Story, L, Sieling, B, Chen, WL, Petro, MS and Story, J (1984). Hypocholesterolemic effects of oat bran and bean intake in hypercholesterolemic men. Am J Clin Nutr, 40, 1146
17. Sacks, FM, Castelli, WP, Donner, A and Kass, EH (1975). Plasma lipids and lipoproteins in vegetarians and controls. N Engl J Med, 292, 1148
18. Kritchevsky, D, Tepper, SA and Goodman, G (1984). Diet, nutrient intake and metabolism in populations at high and low risk for colon cancer. 7. Relation of diet to serum lipids. Am J Clin Nutr, 40, 921
19. Schneeman, BO and Lefevre, M (1986). Effects of fiber on plasma lipoprotein composition. In Vahouny, GV and Kritchevsky, D (eds.) "Dietary Fiber: Basic and Clinical Aspects". p. 309 (New York, Plenum Press).

Table 1. Influence of stock diet fractions on atherosclerosis in rabbits[*]

Group	Fat (%)[a]	Fiber (%)[b]	Serum cholesterol (mg/dl)	Avg. Atherosclerosis (arch + thoracic/2)
1	CNO (14)	Cellulose (15)	207 ± 36	0.85
2	CNO (12) SF (2)	Cellulose (15)	249 ± 41	0.90
3	CNO (14)	Stock	64 ± 9	0.40
4	CNO (12) SF (2)	Stock	35 ± 2	0.25
5	SF (2)	Stock	40 ± 9	0.15

[*]After Kritchevsky and Tepper [12].
[a] CNO, coconut oil; SF, fat present in stock diet.
[b] Stock - residue after extraction of lipid from stock diet.

Table 2. Serum lipids and dietary fiber intakes in seventh day adventists (SDA)[*]

	Group[a]			
	VEG	LOV	NV	GP
No. Subjects	18	25	25	12
Serum cholesterol (mg/dl)	149 ± 8	192 ± 7	207 ± 7	217 ± 7
Fiber Intake (g/0.02 MJ/day)				
NDF[b]	14.5	15.0	13.5	13.0
Cellulose	2.5	2.0	1.5	2.0
Hemicellulose	11.0	11.5	11.0	10.4
Pectin	7.5	4.5	4.0	4.0
Lignin	0.8	0.7	0.5	0.4

[*] After Kritchevsky et al. [18].
[a] VEG - Vegan SDA; LOV - Lacto-ovovegetarian SDA; GP - General public.
[b] Neutral detergent fiber.

32
Dietary and biochemical studies with textured soy proteins

C.R. Sirtori, A. Canavesi, C. Manzoni, V. Vaccarino
and M.R. Lovati

INTRODUCTION

The hypocholesterolemic activity of vegetable proteins, particularly
from soybean, was suggested early this century from animal studies
(1,2). In more recent years, several Authors have demonstrated that
the substitution of animal proteins with soybean proteins in the
diet, significantly reduces plasma cholesterol levels both in
experimental animals (3) and in man (4). The soybean protein diet
appears to be an effective alternative to drug treatments in adult
type II hypercholesterolemic patients (4,5), the activity being
independent of dietary cholesterol and only partially influenced by
the P/S ratio (6). Unfortunately, the mode of action of textured
vegetable proteins (TVP) from soy has remained quite elusive. Part
of the difficulty in the clarification of the mechanisms, probably
lies in the selective activity of the diet in spontaneously hypercholesterolemic patients and in diet induced hypercholesterolemic
animals (7,8), with little or no activity in normolipidemic animals
and humans (9).

In view of the significant activity of the diet in type II patients
and of the uncertainties about the mode of action, interest is
currently very high on this topic (10). The soybean diet may, in
fact, represent a means of reducing the diet-linked atherogenic
risk. The object of this presentation will be to review some recent
studies on: a) a study in children, where the soybean diet may
represent a choice treatment for hypercholesterolemia; b) data from
animal studies, as well as preliminary data from humans, on the
regulation of low density lipoprotein (LDL) receptors following this
regimen.

EVALUATION OF THE L-TVP DIET IN TYPE II CHILDREN

Hypercholesterolemia poses a serious therapeutic problem in childhood, since the physician may not be willing to prescribe long-term drug therapies in pre-pubertal children. We, therefore, elected to evaluate the soybean diet regimen in a group of 16 children with familial type II disease, within a multi-center study (11).

After 4 weeks of a traditional low lipid-low cholesterol diet, the L-TVP diet was prescribed to the children within a program, allowing an adequate calorie intake for normal growth. All 16 children and their families started the protocol with good compliance. Unfortunately, due to intercurrent illness or movement out of town, only 12 children completed 2 months or more of treatment. The results clearly showed that the initial low lipid diet did not achieve any remarkable change in the plasma lipid/lipoprotein levels. A significant reduction of total cholesterol was, instead, recorded already after 2 weeks of the L-TVP diet. At the fourth week, the mean cholesterol in all 16 subject was reduced to -19.2% vs baseline ($p < 0.001$); LDL-cholesterol levels were also reduced by 19.7% ($p < 0.001$), triglyceridemia increased slightly, as also did HDL-C (from 35.6 ± 6.4 to 36.8 ± 6.5 mg/dl). After 18 weeks, when the study was considered as completed, the 12 children still participating showed the stabilization of their cholesterolemia, with a mean reduction of 21.6%, while a further rise of HDL-C could be recorded (to 37.0 ± 8.6 mg/dl at the end of the treatment, p: ns vs baseline). Most of the children have followed the regimen for more prolonged periods of time (up to 4 years), with complete maintenance of their biochemical improvement and normal growth. One child with homozygous receptor-deficient hypercholesterolemia had a dramatic (-33%) cholesterol reduction (Fig. 1) when the soybean diet was given as an in-patient. Follow-up was characterized by a progressive rise of cholesterolemia, due to inadequate compliance. Treatment with anion exchange resin gave similar results as the dietary regimen.

The soybean diet may, therefore, offer a satisfactory alternative to drug treatments in pre-pubertal children. Similar findings have been recently reported widhalm by (12), who tested the regimen in 11 children with familial disease, starting at age 2 y. This Author reported a reduction of 32% in total cholesterol and 37% in LDL-cholesterol levels vs baseline (on a free diet).

ACTIVITY OF THE SOYBEAN PROTEIN DIET ON LIPOPROTEIN RECEPTORS

The discrepant results between animal and human studies in terms of

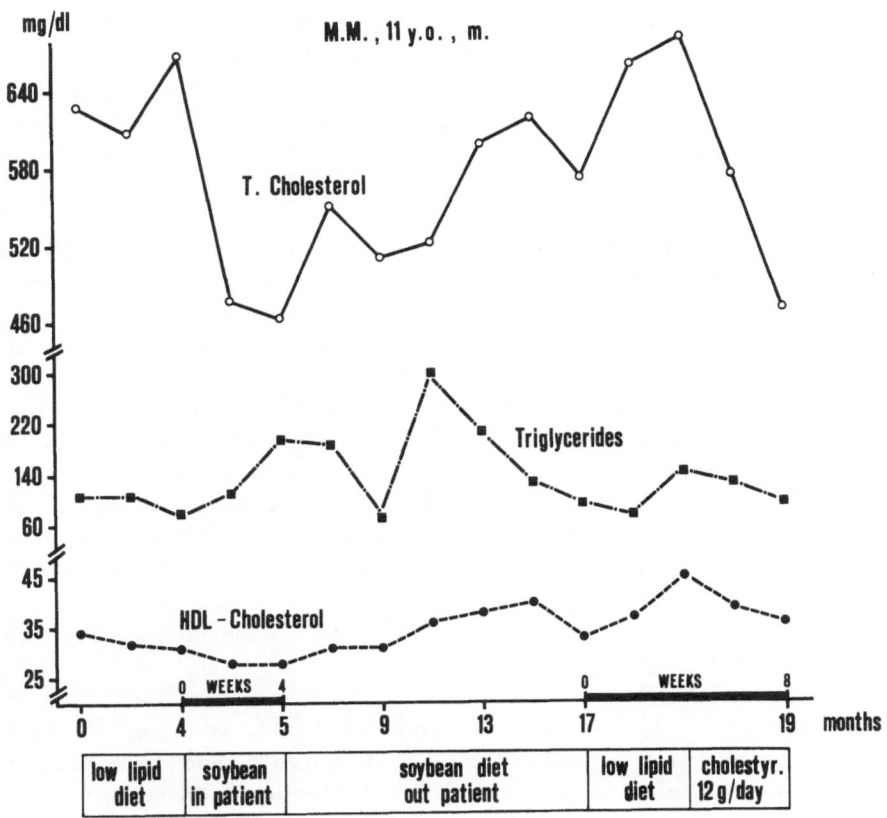

FIGURE 1   Response a child with homozygous receptor-deficient type
II hyperlipoproteinemia to the soybean diet. Treatment, started
as an in-patient resulted in a 33% reduction of total
cholesterolemia.   During a 12 month follow-up at home, a
progressive re-increase of cholesterolemia took place, due to
poor compliance. Interestingly, later administration of an
anion exchange resin, gave similar results as the experimental
diet.

fecal steroid excretion (increased excretion in animals, no change
in humans), have raised interest in the receptorial regulation of
lipoprotein metabolism during different diets.   This topic is of
particular significance, after a recent study indicating that the
addition of cholesterol to a human diet is hypercholesterolemic only
when the diet contains animal proteins, not when dietary proteins
are represented by soy (13).

We evaluated in two different studies, the activity of liver lipo-protein receptors in rats, when exposed to cholesterol-rich regimens with two different dietary proteins. In the first study, two groups of female rats were fed on a 2% cholesterol diet with either casein or soy protein. There was, as expected (8), a clear difference between the cholesterol response to the two diets, with an approximate doubling of total cholesterol and a 12-fold increase of very low density lipoprotein (VLDL) associated cholesterol in rats given casein.

In this experiment, the binding of lipoproteins to liver cells was tested by means of the separated ß-VLDL fraction from blood of male rabbits fed for 4 weeks on a 2% cholesterol regimen. The receptorial activity was determined by incubating rat liver membrane preparations (14) in the presence of ^{125}I-labelled rabbit ß-VLDL. In spite of the significant cholesterol load administered to these animals, the binding of ß-VLDL to liver membranes from soybean fed rats did not differ from that of control animals, whereas it was markedly reduced in the case of animals receiving casein as the major dietary protein (15). The evaluation of the enzymes, involved in the receptorial pathway, provided data consistent with a moderately reduced receptorial activity in the case of the soy-cholesterol fed rats and in a total suppression for the casein-cholesterol group.

In the second study, a turnover experiment with autologous ß-VLDL from rats was carried out. Recipient animals had received, as before, soy+cholesterol and casein+cholesterol. There was clear evidence, in this second experiment, of an accelerated catabolism of ß-VLDL after the soy protein regimen (16) (Fig. 2). This finding complements data from the previous experiment and indicates that some component/s of soy protein may modulate liver receptorial activity, when this is suppressed by cholesterol (17).

Recently in a clinical study, the LDL receptorial activity was examined in freshly isolated mononuclear cells from type II patients, receiving either a low lipid diet with animal proteins or an identical diet (in terms of cholesterol and lipid content) with TVP. The results of this study, currently being evaluated, definitely suggest that the receptorial activity is dramatically increased after the soybean protein regimen in these patients with type II hyperlipoproteinemia.

CONCLUSIONS

The experience gained in the past 14 years clearly indicates that

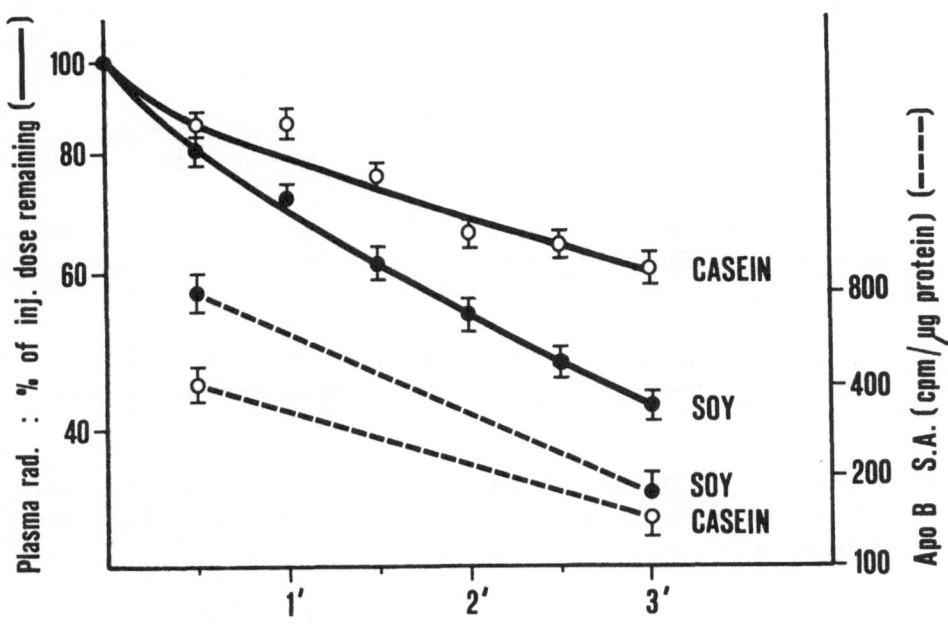

FIGURE 2   Early radioactivity decay of labelled homologous ß–VLDL
in rodents, given cholesterol-rich diets with either soy or
casein.   Both total decay and apo B specific activities (S.A.)
show a markedly accelerated catabolism after soy proteins,
consistent with an improved liver receptorial expression (16).

the soybean protein regimen is therapeutically very effective in
patients with type II hyperlipoproteinemia. A similar activity is
exerted in animal models with diet induced hypercholesterolemia.
Apparently, the available data suggest a different regulation of the
high affinity receptors for lipoproteins, when the soybean diet is
either administered in the presence of high cholesterol loads (e.g.,
animal studies) or per se to type II patients. The mechanism of
the change in the lipoprotein receptor regulation needs further
study.

These studies were supported by the Consiglio Nazionale delle
Ricerche of Italy and by a Grant-in aid from Gipharmex SPA, Milano,
Italy

REFERENCES

1. Ignatowski, A (1909). Uber die Wirkung der tierischen Eiweisses auf die Aorta und die parenchymatosen Organer der Kaninchen. Virchows Arch 198, 248

2. Meeker, DR and Kesten, HD (1940). Experimental atherosclerosis and high protein diets. Proc Soc Exp Biol Med 45, 543

3. Terpstra, AHM West, CE Fennis, JTCM, et al. (1984). Hypocholesterolemic effect of dietary soy protein versus casein in rhesus monkeys. Am J Clin Nutr 39, 1

4. Sirtori, CR Agradi, E Conti, F et al. (1977). Soybean protein diet in the treatment of type II hyperlipoproteinaemia. Lancet i, 275

5. Descovich, GC Ceredi, C Gaddi, A et al. (1980). Multicenter study of soybean protein diet for outpatient hypercholesterolaemic patients. Lancet ii, 709

6. Sirtori, CR Gatti, E Mantero, O et al. (1979). Clinical experience with the soybean protein diet in the treatment of hypercholesterolemia. Am J Clin Nutr 92, 1645

7. Kim, DN Lee, KT Reiner, JM et al. (1978). Effect of a soy product on serum and tissue cholesterol concentrations in swine fed high-fat, high-cholesterol diets. Exp Mol Pathol 29, 385

8. Terpstra, AHM van Tintelen, G and West, CE (1982). The hypocholesterolemic effect of dietary soy protein in rats. J Nutr 112, 810

9. Van Raaij, JAM Katan, MB West, CE et al. (1982). Influence of diets containing casein, soy isolate and concentrate on serum cholesterol and lipoproteins in middle-aged volunteers. Am J Clin Nutr 35, 925

10. Gibney, MJ Kritchevsky, D (1983). Animal and Vegetable Proteins in Lipid Metabolism and Atherosclerosis. Alan R Liss Inc, New York

11. Gaddi, A Descovich, GC Noseda, G et al. (1987) Hypercholesterolaemia treated by soybean protein diet. Arch Dis Child, in press

12. Widhalm, K (1986). Pediatric guidelines for lipid reduction. In: Lipoproteins and Atherosclerosis - Current Views, Future Trends, Helsinki, Finland, Abs 11

13. Meinertz, H Nilausen, K Faergeman, O (1984). Effects of dietary soy protein and casein on plasma lipoproteins in normolipidemic subjects. Circulation 70, 1161 (Abstr)

14. Kovanen, PT Brown, MS Goldstein, JL (1979). Increased binding of low density lipoprotein to liver membranes from rats treated with 17 α-ethinyl estradiol. J Biol Chem 254, 11367

15. Sirtori, CR Galli, G Lovati, MR et al. (1984). Effects of dietary proteins on the regulation of liver lipoprotein receptors in rats. J Nutr 114, 1493

16. Lovati, MR Allievi L and Sirtori, CR (1985). Accelerated early catabolism of very low density lipoproteins in rats after dietary soy proteins. Atherosclerosis 56, 243

17. Redgrave, TG (1984). Dietary proteins and atherosclerosis. Atherosclerosis 52, 349

33
Fats from marine animals in human nutrition and prevention of cardiovascular diseases
J. Dyerberg

INTRODUCTION

In preventive medicine much insight can be obtained from epidemiological observations. Even if epidemiological data can provide a basis for controlled intervention studies only, the impact of such data can be of a magnitude that they influence an area of research for a considerable period of time. The coincidence of epidemiological observations of a combination of a high seafood intake with low coronary mortality and the insight obtained in eicosanoid metabolism are examples of such driving forces in present preventive cardiovascular medicine. Beside from adding to the clarification of many hitherto unsolved biological problems, one should, however, be avare of the risk of overfocusing on single aspects in the multifactorial complex of atherothrombotic disorders.

EPIDEMIOLOGICAL DATA

Much of the present interest in seafood, particularly n-3 polyunsaturated fatty acids (PUFAs), originates in our observations of Greenland Eskimos (1) in the 1970's. These studies were based on observations of a low incidence of cardiovascular diseases among Eskimos (2,3), documented by statistical analyses of mortality data from Greenland, table I. In an examination of morbidity in a 25-year period in a northern district of Greenland Kromann et al. (4) found a 1:10 incidence of acute myocardial infarction compared to Danish morbidity data adjusted for age and sex, wheras the stroke incidence was twice that of the Danish incidence. In the same survey psoriasis, diabetes, bronchial asthma and polyarthritis chronica were relatively lower among Eskimos. The low incidence of ischemic heart disease has since been confirmed in other fish-eating communities, especially in Japan, where seafood consumption traditionally is high (5,6). It is in that respect interesting to note that hand-in-hand with westernized dietary habits in Japan, westernized disease patterns have occurred, including increased deaths from heart diseases (7,8).
Of considerable interest are the recent calculations by Kromhout et al. (9) of the relationship between fish intake and coronary deaths

over a 20-year period in 852 middle-aged men studied in Holland and
whose dietary habits for the study period were known. To compare relative risk as a function of the amount of fish consumed, individuals who ate no fish were assigned a risk level of 1.0. The risk ratios for those consuming 1-14 g, 15-29 g and 30-144 g of fish per
day were 0.64, 0.56 and 0.36 respectively with a significant inverse
relationship between fish consumption and coronary death risk. This
has been confirmed in other studies (10), but not from areas in the
world where fish consumption traditionally is high (11,12). Of special interest is the inverse relationship between a relatively low
level of fish intake and CHD. This makes nutritional advices on sea-
food, compared to the situation based on data from Greenland and Japan, much easier to give and accept. At the same time it gives rise
to new questions in that biological consequences of such a diet are
not easy to measure.

Table I.

5-year mortality of ischemic heart disease in persons aged 45-64
years in Greenland 1974-78 (incl.). Values are per cent of all
deaths. Values in brackets are 95% confidence limits.

IHD deaths (%)

males	9	(6-13)
females	7	(4-12)
both sexes	8.4	(6-12)

BIOLOGICAL INFLUENCES OF A SEA-FOOD DIET

The Eskimos eat a diet with aprox 40 energy% of fat which is about
equal to many western type diets, but the content of polyunsaturated fat is approx. one fifth of the total fat, which is 50% more
than in a typical Danish diet. Saturated fat is correspondingly lower also due to a high content of monounsaturated fat. The P/S ratio
is approx 0.8, but cholesterol intake is nearly twice that of Danish
avarage (0.79 versus 0.42 g/day). When examining the plasma lipid levels of Eskimos (13), we found a remarkable difference compared to
Danes with a favourable lipid profile in Eskimos (table II).

Table II

Avarage differences in plasma lipid and lipoprotein concentration
between Danes and Eskimos.

	Cholesterol mmol/l	Triglyc. mmol/l	LDL g/l	VLDL g/l	HDL g/l
females	1.38	0.59	0.87	0.66	-0.10
males	0.92	0.73	0.66	1.05	-1.23

Of major interest is, however, that when trying to compute the difference between cholesterol levels in Danes and Eskimos as a function of their dietary habits, and using well established formulas for such calculations we could only account for half of the observed difference (14). Accordingly we ascribed the hypocholesterolemic and even more the marked hypotriglyceridemic effect of the Eskimo diet to the effect of PUFA's, belonging to the n-3 family constituting approx. 80% of the dietary PUFAs. This marked hypolipidemic effect of n-3 PUFAs, much more pronounced than the effect of n-6 PUFAs especially lowering plasma VLDL, has since been verified both in normals and in patients (15,16). It constitutes a major reason for including n-3 PUFAs in dietary advices, and is beside this a break-through for a more differentiated look on polyunsaturated fats, which has hitherto been considered as an undifferantiated dietary component. In fact, the ability of 4 g of n-3 PUFAs, in normolipemic volunteers, to lower VLDL by 30%, compared to no effect of 4 g of n-6 PUFAs (17), is to be compared with highly efficient hypolipidemic drugs.
The major reason for the interest in n-3 PUFAs stems from their effect on eicosanoid production and hemostasis. In in vitro experiments and in in vivo examinations of Eskimos (18,19) we showed that n-3 PUFAs influence hemostasis in a way expected to be antithrombotic. Our hypothesis, which since has been confirmed on substantial points, suggested that eicosapentaenoic acid (EPA) 20:5, n-3 inhibits thromboxane A_2 (TXA$_2$) formation in the platelets, and generates the formation of TXA$_3$, which is a very week platelet aggregator. Also EPA in the vessel wall shifts the production of PGI$_2$ (prostacyclin) to PGI$_3$, which is as potent an antiaggregator as PGI$_2$. This would shift the hemostatic balance so that thrombi would not form as easily when EPA is substituted for arachidonic acid (AA) in cell membrane lipids. We found in the Eskimos a prolonged cutaneous bleeding time compared to Danes (8.1 versus 4.7 min) and an inhibited platelet aggregation, which was parallelled by an enrichment of platelet lipids with EPA (8.0%) on the expence of AA (8.5%) in contrast to the corresponding values in Danes (0.5 and 22.1% respectively). Inhibition of platelet aggregation and prolongation of cutaneous bleeding time by feeding fish oils, fish diets or fish oil concentrates, has since been reported in several studies in human volunteers (17,20,21), even though the effect obtained must be considered as moderate. Much debate has recently concentrated on whether prostaglandins (PG) of the 3-family actually are formed in humans or whether n-3 PUFAs exert their effect only by inhibiting the formation of PGs of the 2-family from AA. In contrast to the rat, it seems as humans do form prostaglandins of the 3-family and that intake of n-3 PUFAs do not inhibit PG-2-family production (22). We have in collaboration with others, been able to demonstrate that the Eskimos, who take n-3 PUFAs instead of n-6 PUFAs and not as in many volunteer studies as a supplementum to their diet, and who have obtained a steady state equilibrium of membrane fatty acid profile do not have a depressed total PG-metabolite excretion in the urine (23). Furthermore, their ratio of prostacyclin metabolites over thromboxane metabolites in 24 hour urine samples was significantly higher than that of Danes (0.42 versus 0.14 respectively p<0.01) (24). These findings do support the recommandation of a higher sea

food intake but do not themselves constitute a scientific basis for accepting n-3 PUFAs as antithrombotic agents. Another important role of n-3 PUFAs in atherothrombotic disorders may be their effect on metabolism of leucotrienes and other lipoxygenase products. Leucotrienes of the 5-series, originating from EPA, have a different profile of biological activities than the 4-series from AA and may alter host responce to proinflammatory stimuli (24). Inflammatory responces may be a critical factor in plaque formation following endothelial injury. The procoagulant activity exposed by invading cells, especially the monocyte, may further be attenuated due to altered lipid composition of the cell membrane as a consequence of dietary n-3 PUFAs (25). Thus n-3 PUFAs and especially EPA as a critical metabolic substrate have a potential for modulating the hemostatic/inflammatory reaction in the very initial phases of thrombosis formation.

n-3 PUFAs have other effects that should be considered carefully from a thrombopreventive point of view. Due to their high unsaturation index they may influence blood viscosity and erythrocyte deformeability (26,27) faciliating microcirculation.

We found that Eskimos had unexpectedly high levels of antithrombin III, which also increased in volunteers given fish oil concentrates (28). An even greater effect was obtained after dietary n-6 PUFA intake (17). Whether this effect has any bearing on the development of arterial thrombi, as it has in venous thrombi, remains to be clarified.

We noticed a slight but significant fall in systolic blood pressure in volunteers given fish oil concentrate (17), which also has been noticed in patients with mild essential hypertension (29,30). We believe that this might be a consequence of a shift in thromboxane/prostacyclin balance in favour of prostacyclin, influencing peripheral vascular resistance. The effect of a slight decrease in blood pressure on the development of atherosclerosis is difficult to assess, but at least it points in the right direction. Any antithrombotic effect of n-3 PUFAs or fish oil, which is the only natural scource of long-chained n-3 PUFAs, has a destinct multifactorial outlook. A review of marine oils and thrombogenesis is given in (31).

INTERVENTION STUDIES

Animal experiments have shown indisputably that a diet rich in fish oils can inhibit experimental thrombosis and atherosclerosis significantly (32,33,34,35). One reason for not directly extrapolating these findings to the situation in humans is that there are profound differences among species in the impact of n-3 PUFAs feeding on eicosanoid production (36). The situation in humans is far from clarified. As dealt with above numerous biological effects of n-3 PUFAs have been demonstrated to be considered as likely antithrombotic factors, but controlled clinical studies are still lacking. A 16-year study initiated in the 1950's by Nelson was reported to result in a four-fold greater incidence of fatal heart attacks in controls compared to the diet groups adviced to consume fish as a main course three times a week (37). The study design does not, however, full fill present demands to clinical trials, and the results can only be considered indicative along with the epidemiological findings. Saynor (38) in an open study gave fish oil concentrates to patients with effort angina. He found an impressive decline in GTN consumption following fish oil supplementation. However, we were not able to confirm these findings in a controlled study measuring anginal attacks and GTN consumption in groups of patients allocated to either fish oil or placebo-oil supplementation, even if a fall in GTN consumption in the fish oil group per se was significant (39). Effort angina is obviously not the ideal model for studing the effect of antithrombotic measures. Presently other clinical trials are on-going without results to be disclosed yet.

CONCLUSION

n-3 polyunsaturated fatty acids have caught attention to themselves as potential antithrombotic agents and as candidates for influencing other cellular responces to noxious stimuly beneficially. The investigations initiated by epidemiological examinations of exotic populations have led to an establishment of n-3 PUFAs as food components with their own spectrum of biological effects, different from that of the n-6 PUFAs abudant in vegetable oils and in food products made from these. The biological effects of n-3 PUFAs seem to be related to the long-chained members of the fatty acid family, the only natural source of which are marine oils.

A more general use of fish oils or fish oil products in preventive cardiology must await the outcome of clinical studies, but the many, until now disclosed, beneficial effects of these oils, justify a recommandation of a wider use of fish products and sea-food in the diet than presently is enjoyed in many western and westernized countries.

References

1.   Bang, HO and Dyerberg, J (1980). Lipid metabolism and ischemic heart disease in Greenland Eskimos. In: Draper, HH (ed.) "Advances in nutritional research" vol. 3 p. 1-23 (New York: Plenum Press).

2.   Rodahl, K (1954). Diet and cardiovascular disease in the Eskimos. Am J Cardiol, 4, 192-197.

3.   Ehrström, MC (1951). Medical studies in North Greenland 1948-1949. VI. Blood pressure, hypertension and atherosclerosis in relation to food and mode of living. Acta Med Scand 140, 416- 422.

4.   Kromann, N and Green, A (1980). Epidemiological studies in the Upernavik district, Greenland. Acta Med Scand 208, 401-406.

5.   Hirai, A, Hamazaki, T, Terano, T, Nishikawa, T, Tamura, Y, Kumagai, A and Sajiki, J (1980). Eicosapentaenoic acid and platelet function in Japanese. Lancet ii, 1132.

6.   Hirai, A, Terano, T, Saito, H, Tamura, Y, Yoshida, S, Sajiki, J and Kumagai, A (1984). Eicosapentaenoic acid and platelet function in Japanese. In: Lowenburg, W and Yamori, Y (eds.) "Nutritional Prevention of Cardiovascular Diseases". p.231-239 (London: Academic Press).

7. Kagawa, Y (1978). Impact of westernization on the nutrition of Japanese: Changes in physique, cancer, longevity and centenarians. Preventive medicine 7, 205-217.

8. Goto, Y and Homma, Y (1984). Recent trends of coronary heart disease in Japan in relation to dietary alterations. In: Lowenburg, W and Yamori, Y (eds) "Nutritional Prevention of Cardiovascular Diseases". p.73-85. (London: Academic Press).

9. Kromhout, D, Borschieter, EB and Coulander, C (1985). The inverse relation between fish consumption and 20-year mortality from coronary heart disease. N Engl J Med 312, 1205-1209.

10. Shekelle, RB, Missell, L, Paul, O, Shyock, AM and Stamler, J (1985). Fish consumption and mortality from coronary heart disease. N Engl J Med 313, 820.

11. Curb, JD and Reed, DM (1985). Fish consumption and mortality from coronary heart disease. N Engl J Med 313, 821.

12. Vollset, SE, Hench, I and Bjelke, E (1985). Fish consumption and mortality from coronary heart disease. N Engl J Med 313, 820-821.

13. Bang, HO and Dyerberg, J (1972). Plasma lipids and lipoprotein in Greenland West Coast Eskimos. Acta Med Scand 192, 85-94.

14. Bang, HO, Dyerberg, J and Sinclair, HM (1980). The composition of the food in north western Greenland. Am J Clin Nutr 33, 2657-2661.

15. Dyerberg, J (1981). Platelet-vessel wall interaction: influence of diet. Phil Trans R Soc Lond B294, 373-381.

16. Phillipson, BE, Rothrock, DW, Connor, WE, Harris, WS and Illingworth, DR (1985). Reduction of plasma lipids, lipoproteins and apoproteins by dietary fish oil in patients with hypertriglyceridemia. N Engl J Med 312, 1210-1216.

17. Mortensen, J, Schmidt, EB, Nielsen, AH and Dyerberg, J (1983). The effect of n-6 and n-3 polyunsaturated fatty acids on hemostasis, blood lipids and blood pressure. Thromb Haemostas (Stuttgart) 50, 543-546.

18. Dyerberg, J, Bang, HO, Stoffersen, E, Moncada, S and Vane, JR (1978). Eicosapentaenoic acid and prevention of thrombosis and atherosclerosis? Lancet ii, 117-119.

19. Dyerberg, J and Bang, HO (1979). Haemostatic function and platelet polyunsaturated fatty acids in Eskimos. Lancet ii, 433-435.

20. Sanders, TAB and Rosshanai, F (1983). The influence of different types of n-3 polyunsaturated fatty acids on blood lipids and platelet function in healthy volunteers. Clin Science 64, 91-99.

21. Siess, W, Roth, P, Scherer, B, Kurzmann, I, Böhlig, B and Weber PC (1980). Platelet-membrane fatty acids, platelet aggregation and thromboxane formation during a mackerel diet. Lancet i, 441-444.

22. Fisher, S and Weber, PC (1984). Prostaglandin I_3 is formed in vivo in man after dietary eicosapentaenoic acid. Nature 307, 165-168.

23. Zuccato, E, Hornstra, G and Dyerberg, J (1985). Long term "marine diet" in Eskimos is not associated with altered urinary excretion of total tetranor prostaglandin metabolism. Prostaglandins 30, 465-477.

24. Lee, TH, Mencia-Huerta, J-M, Shih, C, Cosey, EJ, Lewis, RA and Austen, KF (1984). Effects of exogenous arachidonic, eicosapentae

noic and docosahexaenoic acids on the generation of 5-lipoxygenase pathway products by ionophore-activated human neutrophils. J Clin Invest, 74, 1922-1933.
25.   Dam-Mieras, MCE, Muller, AD, Rand, ML and Hornstra, G (1986). Dietary lipids and macrophage procoagelant activity. Thromb Res 1986, 1, 133-137.
26.   Kobayashi, S, Hirai, A, Terano, T, Hamazaki, T, Tamura, Y and Kumagai, A (1981). Reduction in blood viscosity by eicosapentaenoic acid. Lancet ii, 197.
27.   Woodcock, BE, Schmidt, E, Lambert, WB, Jones, WM, Galloway, JH, Greaves, M and Presston, FE (1984). Beneficial effect of fish oil on blood viscosity in peripheral vascular disease. Br Med J, 288, 592- 594.
28.   Stoffersen, E, Jørgensen, KA and Dyerberg, J (1982). Anti-thrombin III and dietary intake of polyunsaturated fatty acids. Scand J Clin Lab Invest, 42, 83-86.
29.   Singer, P, Wirth, M, Voigt, S, Richter-Heinrich, E, Gödicke, W, Berger, I, Neumann, E, Listing, J, Hartrodt, W and Taube, C (1985). Blood pressure- and lipid-lowering effect of mackerel and herring diet in patients with mild essential hypertension. Atherosclerosis, 56, 223-235.
30.   Norris, PG, Jones, CJH and Weston, MJ (1986). Effect of dietary supplementation with fish oil on systolic blood pressure in mild essential hypertension. Br Med J, 293, 104-105.
31.   Dyerberg, J and Jørgensen, KA (1982). Marine Oils and Thrombogenesis. Prog Lipid Res, 21, 255-269.
32.   Hornstra, G (1980). Dietary Fats and Arterial Thrombosis. University of Maastricht, The Netherlands. 311.
33.   Black, KL, Culp, G, Madison, D, Randall, OS and Lands, WEM (1979). The protective effects of dietary fish oil on focal cerebral infarction. Prostaglandins and Medicine, 3, 257-268.
34.   Culp, BR, Lands, WEM, Lucchesi, BR, Pitt, B and Romson, J (1980). The effect of dietary supplementation of fish oil on experimental myocardial infarction. Prostaglandins 20,1021-1031.
35.   Weiner, BH et al (1986). Inhibition of atheroscloerosis by cod -liver oil in a hyperlipidemic swine model. N Engl J Med 315, 841-846.
36.   Morita, I, Takahashi, R, Saito, Y and Murota, S (1983). Effects of eicosapentaenoic acid on arachidonic acid metabolism in cultured vascular cells and platelet-species difference. Thromb res, 31, 211- 217.
37.   Nelson, AM (1972). Diet therapy in coronary disease. Effect on mortality of high-protein, high-seafood, fat controlled diet. Geriatrics, 27, 103-116.
38.   Saynor, R, Verel, D and Gillot, T (1984). The long-term effect of dietary supplementation with fish lipid concentrate on serum lipids, bleeding time, platelets and angina. Atherosclerosis, 50, 3-10.
39.   Kristensen, SD, Schmidt, EB, Andersen, HR and Dyerberg, J. Fish oil in angina pectoris. Atherosclerosis in press.

34
The influence of diet and drugs of cholesterol metabolism in the liver

L. Barbara, E. Roda, M. Malavolti, P. Simoni,
G. Mazzella, G. Borghi and A. Roda

The liver plays a central role in lipoprotein metabolism.
There is a close relationship between the level of LDL cholesterol
and the development of atherosclerosis (1).
In man and in several experimental animals low density lipoproteins
can be degraded by specific receptors; LDL cholesterol can also be
cleared by a LDL receptor independent mechanism, this pathway accounts usually   for about 20% of the total cholesterol uptake(1,
2). The receptor dependent uptake of LDL can be increased by drugs
as cholestiramine that causes a fecal loss of Bile Acids and an increased bile acid synthesis which is the principal way of degradation of cholesterol (3,4,5).
The hepatic LDL receptors account for the degradation of more than
50% of the circulating LDL.
In the steady state the circulating level of cholesterol carried in
LDL is determined by the rate of production of this class of lipoproteins relative to the rate at which it is removed from the circu
lation (3,6).
The diet can affect the hepatic control of lipoproteins metabolism.
The LDL receptor in the liver has been shown to be regulated so
that when hepatic cholesterol accumulates, as in cholesterol feeding, the receptor level goes down.
The hepatic LDL receptor level depends also on the type of fat present in the diet and the receptors can be expressed independently
of hepatic cholesterol level (7).
Receptor mediated transport of LDL is suppressed by about one third
in hamsters fed dietary cholesterol with polyunsaturated fat.
In contrast it is suppressed by about 90% in animals fed saturated
oil with an equivalent amount of cholesterol, even though the saturated fat-fed animals have lower liver cholesterol concentrations
than the polyunsaturated fat-fed animals (6,8).
The low plasma LDL cholesterol concentration after feeding with po-

lyunsaturated fats can be explained by a certain degree of insensitivity of the LDL receptors to down regulation.

The degree of regulation of the LDL receptor is a key factor in the tolerance of everyone to dietary cholesterol.

The individual differences in LDL receptor activity could explain the variations in serum LDL cholesterol among patients.

The liver can eliminate the excess of cholesterol in blood by the secretion of cholesterol and bile acids in bile (1,8).

The biliary secretion of an excess of cholesterol relative to bile acids and phospholipids can cause the formation of cholesterol gallstones (9).

In order to dissolve cholesterol gallstones and to increase the amount of solubilizing lipids is widely used the treatment with bile acids.

Chenodeoxycholic, a naturally occurring primary bile acid, has been used in the medical treatment of cholesterol cholelithiasis.

The oral administration of this bile acid decreases cholesterol absorption, suppresses cholesterol and bile acid synthesis; in addition during chenodeoxycholic acid treatment, the uptake of LDL by the specific LDL receptor is decreased and the level of cholesterol in blood increases.

Ursodeoxycholic acid, a bile acid that is used in alternative or in association to chenodeoxycholic acid for the treatment of gallstones in several studies has been shown unable to suppress bile acid synthesis; on the contrary some authors have found an increased bile acid synthesis after ursodeoxycholic acid treatment (11).

To an increase in bile acid synthesis should correspond a higher LDL uptake. This metabolic characteristic could explain the fact that cholesterol in blood does not increase after ursodeoxycholic treatment. (10,12).

Since in occidental society the caloric and cholesterol intake is high appears to be important the study of diets and drugs able to maintain a high degree of activation of the LDL receptor and as a consequence on low level of cholesterol in blood withouth any not tolerable restriction in food intake.

References

1) Brown, MS and Goldstein, JL (1983). Lipoprotein receptors in the liver control signals for plasma cholesterol traffic. J Clin Invest 72, 743.

2) Pittman, RC, Carew, TE, Attie, AD, Witztum, JL, Watanabe, Y and Steinberg, D (1982). Receptor-dependent and receptor-independent degradation of low density lipoprotein in normal rabbits and in receptor-deficient mutant rabbits. J Biol Chem, 257, 7994.

3) Dietschy, JM (1984). Regulation of cholesterol metabolism in man and in other species. Klin Wochenschr, 62, 338.

4) Fromm, H (1984). Gallstones dissolution and the cholesterol - bile acid - lipoprotein axis. Propition effects of ursodeoxycholic acid. Gastroenterology, 87, 229.

5) Witztum, JL, Young, SG, Elam, RL, Careu, TE and Fisher, MI(1985) Cholestyramine - induced changes in low density lipoprotein composition and metabolism. I. studies in the Guinea Pig. J Lipid Res, 26, 92.

6) Spady, DK and Dietschy,JM (1985). Dietary saturated triacylglycerols suppress hepatic low density lipoprotein receptor activity in the hamster. Proc Natl Acad Sci U.S.A., 82, 4526.

7) Schonfeld G, Patsch, W, Rudel, LL, Nelson, C, Epstein, M and Olson RE (1982). The effects of dietary cholesterol and fatty acids on plasma lipoproteins. J Clin Invest, 69, 1072.

8) Rudel, LL, Parks, JS and Carroll, RM (1983). Effects of polyunsaturated versus saturated dietary fat on non-human primate HDL. In: Dietary Fats and Health. Perkins, EG and Visek, WJ, editors. American Oil Chemists' Society, Champaign, IL, 649.

9) Admirand, W, Small, DM (1968). The physicochemical basis of cholesterol gallstone formation in man. J Clin Invest, 47, 1043.

10) Danzinger, RG, Hofmann, AF, Thistle, JL, Schoenfield, L (1973). Effect of oral chenodeoxycholic acid on bile acid kinetics and biliary lipids in women with cholelithiasis, J Clin Invest, 52, 2809.

11) Hardison , WGM, Grundy, SM (1984). Effect of ursodeoxycholate and its taurine conjugate on bile acid synthesis and cholesterol absorption. Gastroenterology, 87, 130.

12) Fromm, H, Roat, JW, Gonzales, V, Sarva, RP, Farivar, S (1983). Comparative efficacy and side effects of ursodeoxycholic and chenodeoxycholic acids in dissolving gallstones. A double blind study. Gastroenterology, 85, 1257.

35
Individuality of the response of serum cholesterol to dietary cholesterol

A.C. Beynen and M.B. Katan

INTRODUCTION

In the numerous studies which have dealt with the effect of dietary cholesterol on serum cholesterol levels in humans a striking variability in individual response was generally found (1). Certain individuals showed negligible changes in the concentration of serum cholesterol (hyporesponders), whereas others developed elevated concentrations (hyperresponders). In the literature the concept of human hyper- and hyporesponders became firmly entrenched (2, 3). However, in almost all studies the dietary challenge was only given once and thus the reproducibility of the individual cholesterolemic response was not known.

Studies with a small number of subjects who participated twice in the same type of experiment, did not provide evidence that human hypo- and hyperresponders exist. In 1942 Messinger et al. (4) fed 4 patients with various diseases a daily supplement of 150 g of egg yolk powder (providing 3750 mg cholesterol) emulsified in milk. Typical increases of 6 to 31% in serum cholesterol were observed, but the individual cholesterolemic responses were not reproducible. In fact, a patient who displayed the highest response in the first experiment, showed the lowest response in the second experiment. We have obtained similar results with healthy subjects who consumed six egg yolks (about 1500 mg cholesterol) per day for 10 days in two successive experiments one year apart (5). Three subjects showed entirely different cholesterolemic responses from one year to another. This lack of reproducibility in certain individuals is not unexpected in view of within-person variability in the level of serum cholesterol, which is of the same order of magnitude (6, 7) as the cholesterolemic responses to dietary cholesterol.

It is important to know whether individuals with a consistently low or high serum cholesterol response to dietary cholesterol do exist. Hypercholesterolemia may of course be due to monogenetic disorders, or occur secondary to other diseases or obesity, but the majority of subjects with mild hypercholesterolemia have no clearly defined defect. Many of the latter could conceivably be persons who are hyperresponsive to an affluent diet.

The subject of hypo- and hyperresponsiveness is of both practical and scientific interest. Patients with hypercholesterol-

emia generally receive dietary advice from clinicians in order to
lower their serum cholesterol levels. Frequently, such advice turns
out to be ineffective. Although lack of compliance may be involved,
it is possible that certain patients are insensitive to cholesterol-
lowering diets and need a different form of therapy. It is assumed
here that subjects hypo- and hyperresponsive to cholesterol-lowering
diets are also hypo- and hyperresponsive, respectively, to hypercholesterolemic diets. From the scientific point of view elucidation
of the mechanism underlying hypo- and hyperresponsiveness may shed
more light on the relations between dietary components and cholesterol metabolism.

CONSISTENT HYPO- AND HYPERRESPONDERS TO DIETARY CHOLESTEROL

We have carried out three controlled dietary trials with the same
subjects to address the question whether individuals do exist with
a consistently high or low serum cholesterol response to dietary
cholesterol (8). In each trial the volunteers successively consumed
a low- and a high-cholesterol diet, the cholesterol component of
the diets (provided by egg yolk) being the only variable. Standardized regression coefficients for individual responses (n=32) in
one experiment as a function of the response in a previous experiment ranged from 0.34 to 0.53 (Fig. 1).

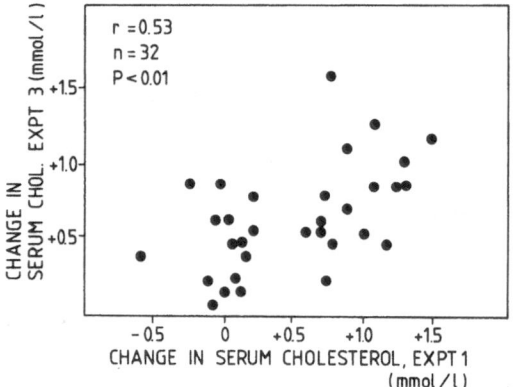

FIGURE 1   Relationship between the individual responses of serum
    cholesterol to dietary cholesterol observed in two different
    experiments. In expt 1 the volunteers successively consumed
    10 and 55 mg of cholesterol/MJ; in expt 3 these values were
    15 and 35 mg/MJ. Reproduced with permission from Beynen et al.
    (9).

Under less controlled conditions we found similar results. In
1976 Bronsgeest-Schoute et al. (10) studied the serum cholesterol

response to cessation of egg consumption in subjects who habitually consumed at least one egg per day. When eggs were eliminated from the diet, daily cholesterol intake decreased from about 800 mg to 300 mg. Mean serum cholesterol fell only slightly (by 3%), but the individual responses varied from -20% to +8%. In 1982, we re-investigated 34 of these subjects (11), and at our request they again eliminated eggs and egg-containing products from their diet. The differences in serum cholesterol response between individuals were partly reproducible; the individual responses in 1976 and 1982 were positively correlated (Fig. 2).

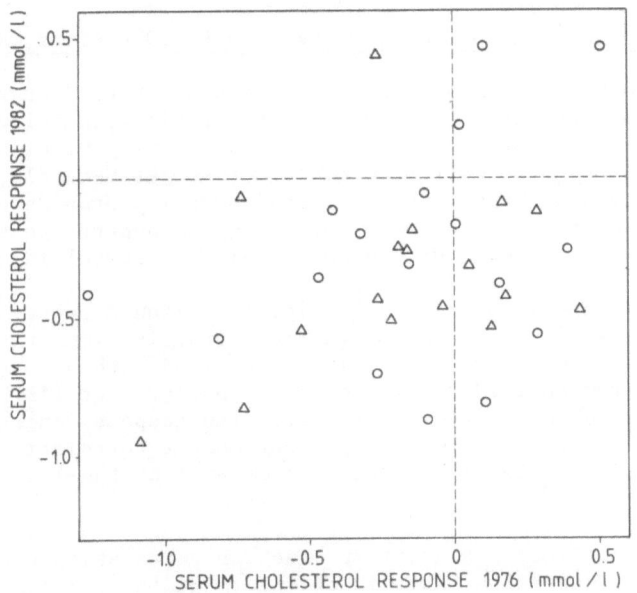

FIGURE 2   Relationship between the cholesterolemic responses to cessation of egg consumption.Subjects participated in a trial in 1976 and again in 1982. The correlation between successive responses was 0.32 (n=34, P<0.05). Reproduced with permission from Beynen and Katan (11).

It could be argued that we observed a consistent response in serum cholesterol because some of our subjects consistently replaced their eggs by low-fat, low-cholesterol foods, and others replaced by cheese or fat-rich meat. Two subjects who were consistently hyperresponsive and four subjects who were consistently hyporesponsive to cessation of egg consumption therefore participated in a follow-up study with strictly controlled diets. The subjects were given 72 mg of cholesterol/MJ for 4 weeks followed by 11 mg/MJ for another 4 weeks; all other nutrients were kept constant. The two hyperresponders and three of the four hyporesponders proved to be also hyper- and hyporesponsive under the controlled conditions (12).

Thus it appears that at least part of the cholesterolemic response to dietary cholesterol in man is individually determined. It is also clear that one will always find subjects who appear hyperresponsive in one experiment and hyporesponsive in another. This is caused by the diet-independent within-person variability of serum cholesterol. Nevertheless, from these repeated experiments with the same subjects it can be concluded that human hypo- and hyperresponders to dietary cholesterol do exist.

CHARACTERISTICS OF HYPO- AND HYPERRESPONDERS TO DIETARY CHOLESTEROL

The characteristics of hypo- and hyperresponders to dietary cholesterol are of interest for several reasons. First, knowledge of the hyperresponder profile may help in identifying beforehand which patients will benefit most from dietary therapy. Secondly, the characteristics of hypo- and hyperresponders may provide clues as to the metabolic basis not only for hypo- and hyperresponsiveness, but also for the effects of diet on serum cholesterol levels in general.

In our controlled trials (8, Fig. 1) we found no relation of responsiveness with age, sex, intestinal transit time, ratio of primary to secondary steroids in the feces and within-subject variability of serum cholesterol while on a constant diet (13). Table 1 shows the variables that did correlate with responsiveness on the basis of the calculated Pearson product-moment correlation coefficients. Both serum total and HDL_2 cholesterol on the low and

Table 1. Statistically significant Pearson correlation coefficients and multiple regression analysis of determinants of responsiveness of serum cholesterol to dietary cholesterol in 32 subjects

Characteristic	Univariate r	Multivariate t value
Serum total cholesterol	0.31	2.1*
HDL_2 cholesterol	0.39	2.2*
Body mass index	-0.50	NS
Body cholesterol synthesis	-0.40	NS
Habitual cholesterol intake	-0.62	5.2**

Responsiveness was defined as the difference in serum total cholesterol level between the high- and low-cholesterol diet period, averaged over three different experiments. *, $P<0.05$; **, $P<0.01$; NS = not significant. Based on Katan and Beynen (13).

high-cholesterol diets were positively associated with responsiveness to dietary cholesterol. It should be stressed that the values for serum total cholesterol and those for calculating the responsiveness variable were based on independent sets of measurements.

Thus hyperresponders tended to have higher levels of serum total, but also of HDL$_2$ cholesterol concentrations than hyporesponders.

Body mass index, total body cholesterol synthesis (based on sterol balance data) and the habitual intake of cholesterol were negatively associated with the cholesterolemic response to dietary cholesterol. Multivariate analysis was performed to take into account the correlations among the variables with predictive value. It then appeared that body mass index and body cholesterol synthesis did not longer contribute significantly to the explanation of variance in responsiveness (Table 1).

In conclusion, our repeated controlled studies suggest that a low habitual cholesterol intake, a high serum HDL$_2$ cholesterol level, or a low body weight do not make one less susceptible to dietary-cholesterol-induced hypercholesterolemia. The negative association of the response of serum cholesterol with body mass index and the positive association with HDL cholesterol were also seen in another cohort, where the effect of cessation of egg consumption on serum cholesterol was studied in subjects who habitually consumed at least one egg/day (11). Similar associations were reported by Oh and Miller (14) who challenged 21 subjects with three eggs/day.

These external validations lend some credence to the relationships that we found. Still we should stress that these relationships were of necessity the product of an extensive exploration of the data, and thus could still turn out to be spurious. Our present aim is to link differences in responsiveness to differences in the nucleotide sequences of the genes that code for proteins involved in cholesterol metabolism. We hope that such studies will in the long term provide a rational explanation of hypo- and hyperresponder phenomena.

ACKNOWLEDGEMENTS

Our studies were supported by the Netherlands Heart Foundation. Thanks are due to I. Zaalmink for typing this manuscript.

REFERENCES

1.   McGill Jr, HC (1979). The relationship of dietary cholesterol to serum cholesterol concentration and to atherosclerosis in man. *Am J Clin Nutr*, 32, 2664

2.   Connor, WE and Connor, SL (1972). The key role of nutritional factors in the prevention of coronary heart disease. *Prev Med*, 1, 49

3.   Reiser, R (1978). Oversimplification of diet: coronary heart disease relationships and exaggerated diet recommendations. *Am J Clin Nutr*, 31, 865

4.   Messinger, WJ, Porosowska, Y and Steele, JM (1950). Effect of feeding egg yolk and cholesterol on serum cholesterol levels. *Arch Intern Med*, 86, 189

5.   Katan, MB and Beynen, AC (1983). Hyper-response to dietary cholesterol in man. *Lancet*, 1, 1213

6.   Keys, A (1967). Blood lipids in man: a brief review. *J Am Diet Ass*, 51, 508

7.   Demacker, PNM, Schade, RWB, Jansen, RTP and Van 't Laar, A (1982). Intra-individual variation of serum cholesterol, trigly-cerides and high density lipoprotein cholesterol in normal humans. *Atherosclerosis*, 45, 259

8.   Katan, MB, Beynen, AC, De Vries, JHM and Nobels, A (1986). Existence of consistent hyper- and hyporesponders to dietary chole-sterol in man. *Am J Epidemiol*, 123, 221

9.   Beynen, AC, Katan, MB and Van Zutphen, LFM (1985). Indivi-duelle Unterschiede der Serumcholesterinreaktion auf Aenderungen der Ernährungsform. *Ernährungs-Umschau*, 32, 356

10.   Bronsgeest-Schoute, DC, Hermus, RJJ, Dallinga-Thie, GM and Hautvast, JGAJ (1979). Dependence of the effects of dietary chole-sterol and experimental conditions on serum lipids in man. III. The effect on serum cholesterol of removal of eggs from the diet of free-living habitually egg-eating people. *Am J Clin Nutr* 32, 2193

11.   Beynen, AC and Katan, MB (1985). Reproducibility of the variations between humans in the response of serum cholesterol to cessation of egg consumption. *Atherosclerosis*, 57, 19

12.   Beynen, AC, Katan, MB and Van Gent, CM (1986). Endogenous cholesterol synthesis, fecal steroid excretion and serum lanosterol in subjects with high or low response of serum cholesterol to dietary cholesterol. *Clin Nutr*, 5, 151

13.   Katan, MB and Beynen, AC (1987). Characteristics of human hypo- and hyperresponders to dietary cholesterol. *Am J Epidemiol*, in press

14.   Oh, SY and Miller, LT (1985). Effect of dietary egg on variability of plasma cholesterol levels and lipoprotein chole-sterol. *Am J Clin Nutr*, 42, 421

36
Familial hypercholesterolemia in Italy; plasma cholesterol evaluation and diagnostic insight

A. Gaddi, A. Braiato, M. Marra, G.L. Magri,
M. Mezzetti, A. Minardi, Z. Sangiorgi and
G.C. Descovich

INTRODUCTION

Familial Hypercholesterolemias (FH), well characterized from the genetic and clinical points of view, actually represent a "diagnostic problem" for the general practitioner.
In fact, the undoubted diagnosis can be drawn on the basis of skin fibroblast (or, perhaps, lymphocyte and lymphoblastoid cell) B-E receptor activity assay [1,2]. This assay is very expensive and requires advanced technologies, thus resulting not available for the large majority of people.
Obviously, if homozygous FH is suspected, B-E receptor analysis is imperative; but this method is not always useful or nearby in heterozygous patient detection. However, heterozygous FH are a relevant social problem both for the high prevalence (1/250 - 1/500) and for the close linkage with premature CHD, particularly in males.

In the last few years several diagnostic criteria have been proposed, other than direct receptor assay: xantomata and/or xantelasma occurrence, Achilles tendon thickness evaluation, premature atheromasia in coronary or other vascular districts, pedigree analysis; several total- and/or LDL- cholesterol cut-off points were also suggested, and within analysis for other hyperlipidemias exclusion (Tab. I) [1-5].
The pedigree analysis seems the better, even if its diagnostic sensibility and specificity are closely related to the number of relatives undergoing plasma cholesterol evaluation.
On the contrary, other diagnostic criteria (particularly, the presence of skin or artery cholesterol depositions) will be regarded with criticism: in fact, if these are assumed as "diagnostic", we cannot define the clinical picture really exhibited by heterozygous FH of different races.

Thus, a research programme started in 1986, under the patronage of the Emilia Romagna Region, to define the prevalence and clinical picture of FH in our country, and to identify the best criteria for inheritance pattern analysis and the sensibility and specificity of different laboratory diagnostic procedures.
In this paper, the significance of total and LDL cholesterol evaluation in plasma will be discussed regarding the definition of an exact "diagnostic" confidence range, both for each individual and for the whole .family, thus decreasing the number of false positive or negative patients who will undergo more extensive and expensive diagnostic procedures.

SUMMARY OF METHODS

A-PATIENTS: among 550 subjects (60 families) with primitive stable hypercholesterolemia, 247 subjects of the Emilia Romagna Region were recruited (m= 128, f= 119 ; age mean m= 39.9, f= 45.6 yr; age I generation= 67.6 +- 12.3, IV generation= 17.7 +- 6.3; number of families= 29, generation/family= 3.1; subjects/family= 8.5). The enrolment criteria were the following:
1- 50% of relatives for each family (absolute number approximation to 50% evaluated by non parametric tests) with: LDL-C > 230 mg/dl, VLDL-TG < 120 mg/dl, HDL-C between the 5th and the 95th percentile of control populaton of the same geographical area, AND
2- LDL-C bimodal distribution in each family, AND
3- clearly evident vertical transmission of the trait.
Moreover, B-E receptor activity was evaluated on fibroblasts in selected patients (data to be published).

B- CONTROLS: unaffected relatives (+/+) of FH patients (+/Rb×) and several Emilia Romagna free living population samples, already screened for epidemiologic studies on atherosclerosis risk factors [6-7].

C- LABORATORY: blood sampling, plasma separation and storage as described elsewhere [8].
- Total plasma cholesterol (TC), triglycerides (TG), HDL cholesterol (HDL-C) evaluation by methods advised by Italian Lipid Clinics, by National Research Council (NRC) of Italy and by NHI [9-10].
- Preparative ultracentrifugation and lipid - lipoprotein analysis as described in [11].
- Plasma apo AI and B by radial immunodifusion.
- Apoprotein isoform patterns by isoelectrofocusing and bi-dimensional PAGE electrophoresis.

- Skin fibroblasts cultures and B-E receptor analysis by
I labeled LDL.

Standardization and quality control: according to other
Italian Lipid Clinics and WHO Lipid Reference Center of
Prague.
Anamnestic records (smoking, physical activity, stress,
history of angor, TIA, stroke, AMI) and clinical,
anthropometric and instrumental (EKG) determinations were
collected as previously reported [6-8] according to the
Italian National Research Council (NRC) standardized
procedures. Nutritional habits, drug consumption by NRC
questionnaires and by seven day record.
Fatal and non fatal new events (propositus, living
parents and offsprings) were classified according to WHO
(8th ICD revision) or (ancestors) on the basis of hard
diagnostic criteria, supported by hospital record, as
described elsewhere [12].

Statistical analysis was performed by BA & S Cumputer
Hard Programme Systems.

RESULTS AND DISCUSSION

Several cut-off points were recently adopted in diagnosis
of FH heterozygous (+/Rb^x: x= "o", or "-" or "i=o")
patients: TC > 250 mg/dl [3], > 273 [13], > 300 [14-15],
or LDL-C >220 mg/dl [13], > 250 mg/dl [15], etc..
In childhood, LDL-C > 148 mg/dl is regarded as expressive
of high CHD risk [16] and possibly related to FH gene.
Table I shows TC mean values in FH (+/Rb^x) of different
Countries; TC cut off points adopted, even if not always
clearly reported by Authors, are deducible by range or by
SD.
It is possible that differences observed among several
studies (Tab I) are actually related to race differences
(as example in LDL production rate), as described for
multigenic hypercholesterolemias [17]; perhaps, in some
studies, patients affected by other, recently described,
hypercholesterolemias may also exist [18-19].
But, more probably, differences in diagnostic criteria
adopted (clinical, instrumental, biochemical, etc) can
explain discordances in mean values and ranges of total
plasma cholesterol. Thus, data are not clearly comparable
and the real influence of race is not exactly definable.

TABLE I: TOTAL PLASMA CHOLESTEROL MEAN VALUES IN SEVERAL STUDIES
ON FAMILIAL HYPERCHOLESTEROLEMIC HETEROZYGOUS PATIENTS

COUNTRY (**)	AGE (year)	SEX	n	TC (mg/dl) mean	SD	range	YEAR	AUTOR	REFERENCE
Australia	51-80	m+f	9	381	89	273-501	1983	Simons LA	(13)
Belgium	34-60	m+f	5	383	58	319-472	1985	Malmendier CL	(15)
China	adults	m+f	--	270	--		1985	Hai-Jiang Cai	(20)
Germany	adults	m+f	10	374	81		1985	Weisweiler P	(21)
Italy	20-60	m+f	30	410	72	310-550	1984	Gaddi A	(8)
Italy	2-78	m+f	247	380	60	> 280	1987	This study	(-)
Israel	2-17	m+f	67	211	52		1979	Heldenberg D	(16)
Japan	adults	m	44	329	64		1985	Yoshimura A	(22)
Japan	adults	f	17	360	65		1985	Yoshimura A	(22)
Japan	5-67	m+f	68	369	100	255-684 (*)	1977	Mabuchi H	(3)
Japan	36-61	m+f	10	378	44	315-469	1983	Mabuchi H	(14)
Netherlands	22-69	m+f	43	440	77	326-629	1986	Mol MJT	(4)
South Africa	25-58	m+f	19	351	57	251-501	1984	Westhuyzen DR	(2)
United Kingdom	14-56	m+f	11	381	54		1985	Durrington PN	(5)
United States	< 2	m+f	6	212	60		1980	Gluek CJ	(23)
United States	2-7	m+f	16	312	32		1980	Gluek CJ	(23)
United States	>= 20	m+f	105	368	70		1974	Kwiterovich PO	(1)
United States	< 19	m+f	88	299	63		1974	Kwiterovich PO	(1)

(*) Two patients aged <10 yr (8 yr: 283 mg/dl; 6 yr: 684 mg/dl).
(**) More exhaustive indications about TC mean values in different populations of FH in
Goldstein JL and Brown MS review [1].

To avoid the possibility of misleading diagnosis, we
assume: a) that the gene inheritance pattern has the most
diagnostic power, b) that the diagnosis must be directed
at the families and not only the individuals, c) that in
each family the presence of all the other hyperlipidemias
(including heavy multigenic hypercholesterolemias, even
very frequent) must be excluded.
In this manner, obviously also supported by several
laboratory determinations (see C), among 60 families in
which TC levels were higher than 300 mg/dl in about 50%
of members, only 29 kindred were selected, without
considering the clinical picture or CHD history.
On the basis of the data collected in these 29 families,
for our population a TC limit (280 mg/dl) was defined
discriminating between "more probable" FH patients and
"more probable" non-FH cases. This CT cut-off point
represents the mid point between the modal CT values of
FH (+/Rb^x) and of unaffected relatives (+/+) (Figure 1)
(+/+ subjects showed the same CT distribution as in the
control population).
This criterion, according to Murphy [24] identifies the

point at which the risk of mistakes (due to false negatives or false positives) is the lowest.
Obviously, if the 280 mg/dl cut is adopted for the identification of a single FH patient, a residual misleading possibility will exist (10% or more).

FIGURE 1

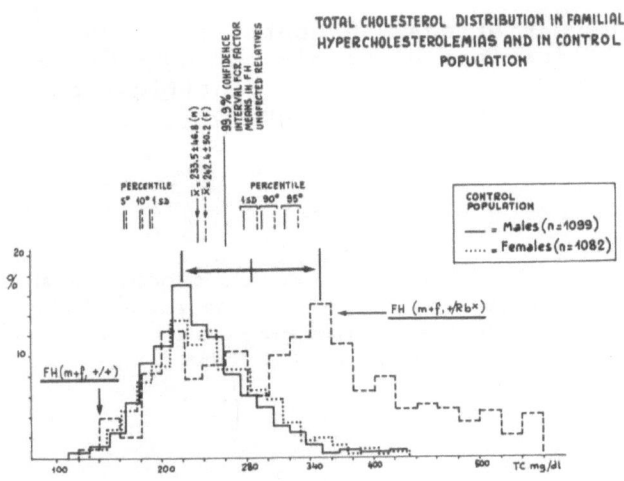

However, in families of few or no cooperating members, in which pedigree analysis is not possible, this cut-off point should be truly diagnostic, particularly if at least two affected relatives are identified; for small families, in which only one suspected +/Rb× patient is present, diagnosis must not be drawn.
On the contrary, in large - really FH - families (6-8 subjects or more) if CT mean values of all +/Rb× (>280 mg/dl) are compared to those of +/+ subjects (<= 280 mg/dl), the discriminative power of this cut-off point results very high (Figure 2), and the probability of an erroneous diagnosis is lower than 0.001. Perhaps, if at the same time a multigenic inheritance for hypercholesterolemia is present, the "blank" area around 280 mg/dl (Fig. 2) will be reduced or lacking, thus increasing the misleading diagnosis probability, but also suggesting (if TC modal and mean values of the family are both higher than 280) the presence of two combined genetic defects (autosomic dominant + multigenic).
This cut-off point might also be adopted for +/Rb× patients showing concurrent apo E2 allele (heterozygous and, perhaps, homozygous too). In fact, as previously

reported [25], +/Rb˟ E3/E2 patients show a TC mean value lower than other E genotypes (377.3 +- 22.6 mg/dl versus 389.2 +- 12.7 mg/dl in E3/E3 and 430.4 +- 27.9 mg/dl in E3/E4), but always much higher than 280 mg/dl.
In any case, the identification of: a) surely "FH-only" families, and b) families with FH + severe multigenic inheritance for hypercholesterolemia, and c) surely multigenic inheritance families (or other IIa phenotype causes) can be easily obtained (examples in Figure 2), and the border-line cases will be reduced to a very small number.
Age-related variations, spontaneous and/or therapy induced modifications of total- and LDL- cholesterol, and R^(b--o) or R^(b--) heterozygous identification will be described in a forthcoming paper.

FIGURE 2

TC mean values and 99.9% intervals of confidence (ic), calculated in all affected relatives (+/Rb˟) or unaffected relatives (+/+) in each FH kindred (n=29). Interrupted lines (99.9 ic) delimit a "blank" area around 280 mg/dl. TC mean values in multigenic hypercholesterolemia families are also shown.

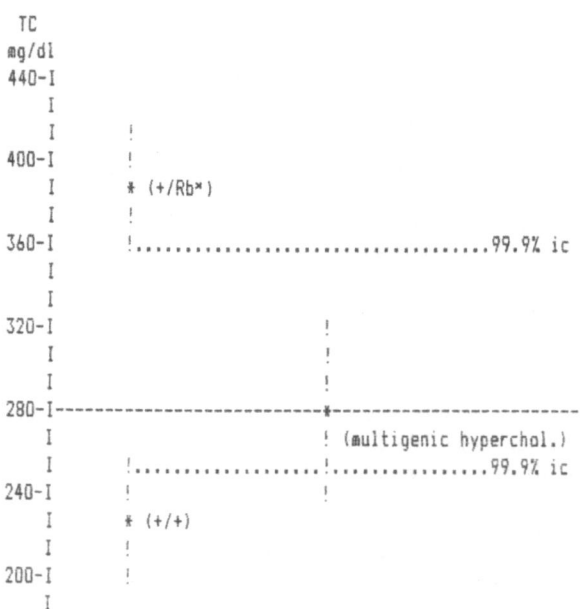

This study was partially supported by a grant of Health Dept. of Emilia Romagna Region and of Bologna University. We gratefully acknowledge Prof. G. Ghiselli (Baylor College of Medicine, Houston) and Prof. D. Grafnetter (WHO Lipid Reference Centre, Prague) for their continuous support in method standardization and quality control; Prof. S. Calandra and Prof. R. Tiozzo-Costa (Institute of General Pathology, Modena University) for skin fibroblast analysis; Prof. Cavicchi (Institute of Genetics, Bologna University) for the suggestions on data analysis and Dr. Giulia Gaddi for help in translation.

REFERENCES

1- Goldstein JL, Brown MS (1983). Familial Hypercholesterolemias. In: Stanbury JB, Wyngaarden JB, Fredrickson DS, Goldstein JL, Brown MS (eds) Metabolic Basis of Inherited Diseases. Mc Graw-Hill BC, pag 675.

2- Van der Westhuyzen DR, Coetzee GA, Demasius IP, Harley EH, Gevers W, Baker SG, Seftel HC (1984). Low density lipoprotein receptor mutations in South African homozygous familial hypercholesterolemic patients. Arteriosclerosis, 4 (3), 238.

3- Mabuchi H, Ito S, Haba T, Ueda R, Tatami R, Kametami T, Koizumi J, Otha M, Miyamoto S, Takeda R, Takegoshi T (1977). Discrimination of familial hypercholesterolemia and secondary hypercholesterolemia by Achilles' Tendon thickness. Atherosclerosis 28, 61.

4- Mol MJTM, Erkelens DW, Gevers Leuven JA, Schouten JA, Stalenhoef AFH (1986). Effects of synvinolin (MK-733) on plasma lipids in familial hypercholesterolemias. Lancet ii, 936.

5- Durrington PN and Miller JP (1985). Double-blind, placebo-controlled, cross-over trial of Probucol in heterozygous familial hypercholesterolemias. Atherosclerosis 55, 187.

6- Descovich GC, Gaddi A, Mannino G, Lenzi S (1981). L' indagine di Brisighella. I Fattori di Rischio Metabolici. Giorn It Cardiol 11, 1591.

7- National Research Council Atherosclerosis Research Group (1981). Atherosclerosis risk factors in nine italian population samples. Am J Epidemiol 11, 368.

8- Gaddi A, Lenzi S, Magri GL, Sangiorgi Z, Descovich GC (1984). Improvement in the Mediteranean diet for hypercholesterolaemia correction using soy bean protein. In: Lenzi S, Descovich GC, (eds) "Atherosclerosis and Cardiovascular Diseases". Lancaster-Boston-The Hague: MTP Press, 456.

9- National Research Council (1977). Laboratory Methods in Atherosclerosis Risk Factor Study. Ed. Dedalo, Bari, Vol I, pag 1.

10- Manual of Laboratory Operations, Lipid Research Clinic Programme: Lipid and Lipoprotein Analysis (1974). DHEW Public, no (NHI) 75, 628.

11- Lindgren FI, Jensen LC, Hacth FT (1972). The isolation and quantitative analysis of serum lipoproteins. In: Wilson G (ed) "Blood Lipids and Lipoproteins", Wiley e Sons Inc, pag 181.

12- Mezzetti M, Gaddi A, Rimondi S, Descovich GC, Lenzi S (1987). Familial Hypercholesterolemias in Emilia-Romagna Region. In: Lenzi S, Descovich GC (eds): "Atherosclerosis and Cardiovascular Disesas prevention and therapy". Ed. Compositori, Bologna, in press.

13- Simons LA, Balasubramaniam S, Holland J (1983). Low density lipoprotein metabolism in the normal to moderately elevated range of plasma cholesterol: comparisons with familial hypercholesterolemias. J Lipid Res 24, 192.

14- Mabuchi HM, Sakai T, Sakay Y, Yoshimura A, Watanabe A, Wakasugi T, Koizumi J, Takeda R (1983). Reduction of serum cholesterol in heterozygous patients with familial hypercholesterolemias. New Engl J Med, 308, 609.

15- Malmendier CL, Delcroix C (1985). Effects of Fenofibrate on high and low density lipoprotein metabolism in heterozygous familial hypercholesterolemia. Atherosclerosis 85, 21.

16- Heldenberg D, Tamir I, Levtow O, Burnstein Y, Werbin B. (1979). Lipoprotein measurements - a necessity for precise assessment of risk in children from high risk families. Arch Dis Child 54, 695.

17- International Collaborative Study Group (1986). Metabolic epidemiology of plasma cholesterol. Mechanisms of variation of plasma cholesterol within populations and between populations. Lancet, ii, 991.

18- Vega GL, Grundy SM (1986). In vivo evidence for reduced binding of LDL to receptors as a cause of primary moderate hypercholesterolemia. J Clin Invest 78 (5), 1410.

19- Levy RA, Ostlund RE jr, Semenkovich CF, Witztum JL (1986). Diversity in expression of heterozygous familial hypercholesterolemia. Characterization of a unique kindred. J Clin Invest 78 (1), 96.

20- Hai-Jiang Cai (1985). Homozygous familial hypercholesterolemic patients in China. 7th Int Symp on Atherosclerosis, Melbourne, October 1985, (n' 8).

21- Weisweiler P, Merk W, Jacob B, Schandt P (1985). Effect of combined treatment with Fenofibrate and Colestipol in familial hypercholesterolemias. 7th Int Symp on Atherosclerosis, Melbourne, October 1985, (n' 453).

22- Yoshimura A, Wakasugi T, Nakayama A, Mabuchi H, Genda A, Takeda R (1985). Coronary angiographic characteristics in patients with familial hypercholesterolemias. 7th Int Symp on Atherosclerosis, Melbourne, October 1985, (n' 37).

23- Glueck CJ, Tsang RC, Mellies MJ (1980). Long-term (2 to 6 yr) therapy of familial hypercholesterolemias and hypertriglyceridemias in childhood. In: Lauer RM, Shekelle RB (eds) "Childhood prevention of atherosclerosis and hypertension", Raven Press, New York, pag 155.

24- Murphy EA and Kwiterovich PO (1977). Genetics pf the hyperlipoproteinemias. In: Rifkind BM, Levy RI (eds) "Hyperlipidemia, diagnosis and theraphy", Grune & Stratton, New York, pag 217.

25- Gaddi A, Sangiorgi Z, Perini P, Ghiselli G, Descovich GC (1987). Hypocholesterolemic effects of soy protein diet and apoprotein E isoforms. Eur Rew Med Pharmac Sci, in press.

EXTRA CORONARY ATHEROSCLEROTIC VASCULAR DISEASES

37
Do atherosclerotic plaques regress spontaneously in humans?

U. Senin, G. Lupattelli, L. Parnetti, A. Susta
M. Mercuri, G. Ciuffetti and A. Ventura

INTRODUCTION

While human atherosclerosis is generally a progressive disease, it has been observed that regression may also occur.

The angiographic literature on regression has shown that besides being induced by therapies treating major atherosclerosis risk factors (1, 2), regression may occur "spontaneously" in rare cases (3, 4, 5). This phenomenon was observed more recently by Hennerici et al.(1985) using an ultrasound imaging system which, as we know, overcomes in part the limitations inherent in the angiographic methods used in the earlier studies cited.

Our aim in this present project was to contribute to the pool of the knowledge available today on the natural evolution of atheromasic lesions and on spontaneous regression in particular. We report here the results of a two year follow-up on atheromasic lesions of the extracranial carotid tract.

MATERIALS AND METHODS

This study was carried out on 118 extracranial carotid tract lesions observed in 70 patients(59 males, 11 females, average age 61+7 years) referred to our Centre for Non Invasive Vascular Diagnosis for TIA, CHD, PAD, cervical bruits. 19 patients were affected by one of these conditions, 51 patients by two or more. 61 patients were suffering from one or more of the major atherosclerosis risk factors(hypercholesterolemia, diabetes mellitus, hypertension, cigarette smoking).

Exclusion criteria were atherosclerotic lesions causing a degree of vascular stenosis greater than 60% and cholesterol levels > 300 mg/dl because those patients were admitted to pharmaceutical and/or surgical trials. We have also excluded lesions with a stenosis degree of less than 15% because, in our experience, their echo-

Acknowledgements: The authors would like to thank Mrs GA Boyd Mancinelli BA (Hons) for her help in the translation of this paper.

structure could not always be well defined. Treatment of the patients admitted to our follow-up was left to the discretion of the referring physician.

Instrumental Equipment

The echotomographic analysis of the lesions was carried out using a Biosound with an electromechanical probe of 4 cm/8MHz, the axial resolution being 0.3 mm and the lateral resolution 0.5 mm. During the two year follow-up ultrasound studies were carried out at least every 6 months. The patient's position and the scanning planes used were standard for the ultrasound imaging of the carotid bifurcation (7).

Lesions Characteristics Monitored: echogenicity, surface aspects and stenosis degree.

Echogenicity:plaques were subdivided into 4 echogenic patterns, "soft", "intermediate", "mixed", "hard". The "soft" were low-reflecting lesions, the "intermediate" reflected moderately, the "mixed" showed a non homogeneous echogenicity with or without a shadow cone, the "hard" were extremely high-reflecting accompanied by a black shadow cone.

Surface aspects: regular or irregular.

Stenosis degree: this was calculated using the following formula

$$\frac{D_t - D_r}{D_t} \times 100$$

where D_t= the total diameter of the vessel lumen and D_r= the residual diameter, both being calculated at the maximal extrinsec point of the lesion. The lesions were then subdivided into three classes of stenosis: 15 - 30%, 31 - 50%, 51 - 60%.

Validation Study of Real-time (B-Mode) Ultrasound

This method for defining the stenosis degree was validated by a comparison with both angiographic findings (8), and histomorphometric tests on endoarterectomy samples (9, 10). Intra- and interobserver reliability for both the stenosis degree and the echogenic characteristics of the lesions, through 'blind' readings of the video echographic images was calculated using the variation coefficient.

Evolution index

Lesions were considered modified if the percentage variation of the stenosis degree was at least $\pm$ 8% (intra- and interobserver variation coefficient for the stenosis degree: $\pm$ 5%) and/or if the echogenic pattern changed.

RESULTS

The following behaviour pattern in stenosis degree was observed after our two year follow-up. 80 (=68%) of the lesions remained unchanged, 38 (=32%) progressed, but none regressed.

Separate analyses were therefore performed on the behaviour patterns of the three parameters monitored (echogenicity, surface characteristics and initial stenosis degree) compared to the modifications in the stenosis observed at the end of the two year follow-up. "Mixed" and "hard" lesions resulted more prone to progression (Table 1 A), while plaques with an irregular surface showed a greater progressive tendency than those with a regular surface (Table 1 B). An initial stenosis degree of less than 50% did not appear to influence atheromasic plaque progression (Table 1 C).

TABLE 1: CAROTID STENOSIS MODIFICATIONS AFTER A TWO YEAR FOLLOW-UP ACCORDING TO: A) ECHOGENIC PATTERN, B) SURFACE CHARACTERISTICS, C) VASCULAR STENOSIS, AS OBSERVED AT THE BEGINNING OF THE STUDY.

At the beginning		After two years	
A) Echogenic pattern		Stenosis	
		unchanged	progressed
	N.		
soft	20	13 (65%)	7 (35%)
intermediate	56	45 (81%)	11 (19%)
mixed	28	15 (54%)	13 (46%)
hard	14	7 (50%)	7 (50%)
B) Surface		Stenosis	
		unchanged	progressed
	N.		
regular	94	68 (73%)	26 (27%)
irregular	24	14 (59%)	10 (41%)
C) Stenosis		Stenosis	
		unchanged	progressed
	N.		
15 - 30%	56	38 (68%)	18 (32%)
31 - 50%	56	39 (70%)	17 (30%)
51 - 60%	6	3 (50%)	3 (50%)

The analysis of the results was completed by observing the evolution of the echogenic pattern during the follow-up. The general tendency of all the echogenic classes studied is to evolve towards higher level echoes. Regression to lower level echoes was limited to a movement from the hard class to the mixed (Table 2)

TABLE 2:ECHOGENIC PATTERN MODIFICATION OF CAROTID PLAQUES AFTER A TWO YEAR FOLLOW-UP.

At the beginning		After two years			
	N.	soft	intermediate	mixed	hard
soft	20	6	11	3	0
intermediate	56	0	43	4	9
mixed	28	0	0	26	2
hard	14	0	0	3	11

No correlation was documented between changes in the echogenic pattern and modifications in the stenosis degree, which increased in approximately 30% of the plaques monitored whether or not changes occurred in the echogenic pattern.

CONCLUSIONS

Modifications in the degree of vessel stenosis were observed in 32% of the lesions studied. In fact they progressed, while 68% remained unchanged.

A profile of the lesion most prone to progression emerged from an analysis of the intrinsic plaque characteristics (echogenicity, surface, initial vessel stenosis): it has an irregular surface; it is either a "mixed" with a non homogeneous echogenicity or else a "hard" highly reflecting plaque. These echogenic patterns most probably reflect complicated atherosclerotic lesions with internal calcifications, thrombi and haemorrhages (11, 12). The irregular surface especially if ulcerated, might cause the development of thrombi and therefore lesion progression. The initial degree of vessel stenosis does not seem to be a determining factor in progression, probably because of the fact that the majority of lesions we studied - 112 out of 118 - had a stenosis degree of less than 50%. However 3 of the remaining 6 lesions, where the stenosis degree was greater than 50%, progressed during the follow-up and the significance of this fact certainly should not be underestimated. In fact earlier studies have shown the importance of the advanced initial stenosis degree in the development and progression of the lesion(13).

Modification in the echogenic patterns, our other evolution index, was observed in 27% of the lesions. These modifications were not, however, correlated with stenosis degree progression. An analy-

292

sis of the trend observed in these modifications would seem to indicate the natural evolution of lesions:they always progress· towards
higher echogenic levels, and no possibility exists of returning to
lower levels. "Soft" plaques, probably of recent formation and high
lipid content, modify their echogenic pattern mainly towards the
"intermediate" class as their fibrous content increases.

The majority of "intermediate" plaques remain stable.· Where modifications occurred they could only be the reflection of complications - intra-plaque thrombi, haemorrhages and calcifications - and
the " intermediate" then become "mixed" or "hard". A reciprocal
inter-change may occur in these last two classes. In fact when the
calcified content of the "mixed" increases they may become"hard",
and the "hard" may undergo modifications because of the high level
of vascularization existing in calcified plaques,as ·Beeuwkes has already observed.

The fact that no case of spontaneous regression was documented
may be due to the relative rarity of the phenomenon even in studies
on larger number of patients than ours (3,4),and in studies analysing
larger numbers of vascular segments (5);a longer period of follow-up
may perhaps also be necessary to observe regression of atherosclerotic lesions in the extracranial carotid tract. Finally, another
factor may have been our exclusion of minimal lesions (stenosis degree < 15%); in fact the cases of spontaneous regression documented
by Hennerici using an analogous instrument to ours (high resolution
- 10MHz - ultrasound Duplex system) were all observed in minimal lesions.

On the other hand we would like to underline the fact that an
observed regression ·may not signify a stable and definitive stage in
lesion evolution: regression mechanisms are multiple and complex and
may indicate only a further step towards progression. The most obvious examples of a "false" regression may be the result of a discharge of atheromatous material from an ulcerated plaque into the
lumen, or the incorporation of thrombi into the vessel wall where
they are organized and retracted. In both the above mentioned examples the degree of vessel stenosis is reduced, but again in both
cases the next stage is a superimposed thrombus which continues the
process of lesion progression.

We hope that the continuation of our follow-up on an even greater
number of patients and of lesions may provide some of the answers
to the problems we have raised.

REFERENCES

1· Malinow,MR (1981).Regression of Atherosclerosis in Humans:Fact
or Myth? Circulation, 64, 1.
2. Olsson, AG, Erikson, U, Helmius, G, Hemmingsson, A, Holme, I

and Ruhn, G (1986). The effect of pronounced serum lipid lowering
for one year on the development of femoral atherosclerosis in
asymptomatic hyperlipoproteinemia. In: Fidge, NH and Nestel, PJ
(eds.) "Atherosclerosis VII".p.89. (Amsterdam Excerpta Medica).

3. Gensini, GF, Esente, P and Kelly,A (1974). Natural history of
coronary disease in patients with and without coronary by-pass
graft surgery. Circulation, 49, 98.

4. Bruschke, AVG, Wijers, TS, Kolsters, W and Landmann,T (1981).
The anatomic evolution of coronary artery disease demonstrated
by coronary arteriography in 256 Nonoperated patients.Circula-
tion, 63, 527.

5. Brown, BG, Bolson,EL, Pierce, CD, Peterson, RB and Dodge, HT
(1984). Regression of atherosclerosis in man:current data and
their methodological limitations. In:Malinow, MRand Blaton,VH
(eds.)" Regression of atherosclerotic lesions".p.289.(New York:
Plenum Press).

6. Hennerici, M, Rautenberg, W, Trockel, U, Kladetzky, RG (1985).
Spontaneous progression and regression of small carotid atheroma,
Lancet, 1, 1415.

7. Wolverson,MK,Bashiti,HM and Peterson GJ (1983).Ultrasonic tissue
characterization of atheromatous plaques using a high resolution
real time scanner.Ultrasound Med Biol, 9, 599.

8. Senin,U,Mannarino,E,Susta,A,Ciuffetti,G,Parnetti,L,Floridi,P,
Pelliccioli P and Signorini,E (1986).Echotomographic extracranial
carotid evaluation in amaurosis fugax,hemispheric TIA and stroke
patients.In:Ventura,A,Crepaldi, and Senin,U(eds.)"Extracoronary
atherosclerosis".p.94.(Basel:Karger).

9. Tanganelli,P,Bianciardi,G,Cao,PG,Centi,L,Moggi,L,Novelli,MT,Pel-
liccioli,G,Senin,U,Signorini,E,Susta,A,Tazza,D and Toti,P(1986)
Carotid atherosclerotic lesions:comparative evaluation of echographic,histomorphometric and angiographic data of endoarterectomy samples.In:Ventura,A,Crepaldi,G,andSenin,U.(eds.)"Extracoronary atherosclerosis".p.189.(Basel:Karger).

10. Weber,G,Bianciardi,G,Centi,L,Novelli,MT,Reri,L,Salvi,M,Toti,P
and Tanganelli,P (1986).Comparative studies of cerebral athero-
sclerosis:observations on endoarterectomy in man.In:Fidge,NH and
Nestel,PJ (eds.)"Atherosclerosis VII".p.593.(Amsterdam:Exc.Med.)

11. Reilly,LM,Lusby, RJ,Hughes,L,Ferrel,LD,Stoney,RJ and Ehrenfeld,
WK(1983).Carotid plaque histology using real-time ultrasonogra-
phy.Am J Surg, 146, 188.

12. Wolverson,MK,Heiberg,E,Sundaram,M,Tantanasirviongse,S,Shields,JB
(1983).Carotid atherosclerosis:high resolution real-time sono-
graphy correlated with angiography.AJR, 140, 355.

13. Malinow,MR(1984).Atherosclerosis:progression,regression and resolution. Am Heart J, 108,1523.

38
Pathogenetic mechanisms of transient brain ischaemic attacks
F. Zacà, M.S. Benassi and M. Trianni

INTRODUCTION

When a focal neurological deficit occurs there is a high possibility to be in the presence of an ischemic event.

When the ischemic origin is verified we must search for the reasons of it.

We may have several pathogenetic mechanisms, such as : ipoperfusion, thrombosis, spasm, embolism, and the latter appears to be the most important phenomenon.

The embolous origins from the heart or arteries and it is made of thrombotic material or atheromasic debris.

The aim of our study is to verify if the plaque unable to induce hemodinamically si_gnificant stenosis and not having ulceration, in its contest can cause neurological phenomenons directly by the releasing of some chemical vasoconstrictive substances or indirectly by platelet activation.

MATERIALS AND METHODS.

The present study was carried out on 182 patients (132 males and 50 females), aged from 55 to 65, selected for carotid endoarteriectomy.

The angiographyc evaluation revealed in all patients a carotid ATS plaque. 162 of the 182 patients had a neurological ischemic disease as TIA, TIA-IR and Stroke.

All patients were also submitted to echotomography with ATL Mark V and 7.5 Mhz Duplex Scanner probe.

- Tissue histamine (H) (1), serotonin (S) (2) and heparansulfate (HS) (3) have been evaluated in non ulcerate fibrous-lipid plaque and in the adjacent tissue area, in 20 patients with previous TIA and in 20 asymptomatic patients. The adiacent area was subdivided into an artery wall area before stenosis, corrisponding to common carotid (c.c.) and into an artery wall area after stenosis, corrisponding to in_ternal carotid (i.c.). The biochemical data have been compared with those obtained from carotids of 20 subjects, sex and age mached, and dead for non cerebrovascular diseases, with no atherosclerotic (ATS) lesions.

- In 8 patients with ATS plaque and previous TIA the plasma H (4) and S (5) levels and platelet activity (6) has been evaluated before and after stenosis areas: the blood was taken in common and internal carotid respectively, before endoarteriectomy .

- 10 patients with haemodinamically non significant and non ulcerate plaque have been submitted to histamine test. A pace-maker has been always used to mantain the same frequency (100/min.). After evaluation of cardiac, common and internal carotid output by Doppler examination we have administrated 20 μg/min. H e.v. for a period of 3 minutes. If the pressure values did not reach those obtained by a previous administration of 10 μg/min. TNG, a further more injection of 4 μg/min. H was done.

The data were analyzed on personal computer IBM utilizing STATIS program (7).
RESULTS AND COMMENT.

As appear in Tab. 1, 75 of the 162 patients with neurological deficit have a carotid stenosis < 70% and 87 ≥ 70%.

A further subdivision of ATS plaque in ulcerate and non ulcerate shows that in the patients with stenosis < 70% the percentage of ulcerate lesions (potentially causing embolus) was very high (71%). However a small percentage of patients with stenosis <70% have non ulcerate plaque (29%). The probability that this plaque had played a pathogenetic role to cause ischemia is emphasized by our results on the tissue vasoactive amine concentration such as H and S in fibrous-lipid ATS plaque. The Fig. 1 shows that the tissue H and S mean concentrations are higher in ATS carotids than in non-ATS carotids : this difference appears statistically significant in all the considered area (p < 0.001). Furthermore the tissue H and S mean values are more elevated in neurological patient with ATS carotids than in the asymptomatic ones. The difference is more statistically significant in the adiacent tissue area after stenosis.

In order to examine throughly the importance of H and S increase in ATS carotid we have begun a study to verify the blood vasoactive amine concentration before and after stenosis. In 6 patients of the 8 until now examined, both H and S have a higher plasma level in i.c than in c.c (0.98+0.15 ng/ml vs 0.53+0.11 ng/ml for H and 27+5.2 ng/ml vs 15+3.3 ng/ml for S; p<0.001).

These preliminary findings induce to suppose a release from the ATS plaque of vaso constrictive substances : this process can produce a chemical embolism.

However we cannot exclude that the differences recorded in carotid circulation before and after a stenosis, could be the result of some biochemical processes occurring on ATS artery wall such as the platelet release reaction (8).

The modifications that the H increase cause on the cerebral flow have been shown on 10 patients undergone to H test to verify the induction of coronary spasm (9). A previous injection of TNG (Tab. 2) increases the cardiac output by 46%; the common and internal carotid output rises in comparison with the starting values, but the percentage flow decreases in comparison with the total cardiac output. In the same way the H administration increases the cardiac output, while the c.c and i.c output decreases either in respect to the starting values or as a percentage of total cardiac output.

If we think that the ATS artery wall cells synthetyze and/or make active some vaso active substances causing cerebral spasm, we can also assume (hypotyze) that the abnormal presence or absence in ATS tissue of other substances, constitutes a "message" transmitted from the plaque to the blood, able to change the normal blood features (Fig. 2).

Our experience reveals a pathological platelet activity in plasma after stenosis

(Fig. 3), with an irreversible aggregation in 5 of 8 patients studied.
The evaluation of HS concentration in ATS plaque and in adjacent area after stenosis, shows a significant decrease in the eparin-similar components in comparison
with the control values (27.9+7.4 mg/100 mg and 35.7+5.1 mg/100 mg respectively vs
45.0+4.6 mg/100 mg; p < 0.001).

TAB. 1: Relationship between cerebrovascular diseases and carotid
percentage stenosis.

		TIA	TIA-IR	STROKE	ALL
< 70	No-ulc	18.6%	5.3%	5.3%	19.0%
	Ulc	42.6%	14.6%	13.3%	71.0%
> 70	No-ulc	44.8%	10.3%	4.5%	60.6%
	Ulc	19.5%	11.4%	9.1%	40.4%
	Obstruction	30.0%	15.0%	55.0%	100.0%

TAB. 2: Cardiac, common and internal carotid output modification
after TNG and H test.

	CARDIAC OUTPUT	C.C. OUTPUT	I.C. OUTPUT
BASE	4200	503(11.9%)	337(8.0%)
TNG	6159	578(9.3%)	350(5.6%)
H	6212	357(5.7%)	211(3.3%)

DISCUSSION

The presence of subjects with TIA and stenosis < 70% without ulceration led to study some possible particular pathogenetic mechanisms causing neurological deficit.
The investigation of some blood parameters did not allow to identify the risk
factors for the cerebrovascular diseases. On the basis of these negative results
it came the necessity to examine those aspects of a ATS not haemodinamically signi
ficant and non ulcerate plaque able to induce a neurological fenomenon. Among the
tissue biochemical components histamine and serotonin appear to have an important
pathogenetic role. The increase of H and S levels in ATS carotid plaque and in tis
sue adiacent intima of patients with TIA and the increase of plasma H and S concen
tration in 6 of 8 patients studied, induce to suppose the release of vasoactive a-
mines from the plaque to blood. However we think that the study needs to be examined throughly for what concerns the role of platelets to release H and S.
The action mechanism of H and S is well known :
- H and S can cause vasospam by activation of H1 and SHT2 receptors respectively
(10, 11).
- the density and response degree of H1 receptors increases near the ATS lesions
(12).
- H and S can cause vasodilatation mediated by H2 and SHT1 receptors respectively;
consequently still fenomenons and membrane permeability increase occurs (13,14).
- S increases the platelet aggregation induced by other substances (15).
- the S reduces the cerebral flow increasing the blood viscosity (16).
- the H test shows a reduction of cerebral flow after H administration.
We don't know if such decrease is a consequence of a cerebral resistance increase
(H1) of another district resistance decrease (H2). The first hypothesis is confirmed by studies on the cerebral spasm caused by vasoactive amine activity after
subarachnoid haemorraghe (17).
On the basis of our and literature data, we can underline the possibility that H
and S, if released from the ATS tissue, are able to cause vasospasm : this phenomenon can be defined "chemical embolism". However when the H and S amount released
into the circulation is low, the compensation mechanism are efficients, but over a
"threshold" concentration, probably, these mechanisms are inadequates and the clinical events appear. Some messages, suitable for changing the normal blood features can originate from the ATS plaque   . In our experience an increase of platelet activity occurs in the internal carotid plasma. To exclude that the different platelet activity before and after stenosis is due to haemodinamic factors,
we have caused a hemodinamically significant stenosis with a pressure sleevy : no
biochemical differences are recorded before and after external stenosis.
Therefore it is possible that the "message" coming from the plaque to the blood
is represented by some substances syntetized by damaged endothelium such as platelet activating factor (PAF) : the vasoconstrictive and platelet aggregator effect
of PAF is no balanced by the synthesis of vasodilatative and anti-aggregant substan
ces as prostacyclins. The absence of the normal artery wall components can be also a "message". Our data demonstrate a significant reduction of HS in the plaque
and in the wall area following the plaque; this can cause a reduction of antithrom

bin activity with a consequent increase of the thrombin activity and coagulation process. Chemical embolus, positive messages, negative messages : the plaque if seem as biological material and therefore not inert is able to produce all that. In the adiacent tissue area ATS initial lesions are always present : infact we found some significant biochemical alterations. In our opinion, the same modifications can be present also in initial lesions not necessary close to ATS plaque. This assumption can explain those tIA occurring in patients without heart diseases, without vessel damage, without modifications in coagulation process.

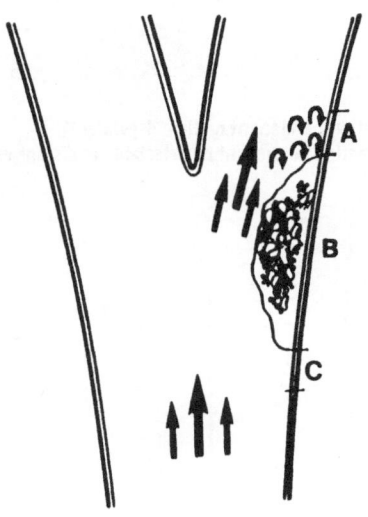

	T I A	NO TIA	CONTROL
STENOSIS %			
Histamine (A)	3.5 + 1.1	2.4 + 0.9**	H= 0.9 + 0.04 μg/mg
Serotonin (A)	3.9 + 1.2	2.7 + 1.1**	
Histamine (B)	6.6 + 2.3	6.3 + 1.9	S= 1.1 + 0.05 μg/mg
Serotonin (B)	4.9 + 0.9	4.1 + 1.0*	
Histamine (C)	2.9 + 1.2	2.0 + 0.9*	
Serotonin (C)	2.1 + 0.5	1.7 + 0.6	

* p 0.05
** p 0.01

Fig. 1: Tissue Histamine and Serotonin mean values in ATS plaque (B) and in adiacent area pre (C) and post (B) stenosis of 20 patients with previous TIA and of 20 patients without previous TIA.
P = statistical significance.

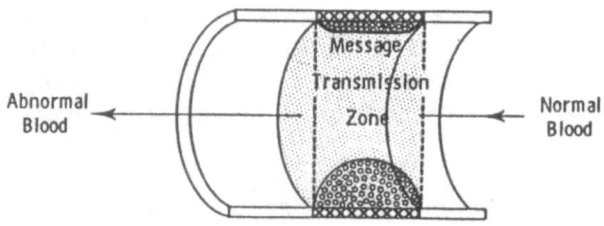

Fig. 2 : Is transformation permanent or time dependent?
Will transformation be present or detectable at distant venous site?

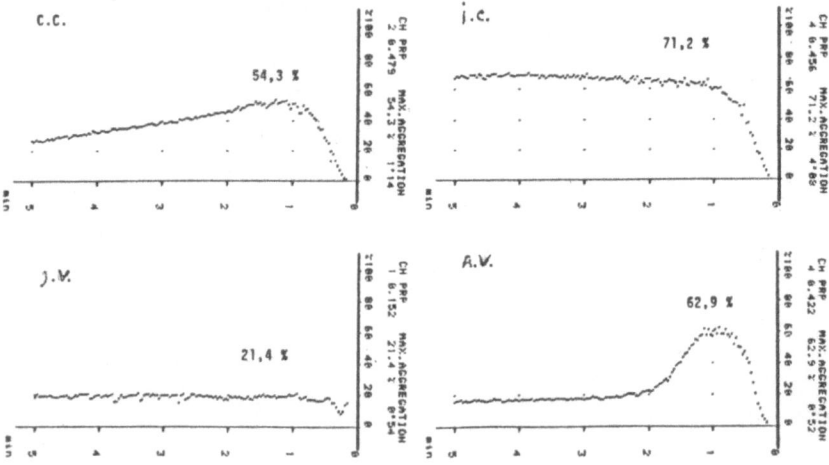

Fig. 3 : platelet aggregation in common carotid (c.c.), internal carotid (i.c.),
jugular (j.v.) and anticubital vein (a.v.).

REFERENCES

1) SKOFITSCH G., SARIA A., HOLZER P. and LEMBECK F. (1981) :
"Histamine in tissue : determination by high performance liquid chromatography
after condensation with o-phthaldialdehyde".
Journal of Chromatography, 226, 53.

2) JACKMAN G.P., CARSON V.J., BOBIK A. and SKEWS H. (1980) :
"Simple and sensitive procedure for the assay of serotonin and catecholamins in
brain by high performance liquid chromatography using fluorescence detection".
Journal of Chromatography, 182, 277.

3) STEVENS R.L., COLOMBO M., GONZALES J.J., HOLLANDER W. and SCHMID K. (1976) :
"The glycosaminoglycans of the human artery and their changes in atherosclerosis".
J. Clin. Inv., 58, 470.

4) LORENZ W., REIMANN M.D., BARTH H., KIRSCHE D., MEYER R., DUENIDEE A. and HERTZEL
M. (1972) :
"A sensitive and specific method for determination of histamine in human whole
blood and plasma".
Physiol. Chem., 353, 91.

5) SOMERVILLE B. and HINTERBERGER H. (1975) :
"Levels of serotonin bound to platelets and free in plasma in jugular and forearm
venous blood as determined by fluorescent OPT assay".
Clinica Chimica Acta, 65, 399.

6) BORN G.V.R. (1962) :
"Aggregation of blood platelets by adenosine diphosphate and its reversal".
Nature, 194, 927.

7) MANNINO G. and GUIDI S. (1978) :
"MIZAR : un programma iterattivo guidato di statistica sanitaria".
In Informatica (Ed. Dedalo), Roma.

8) FUSTER V., CHESEBRO J.H. (1981) :
"Current concepts of thrombogenesis. Role of platelets".
Mayo Clin. Proc., 56, 102.

9) GINSBURG R., BRISTOW M.R., KANTROWITZ N., BAIM D.S. and HARRISON D.C. (1981) :
"Histamine provocation of clinical coronary artery spasm : implications concer-
ning pathogenesis of variant angina pectoris".
Am. Heart J., 102, 819.

10) BRISTOW M.R., GINSBURG R. and HARRISON D.C. (1982) :
"Histamine and the human heart : the other receptor system".
Am. J. Cardiol., 49, 249.

11) VANHOUTTE P.M. (1983) :
"5-hydroxytryptamine and vascular disease".
Federation Proceedings, 42, 233.

12) GINSBURG R., BRISTOW M.R., DAVIS K., DIBIASE A., BILLINGHAM M.E. (1984) :
"Quantitative pharmacological responses of normal and atherosclerotic isolated
human epicardial coronary arteries".
Lab. Inv., 69, 430.

301

13) GINSBURG R., BRISTOW M.R. and DAVIS R. (1984) :
   "Receptors mechanisms in the human epicardial coronary artery".
   Circ. Res., 55, 416.

14) VAN NUETEN J.M. (1985) :
   "Serotonin and blood vessel wall".
   J. Cardiovasc. Pharmacol., 7 (suppl. 7), 549.

15) CLERCK F., DAVID J.L. and JANSSEN P.A.J. (1982) :
   "Inhibition of 5-hydroxytryptamine induced and amplified human platelet aggre-
   gation by ketanserin (R 41 468), a selective 5 H T_z receptor antagonist".
   Agents and Actions, 12, 388.

16) WALKER R.T., MATRAI A., BOGAR L. and DORMANDY J.A. (1985) :
   "Serotonin and flow properties of blood".
   J. Cardiovasc. Pharmacol., 7 (suppl. 7), 535.

17) CHYATTE D. (1984) :
   "Cerebral vasospasm after subarachnoid hemorage".
   Mayo Clin. Proc., 59, 498.

39
Interrelations between the degree of lipid lowering effect and the rate of progression of atherosclerotic cardiovascular disease

P. Rubba, F. Faccenda, P. Pauciullo and M. Mancini

INTRODUCTION

There is extensive evidence that the cholesterol lowering treatment improves the cardiovascular prognosis (1).
While a definite and positive answer can be given to the question if cholesterol lowering treatment is useful, other questions are still open:
a) who should be treated by drugs: asymptomatic people with hyperlipidemia and/or patients with clinical signs of atherosclerotic disease ?

b) how long should they be treated in order to produce demonstrable changes in the arteries?

c) to what extent should the cholesterol concentration be lowered by treatment? Which goal should be chosen for the lipid – lowering regimen ?

Answer to these question is expected to come from some controlled studies, using the progression or regression of atherosclerotic lesions as end-points for the evaluation of the efficacy of lipid lowering treatment (2 -5).

TABLE I

CONTROLLED TRIALS ON ATHEROSCLEROSIS PROGRESSION / REGRESSION			
Author (year)	n	PATIENTS	ANGIOGRAPHY
Duffield RGM (1984)	12T,12C	I. Claudic.	Femoral
Brensike JF (1984)	59T,57C	Clinical CHD	Coronary
Olsson AG (1986)	22T,25C	Asymptomat.	Femoral
Blankenhorn DH (1986)	80T,80C	CABG	Coronary + Femoral

TABLE 1 summarizes the general features of the studies
published so far. The last study, that of Blankenhorn,
had not been completed at the time of this report.

These trials were of small size, involving less than one
hundred patients in the treatment and control group.
In three studies patients with overt ischaemia were
included (intermittent claudication, angina, previous
myocardial infarction); in one case asymptomatic
hyperlipidemia was the criterium for inclusion.
In all the four researches progression/regression of
atherosclerotic lesions was estimated from the results of
repeat angiographies.

The study lasting one year showed (table II) a trend to
less progression, approaching statistical significance.
The other two completed trials, where treatment was
maintained for 19 and 60 months respectively, demonstrated
a reduction of atherosclerosis progression which was
statistically significant.
No evidence of enhanced regression could be obtained.

TABLE II

CONTROLLED TRIALS ON ATHEROSCLEROSIS PROGRESSION

Author (year)	Treatment	Follow-up (months)	LDL chol	Less Progress.
Duffield RGM (1984)	Cholestyr.-NA	19	-25%*	p < 0.001
Brensike JF (1984)	Cholestyramine	60	-26%	p < 0.01
Olsson AG (1986)	Fenofibrate-NA	12	-39%	p= 0.09
Blankenhorn DH (1986)	Colestipol-NA	24	-41%	----

*) total chol

The degree of reduction of Low density lipoprotein (LDL) cholesterol was in the range of 25-41 %.

Some general conclusions can be drawn from these published reports:
- lipid lowering treatment should be prologed for more than one year before significant arterial changes can be demonstrated
- lipid lowering treatment should be aggressive in order to produce a cholesterol lowering effect of at least 25-30 %
- even when lipid lowering treatment is very aggressive, regression seldom occurs. A reasonable aim is that of a slower progression of atherosclerotic lesions.

LIPID LOWERING DRUGS

Only a few lipid lowering drugs are so effective and well tolerated long term that can be used in treatments aiming at the reduction of atherosclerosis progression .
Mevinolin and its derivatives are very promising agents, still being investigated for their toxic effect during prolonged treatment (6).

Cholestyramine effectiveness have been definitely proved
by the Lipid Clinic trial ; however it was also found
that only 50% of the patients were able to take the full
dosage of the drug, because of frequent and umpleasant
side effects (in particular constipation and gastric
discomfort). As expected the protective effect of the
drug against cardiovascular events was directly related
to the dosage taken (7).

Fibrates developed in the last ten years such as
fenofibrate (3,8) are good substitutes of colestyramine;
in cases of refractory hyperlipidemia an associatiation
of cholestyramine with a fibrate might be indicated.

NON INVASIVE EVALUATION OF ATHEROSCLEROTIC LESIONS

A major limitations of the trials using angiography for
the follow up of arterial lesions is that the number of
patients available for study is small and that of
vascular examinations in each patient is also limited ,
because of the invasiveness of this diagnostic procedure.

More recently high-resolution B mode echography and echo-
Doppler has been found very accurate for the detection
and evaluation of lesions in carotid, iliac and femoral
arteries. Differentiation of normal vessels, minor wall
irregularities, non-flow-reducing stenoses and severe
stenoses or occlusion is therefore possible (9,10).
Once a lesion is recognized, it can be followed up by
repeat examinations. This is easily accepted by all
patients because the procedure is completely non
traumatic. The natural history of atherosclerotic disease
can therefore be evaluated and the efficacy of various
therapeutic interventions determined.
Non invasive ultrasound methods have been chosen for an
on going controlled trial aiming at the evaluation of the
effectiveness of lipid lowering treatment in relation to
atherosclerosis progression in man.

REFERENCES

1) Lipid Research Clinics Program, (1984) The Lipid Research Clinics Coronary Primary Prevention Trial Results. I. Reduction in Incidence of Coronary Heart Disease. JAMA, 251, 351-64

2) Duffield R.G.M., Miller N.E., Brunt J.N.H., Lewis B., Jamieson C.W., Colchester A.C.F. (1983) Treatment of hyperlipidemia retards progression of symptomatic femoral atherosclerosis. A randomised controlled trial. Lancet 2, 639-642

3) Olsson A.G., Erikson U., Helmius G., Hemingsson A., Holme I., Ruhn G. (1986) The effect of pronounced serum lipid lowering for one year on the development of femoral atherosclerosis in asymptomatic hyperlipoproteinemia, in Atherosclerosis VII, Fidge N.H. and Nestel P.J. eds., Excerpta Medica, Amsterdam, pag. 89-93

4) Brensike J..F., Levy R.I., Kelsey S.F., Passamani E.R., Richardson J.M., Loh I.K., Stone N.J., Aldrich R.F., Battaglini J.W., Moriarty D.J., Fisher M.R., Friedman L., Detre K.M., Epstein S.E. (1984) Effects of therapy with cholestyramine on progression of coronary arteriosclerosis : results of the NHLBI Type II Coronary Intervention Study, 69,313-24

5) Blankenhorn D.H. (1986) Status of the USC CLAS Study, in Atherosclerosis VII, Fidge N.H. and Nestel P.J. eds., Excerpta Medica, Amsterdam, pag. 75-8

6) Illingworth D.R., Pappu A.S., Bacon S.P. (1986) Metabolic and clinical effects of Mevinolin in Familial Hypercholesterolemia, in Atherosclerosis VII, Fidge N.H. and Nestel P.J. eds., Excerpta Medica, Amsterdam, pag. 611-4

7) Lipid Research Clinics Program (1984) II. The relationship of reduction in incidence of Coronary Heart Disease to cholesterol lowering, JAMA 251,365-74

8) Rubba P., Postiglione A., De Simone B., Lamenza F., Montefusco S., Mancini M. (1985) Comparative evaluation of the lipid lowering effects of fenofibrate and pantethine in type II hyperlipoproteinemia, Curr. Ther. Res., 38,719-27

9) Strandness D.E. (1983) Noninvasive evaluation of arteriosclerosis. Comparison of methods, Arteriosclerosis 3,103-16

10) Rubba P., Postiglione A., De Simone B., Faccenda F., Riccardi G., Mancini M. (1984) Premature development of iliac artery stenosis in asymptomatic type II hyperlipoproteinemia, Arteriosclerosis 4,625-9

Acknowledgement

This work was supported in part by Consiglio Nazionale delle Ricerche (CNR) - Grant no. 8500747.56 - Progetto Finalizzato Medicina Preventiva e Riabilitativa, sottoprogetto Malattie degenerative, Obiettivo 44

40
Results of carotid endarterectomy
M. D'Addato and L. Pedrini

The results of medical and surgical treatment of carotid lesions have been reported by numerous Authors especially at the beginning of the surgical experiences.

A more profound knowledge mostly of the atheromatous lesions,
with the help of ultrasound diagnostic methods, at present allows
the differentiation of lesions which require medical treatment
from those in which surgery is mandatory. The latter lesions likely represent an evolution or the complication of the former ones,
therefore they are more at risk.

The results of the surgical treatment of carotid arteries have
to be evaluated considering both the survival and the prevention
of stable neurological deficits. In addition, from a stricter surgical standpoint, one has also to take into account the appearance
of a restenosis or of occlusions and the hemodynamic effects due
to the carotid revascularization on cerebral parenchyma.

Clinical and vascular conditions and the preoperative paren-
chymal damage deeply influence the early and late results; therefore, they have to be taken into consideration in the evaluation
of the results themselves.

MATERIALS AND METHODS

In the period 1974-1986, 546 carotid operations were performed, in 513 patients between 21 and 84 years old (mean age 59
years) (Tab. 1).

In 82.8% of the cases an endarterectomy (E.A.) has been performed, in 12.8% an EA + saphenous or PTFE patch, while in 4.4%
a vein graft has been implanted.

All of the patients have been treated with antiplatelet agents
in the post-operative period.

The diagnostic and monitoring techniques have modified, in

Tab. 1 – Vascular lesions surgically treated in 513 patients (114 males and 394 females).

VASCULAR LESIONS		
Unilateral stenoses	194	⎫
Bilateral stenoses	204	⎬ 468
Stenoses + obstructions	70	⎭
Obstructions	32	
Kinkings	30	
Aneurisms	12	
Dysplasias	4	
Total operations	546	

these years, the therapeutical indications and the surgical technique which is used.

RESULTS

The survival rate after carotid E.A. is repoi ted in Fig. 1;

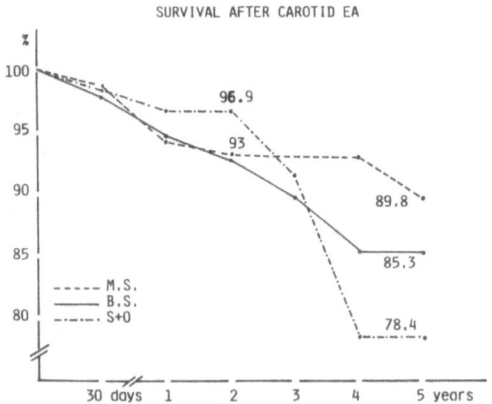

Fig. 1 – Survival rate after carotid E.A. in patients operated for unilateral stenosis (U.S.), bilateral stenosis (B.S.) and stenosis + obstruction (S+O) (Life-table analysis method)

there is a marked difference of the late survival rate depending on the severity of the vascular lesion, while there is no significant difference regarding the surgical risk. Analyzing the survival rate in relation to the age, the result is that age is not a surgical risk factor (4,5), while the survival rate in the group of patients operated on after 75 years old is logically reduced; however, this group is numerically of little importance for a

310

meaningful evaluation from the statistical point of view.
The causes of death, early or late, are reported in Tab. 2.

Tab. 2 - Causes of death after carotid EA (546 operations)

Operative	
Stroke	2
Cerebral hemorrhage	2
Myocardial infarction	1
Late	
Myocardial infarction	6
Asystolia	2
AAA rupture	1
Neoplasm	2
Cerebral hemorrhage	1
Embolism stroke	1
Contralateral stroke	1
Suicide	1

The postoperative neurological follow-up is reported in Fig.
2 and 3. These diagrams, calculated with the Life Table Analysis

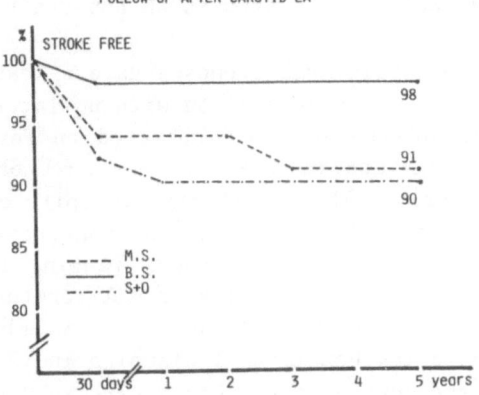

Fig. 2 - Percentage of stroke-free patients, among them submitted
to carotid EA related with their preoperative carotid lesions (Life-Table analysis method).

method, show evident differences among the treated groups regarding both the surgical risk and the late results. The different
behaviours are due either to the preoperative neurological lesion
or to the severity of the vascular lesion; with regard to this it

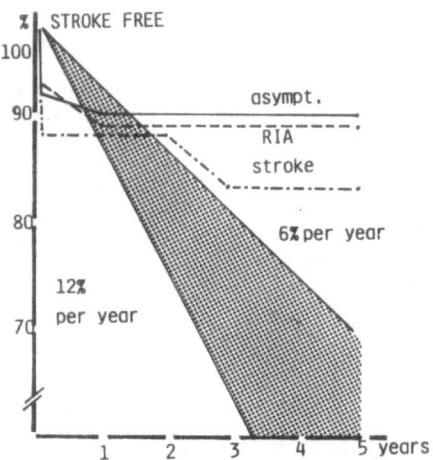

Fig. 3 – Absence of strokes in follow-up period depending on preoperative symptomatology (Life Table analysis method).
The dashed area corresponds to a year 6–12% incidence
yearly incidence of strokes in non-treated patients.

is to be noted that bilateral stenoses have a lesser surgical risk
and a better follow-up in comparison with unilateral ones.

The results of the patients operated on for stroke or for a
stenosis in combination with a contralateral obstruction can be
better foreseen (2,6). These patients, in spite of a higher operative risk, show better late results than non-treated patients, who
present a yearly incidence of strokes ranging between 6 and 12%
(dashed area of Fig. 3), as results from literature demonstrate.

Intraoperative strokes were provoked by embolism, thromboses
or ischemia due to the homolateral clamping in 17 cases (3.1%) and
by ischemia of the contralateral hemisphere in 2 cases (0.36%).

The three late strokes were caused respectively by a cariope-
nic embolism in one case, by an embolism/thrombosis in the second
case and by ischemia of the contralateral hemisphere in the third
one.

One of the newest problems in carotid surgery are the recurrencies (7). The evaluation reported by other Authors and our i-
nitial data were almost always performed in groups of symptomatic
patients or in patients in whom the stenosis found in the follow-

up period cannot be differentiated from a stenosis provoked by a technical defect, not corrected during the operation.

Therefore, in order to know the real incidence of restenoses, a prospectical study has been performed on 50 patients, controlled with anechographic examination in the immediate postoperative period and one year after surgery. The results (Tab. 3) show a 6%

Tab. 3 – Echographical evaluation of the treated carotid in a group of 50 patients controlled in the early postoperative period and after one year; all of the patients were asymptomatic in the follow-up period.

No thickening		24
Intimal thickening $<$ 3 mm.		18
Stenosis $>$ 50%	common c.	2
	internal c.	1
Patch ectasia (unmodified)		2
Recurrencies	= 50%	1
	$>$ 70%	2*

* 1 reoperated

incidence of recurrencies. Carotid restenoses are usually caused by a fibrous hyperplasia and are seldom symptomatic because they do not come up against the classical degenerations of the atherosclerotic plaque, so that they require a reoperation only when they become hemodynamically significant.

The last evaluation which was performed concerns the alterations of the hemispheric perfusion, provoked by the revascularization carotid surgery. This evaluation has been carried out in 15 patients with a cerebral SPECT, using a rotating Gamma camera and, as a tracer, HIPDM I$_{123}$. This examination was performed before surgery and repeated after 7-10 days and again 3 months later. It could show, preoperatively, symptomatic and asymptomatic areas of hypoperfusion either in the hemisphere homolateral to the side of the operation or in the contralateral one and in the cerebellum. Endarterectomy has brought to a normalization of flow in 21% of the areas, to an improvement of it in 63%, while only two areas remained unvaried, which CT showed as infarctual lesions.

CONSIDERATIONS

In conclusion, extra-cranial carotid disobliterating surgery has precise indications, well characterized from the anatomical standpoint, at present, by the combined use of angiography and

high resolution echotomography. As far as we know, the atherosclerotic lesions which require a surgical treatment are the symptomatic lesions stenotizing the carotid lumen for over 50% and
the degenerated plaques with macroscopical ulcerations or sub intimal hemorrhages and the asymptomatic stenoses over 70% or degenerated. The asymptomatic lesions, which have a surgical risk e-
qual to the others, must be treated only in specialized centres
able to offer a low surgical risk (8).

CT and preoperative angiography are mandatory for a correct
evaluation of the patient, in order to exclude from surgery those
who have contraindications (high degree stenoses of the siphon,
stenoses of intracranial arteries, stenoses widespread along the
whole carotid axis, neoplasms or vascular malformations at hemor-
rhagic risk, severe cerebral atrophias).

Late results show, besides a reduced neurological symptomatology, transient or permanent, also an improvement of the cerebral
perfusion, which is important in the global concept of organ preservation.

SUMMARY

Here were reported early and late results of the treatment of
extracranial carotid lesions in 513 patients, in whom 547 operations were performed for a stenotizing or obliterating pathology,
uni or bilateral. Late survival rate is different, depending on
extra-cranial vascular lesions, as different is the influence of
strokes in the post operative period, being lower in those patients with a bilateral stenosis of the carotid arteries, both of
which operated on. The presence of a stroke in the history of a
patient causes a higher surgical risk and the appearance of new
strokes in the post operative period, although with a lower incidence than that presented by the non-treated patients. Late recurrencies, mostly asymptomatic, appear quite precocious and have an
incidence of about 6%. Carotid endarterectomy has brought to a
global improvement of cerebral perfusion, evaluated by SPECT, with
disappearance or reduction of the areas of hypoperfusion, not affected by the outcomes of cerebral infarctions.

REFERENCES

1. Lusby R.J., Ferrell L.D., Ehrenfeld W.K., Stoney R.J., Wylie
E.J. (1982). Carotid plaque hemorrhage. Arch. Surg. 117: 1479-88.
2. Hammacher E.R., Eikelboom B.C., Bast T.J., De Geest R., Vermeu-
len F.E.E. (1984). Surgical treatment of patients with a carotid
artery occlusion and a controlateral stenosis. J. Cardiovasc. Surg.

25:513-7.
3. Riles T.S., Imparato A.M., Mintzer R., Baumann F.G. (1982). Comparison of results of bilateral and unilateral carotid endarterectomy five years after surgery. Surgery 91 (3): 258-62.
4. Plecha F.R., Bertin V.J., Plecha E.J., Avellone J.C., Farrell C.J., Hertzer N.R., Mayda J.I., Rhodes R.S. (1985). The early results of vascular surgery in patients 75 years of age and older: an analysis of 3259 cases. J. Vasc. Surg. 2: 769-74.
5. Rosenthal D., Rudderman R.H., Jones D.H., Clark M.D., Stanton P.E.Jr., Lamis P.A., Daniels W.W. (1986). Carotid endarterectomy in the octogenarian: is it appropriate? J. Vasc. Surg. 3: 782-7.
6. Bardin J.A., Bernstein E.F., Humber P.B., Collins G.M., Dilley R.B., Devin J.B., Stuart S.M. (1982). Is carotid endarterectomy beneficial in prevention of recurrent stroke? Arch. Surg. 117: 1401-7.
7. Colgan M.P., Kingston V., Shanik G. (1984). Stenosis following carotid endarterectomy. Arch. Surg. 119: 1033-5.
8. Chambers B.R., Norris J.W. (1984). The case against surgery for asymptomatic carotid stenosis stroke 15 (6): 964-7.

NEW TECHNOLOGIES AND NEW DIAGNOSTIC AND THERAPEUTIC APPROACHES TO CARDIOVASCULAR DISEASES

41
Haemostatic factors and lipoproteins in atherogenesis
E.B. Smith and G.A. Keen

INTRODUCTION

There is increasing evidence that a hypercoaguable state is a significant risk factor for myocardial infarction (MI), and at autopsy occlusive thrombus has been found in 95% of cases with acute localised infarction[1]. It is not, however, clear if increased tendency to thrombosis is primarily related to the final occlusive event, or if it also plays a significant role in atherogenesis. This paper attempts to bring together recent epidemiological data and studies on haemostatic factors, fibrin and lipoproteins in atherosclerotic lesions.

PLASMA HAEMOSTATIC FACTORS IN RELATION TO CORONARY HEART DISEASE (CHD)

Prospective Studies

In the last three years prospective studies have been published from four centres (Table 1). Raised plasma fibrinogen was significantly associated with subsequent development of fatal and non-fatal MI and with stroke, and frequently showed a higher association than total cholesterol. Meade et al.[5] also found increased Factor VIIc in subjects who subsequently developed fatal MI.

In angiographic studies significantly higher fibrinogen levels (p<0.02) were found in patients with two or three stenosed coronary vessels than in subjects with none or one stenosed vessel[6].

Relation Between Fibrinogen, FVIIc and Other Risk Factors for CHD

Fibrinogen levels show significant positive correlations with plasma cholesterol level[7], age[8], smoking and obesity[7,8] and job grade and stress[9]. Both fibrinogen and FVIIc were raised in patients with hyperlipidaemia, and reduction of triglyceride and cholesterol with diet alone[10] or diet and clofibrate[11] significantly decreased FVIIc, but not fibrinogen. In acute feeding experiments in normal subjects, increased dietary fat led to increased FVIIc (p=0.02) whereas the same calorie supplement eaten as carbohydrate had no effect[12].

Table 1. Prospective studies: levels of haemostatic factors and cholesterol in men who developed CHD compared with healthy survivors

	FVIIc	Fibrinogen	Cholesterol
Wilhelmsen et al, 1984 [2]			
MI (n=92)	-	↑p<0.01	↑p<0.01
Stroke (n=37)	-	↑p<0.01	↑ NS
Stone & Thorp, 1985 [3]	-		
MI, 40-54 y (n=11)	-	↑p<0.001	↑p<0.05
55-69 y (n=29)	-	↑p<0.01	↑p<0.001
Kannel et al, 1985 [4]	-	↑impact on incidence > all	
(n=312)		risk factors except systolic BP	
Meade et al, 1986 [5]			
CHD death <5 ys (n=27)	↑p=0.04	↑p=0.02	↑ NS
whole period (n=68)	↑p=0.03	↑p=0.02	↑p=0.07
non-fatal CHD <5yrs(n=39)	↑ NS	↑p=0.004	↑ NS
whole period (n=60)	↔ NS	↑p=0.002	↑ NS

Many of the major risk factors are, therefore, associated with increased potential for clotting, but no clotting factors were measured in any of the large intervention trials. One can speculate that any beneficial influence on CHD observed following stopping smoking or reduction in lipids may be the result of decreased clotting.

FIBRIN, HAEMOSTATIC FACTORS AND LIPOPROTEINS IN THE ARTERIAL WALL

In 1852 Rokitansky[13] proposed that the atheromatous process (sic) was initiated by deposition on the arterial wall. "The deposit is an endogenous product derived from the blood, and for the most part from the fibrin of the arterial blood." After 100 years of neglect, the idea that fibrin encrustation contributes to the growth of human atherosclerotic lesions was again suggested by Duguid[14]. This stimulated numerous experimental studies which demonstrated conclusively that injected blood clots, fibrin or platelet-rich thrombi, and thrombi produced in situ, became covered with endothelium, invaded by smooth muscle cells (SMC) and collagen, and accumulated lipid so that they became indistinguishable from atherosclerotic plaques [reviewed in Ref. 15].

It is now clear from both histological and quantitative chemical studies that fibrin is present in virtually all atherosclerotic lesions, and is frequently a major component, accounting for up to 30% of the lipid - extracted dry weight[16,17,18]. Its location in lesions is extremely variable; it occurs on the luminal surface, just under the endothelium, deep in the plaque centre, at the shoulders, and distributed diffusely throughout the plaque. It is not clear if it is derived mainly from incorporated mural thrombus, is deposited in situ from fibrinogen within the intima, or if both processes occur. Fibrin stimulates replication of SMCs and fibroblasts by providing a scaffold along which the cells migrate, and it binds fibronectin, which increases cell adhesion[15]. Fibrin encrustations occur quite frequently in human aorta, SMCs are found in the deep layers of the fibrin, and collagen is deposited along the surfaces of the fibrin strands.

Plasma Proteins in Intima

The probable precursors of fibrous atherosclerotic plaques are raised, translucent gelatinous lesions[16,19]; macroscopically, these often look like incorporated fibrin mural thrombi but their fibrin content is variable.

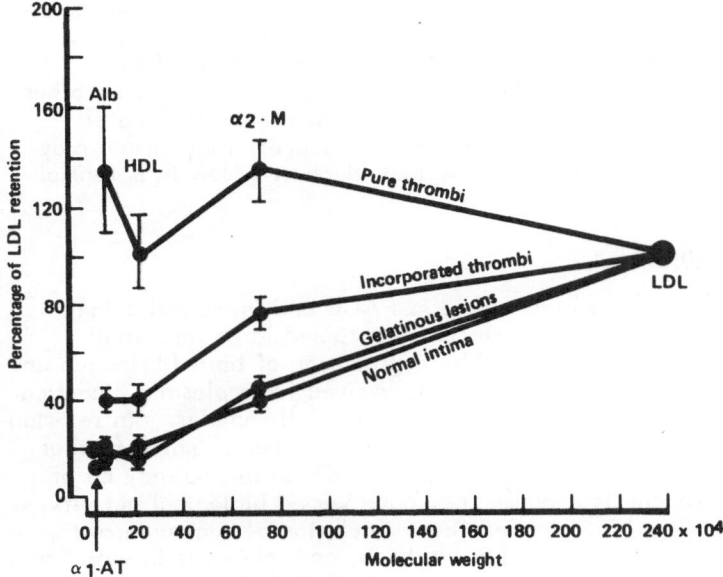

FIGURE 1 Relative retention of plasma proteins in intima and thrombi.
Retention of each protein was calculated as microlitres of the
patient's own plasma and expressed as percentage of LDL retention.

A characteristic feature of aortic intima is a high concentration of plasma proteins which are retained in direct proportion to molecular mass (Mr) and plasma concentration. The almost linear relation with Mr in normal intima and gelatinous lesions is shown in Figure 1; by contrast, "pure" mural thrombi without endothelial cover or SMC invasion contained low concentrations with no consistent gradient on Mr. However, plasma protein retention in partially incorporated thrombi (mainly covered with endothelium and invaded by SMCs and collagen in the base) closely resembled that in gelatinous lesions, suggesting that they may be presursors[20].

Retention of prothrombin in intima is greater than predicted from its plasma concentration and Mr[21]. In the lipid and fibrin rich plaque centres

Table 2.   Prothrombin and antithrombin III in intima

	Prothrombin Concentration: μg/100mg*	Molar ratio: Prothrombin AT III	Concentration:mg/100mg* Soluble FRA	Fibrin
Normal intima	43.4	0.3	3.4	3.5
Gelatinous lesions	72.1	0.4	5.6	4.3
Plaque centres	75.6	1.1	3.2	12.6

* per 100mg lipid-extracted dry tissue

prothrombin concentration was almost twice that in normal intima, but concentration of the thrombin inhibitor antithrombin III fell, so that the molar ratios of inhibitor/prothrombin fell from 3:1 in normal intima to <1:1 in the plaque centres (Table 2).   In striking contrast, we failed to recover measurable amounts of plasminogen from the intimas of all patients dying with MI (n=17) and half the patients (n=37) dying from other causes[22].   Absence of plasminogen was also associated with greater involvement with atherosclerosis.   These results suggest that intima may be high in clotting potential, but in some individuals it is low in potential for removal of fibrin.

Intimal Fibrinogen and FDPs

Intimal extracts have been analysed by SDS-PAGE and immunoblotting; in addition to intact fibrinogen, all samples contained large and small fragments which appear to be derived by degradation of both fibrinogen and cross-linked fibrin[23].   Fragment D-dimer, derived from plasmin digestion of cross-linked fibrin, is a prominent component in all samples.   In relation to this finding, the apparent absence of free plasminogen requires further investigation.   The concentration and type of FDPs in intima may be of significance in atherogenesis because they have varied biological activity, including chemotaxis for blood leukocytes, stimulation of tumour growth, angiogenesis, mitogenesis and collagen synthesis, and increases in vascular permeability and SMC contractility [reviewed in Ref. 15].

Relation Between Low Density Lipoprotein (LDL) and Fibrin in Atherosclerotic Lesions

Cholesterol ester is the major lipid component in intima.   In fatty streaks it is mainly intracellular cholesterol oleate, but in fibrous plaques it is mainly extracellular cholesterol linoleate, which appears to have been derived directly from plasma LDL[24].   Large amounts of LDL are present in the gelatinous lesions that are the probable precursors of fibrous plaques[19,25], but the mechanisms involved in the deposition of lipids from it are not understood.
     If soluble LDL is removed from intima a tightly bound apo-B-containing lipoprotein remains in the tissue, and this can be released by incubation with proteolytic enzymes[26] or detergents[27].   In normal intima and early gelatinous lesions which have not accumulated excess lipid, the bound fraction accounts for 10-15% of total LDL, but in the lipid-rich centres of gelatinous and early fibrous plaques the bound fraction may account for

Table 3. Plasma constituents in thrombi covered with endothelium and in atherosclerotic lesions

	Concentration: mg/100mg dry tissue				
	Free LP	Bound LP	Soluble FRA*	Fibrin	Residual Cholesterol
Partially incorporated mural thrombi (n=4)	10.1	4.3	21.9	47.7	5.3
Gelatinous thickenings: Low lipid (n=25)	13.7	1.8	7.7	4.3	5.4
Gelatinous and fibrous plaques: lipid-rich areas (n=35)	5.4	7.4	7.7	22.7	89.6
Normal intima (n=12)	4.3	0.8	2.2	2.0	3.2

* Fibrinogen and related antigens

more than 50% of LDL (Table 3), suggesting that tight-binding may be a step in the irreversible deposition of the lipid from LDL. The protease that releases LDL most effectively is plasmin; purified collagenase releases much less LDL[26]. The highest concentrations of bound LDL occur in lesions that are rich in fibrin in addition to cholesterol and release of LDL and FDPs appear to occur in parallel (Smith and Keen, unpublished). Together, these findings suggest that fibrin is associated with the binding of LDL, but the relationship is not simple; little LDL is bound by pure fibrin thrombi[18], and in thrombi binding seems to be associated with endothelialisation and collagen invasion (Table 3).

SUMMARY AND CONCLUSIONS

Raised plasma fibrinogen is a major risk factor for CHD, and fibrinogen level is correlated with other risk factors, particularly hypercholesterolaemia, smoking and obesity. Fibrin is a major component of many lesions, and is associated with binding of LDL in lipid-rich fibrous plaques. Fibrin promotes cellular migration and proliferation, thus may initiate formation of focal proliferative lesions. Fibrin/fibrinogen degradation products (FDPs) are present in intima; they may influence plaque development by changing permeability and stimulating cell proliferation and leukocyte chemotaxis.

ACKNOWLEDGEMENTS-

The author's work was supported by grants from the Medical Research Council, British Heart Foundation and Wellcome Trust.

REFERENCES

1. Davies, MJ and Thomas, A (1984). Thrombosis and acute coronary-artery lesions in sudden cardiac ischemic death. N Engl J Med, 310, 1137
2. Wilhelmsen, L, Svardsudd, K, Korsan-Bengtsen, K, Larsson, B, Welin, L and Tibblin, G (1984). Fibrinogen as a risk factor for stroke and myocardial infarction. N Engl J Med, 311, 501

3.   Stone, MC and Thorp, JM (1985). Plasma fibrinogen - a major coronary risk factor. J R Coll Gen Pract, 35, 565

4.   Kannel, WB, Castelli, WP and Meeks, SL (1985). Fibrinogen and cardiovascular disease. Amer Coll Cardiol, 34th Ann Scientific Session (Abstract)

5.   Meade, TW, Brozovic, M, Chakrabarti, RR et al (1986). Haemostatic function and ischaemic heart disease: principal results of the Northwick Park heart study. Lancet ii, 533

6.   Lowe, GDO, Drummond, MM, Lorimer, AR et al (1980). Relation between extent of coronary artery disease and blood viscosity. Brit Med J, i, 673

7.   Korsan-Bengsten, K, Wilhelmsen, L and Tibblin, G (1972). Blood coagulation and fibrinolysis in a random sample of 788 men 54 years old: II. Relations of the variables to "risk factors" for myocardial infarction. Thromb Diath Haemor, 28, 99

8.   Meade, TW, Chakrabarti, R, Haines, AP, North, WRS and Stirling, Y (1979). Characteristics affecting fibrinolytic activity and plasma fibrinogen concentrations. Brit Med J, i, 153

9.   Markowe, HLJ, Marmot, MG, Shipley, MJ et al (1985). Fibrinogen: a possible link between social class and coronary heart disease. Brit. Med J, 291, 1312

10. Elkeles, RS, Chakrabarti, R, Vickers, M, Stirling, Y and Meade, TW (1980). Effect of treatment of hyperlipidaemia on haemostatic variables. Brit Med J 281: 973

11. Simpson, HCR, Meade, TW, Stirling, Y, Mann, JI, Chakrabarti, R and Woolf, L (1983). Hypertriglyceridaemia and hypercoagulability. The Lancet 1, 786

12. Miller, GJ, Martin, JC, Webster, J et al (1986). Association between dietary fat intake and plasma Factor VII coagulant activity - a predictor of cardiovascular mortality. Atherosclerosis, 60, 269

13. Rokitansky, C (1852). A Manual of Pathological Anatomy: Sydenham Society, London, Vol. IV

14. Duguid, JB (1946). Thrombosis as a factor in the pathogenesis of coronary atherosclerosis. J Pathol Bacteriol 58, 207

15. Smith, EB (1986). Fibrinogen, fibrin and fibrin degradation products in relation to atherosclerosis. Clin Haematol, 15: 2, 355

16. Haust, MD (1981). The natural history of human atherosclerotic lesions. In: Moore, S (ed.) "Vascular Injury and Atherosclerosis" p.1. (New York: Marcel Dekker)

17. Woolf, N (1982) "The Pathology of Atherosclerosis". (London: Butterworths)

18. Smith, EB, Staples, EM, Dietz, HS and Smith RH (1979). Role of endothelium in sequestration of lipoprotein and fibrinogen in aortic lesions, thrombi and graft pseudo-intimas. Lancet ii, 812

19. Smith, EB (1983) Identification of the gelatinous lesion. In: Schettler, G, Gotto, AM, Middelhoff, G, Habernicht, AJR and Jurutka, KR (eds) "Atherosclerosis VI". p.170. (Berlin: Springer-Verlag)

20. Smith, EB and Staples, EM (1982). Intimal and medial plasma protein concentrations and endothelial function. Atherosclerosis, 41, 295

21. Smith, EB and Staples, E (1981). Haemostatic factors in human aortic intima. Lancet, i, 1171

22. Smith, EB and Ashall, C (1985). Fibrinolysis and plasminogen concentration in aortic intima in relation to death following myocardial infarction. Atherosclerosis, 55, 171

23. Smith, EB, Keen, GA, Thompson, WD and Snyder, C (in press). Fibrinogen and FDP in intima in relation to atherogenesis. Proc. Fibrinogen Workshop, Giessen, 1986

24. Smith, EB (1974). the relationship between plasma and tissue lipids in human atherosclerosis. Advan Lipid Res, 12, 1

25. Smith, EB and Ashall, C (1983). Low density lipoprotein concentration in interstitial fluid from human atherosclerotic lesions. Biochim Biophys Acta, 754, 249

26. Smith, EB, Massie, IB and Alexander, KM (1976). The release of an immobilized lipoprotein fraction from atheroslcerotic lesions by incubation with plasmin. Atheroslcerosis 25, 71

27. Hoff, HF, Heideman, CL, Gotto, AM and Gaubatz, JW (1977). Apoprotein B retention in the grossly normal and atherosclerotic human aorta. Cicrulation Res 41, 684

42

Comparative evaluation of echographic and histomorphometric data of carotid endarterectomy samples

G. Weber, D. Bertini, G. Bianciardi, L. Centi, L. Moggi,
M.T. Novelli, G. Nuzzaci, C. Pratesi, L. Resi, D. Righi,
M. Salvi, U. Senin, A. Susta, P. Toti and P. Tanganelli

INTRODUCTION

Stroke still represents in many countries one of the most frequent causes of death; atherosclerosis of the large extracranial arteries (chiefly the carotid arteries at bifurcation) has been correlated with cerebral ischemic infarction in a 60% of the cases (1).

Not only in stroke but also in reversible cerebral ischemic attacks the extracranial carotid atherosclerotic lesions seem to be of relevance (cfr. the Italian Multicenter Study by D. Inzitari et al., 2).

The evaluation of arteriosclerotic lesions by "non-invasive" methods presents problems not completely resolved, still requiring further studies into the accuracy and reproducibility of these methods "in vivo" in man.

Comparative studies (and very few indeed) of ultrasound data with anatomical and histological lesions examinations have so far been carried out on autopsy material (open stretched arteries) or on animal arteries having arteriosclerotic lesions due to diet, examined ultrasonically after removal. Recently, studies have been carried out on surgical samples of the carotid obtained by endarterectomy (3,4,5,6,7). As for the rationale of the endarterectomy procedure, we have observed in human disease and in experimental situations in non-human primates and other mammals that cerebral arteries are the last to be affected. The reason for this is still unclear (cfr. also, for human beings, D. Inzitari et al., 2).

A comparison of the informations obtained from the histological samples and from the analysis of ultrasound photographic images, would be a first step in the validation of this non invasive diagnostic technique for measuring the degree, extent and possibly composition and complications of the lesion.

As a Group taking part to the Italian National Research Council Project "Progression and Regression of Atherosclerotic Lesions", we have performed a quantitative morphometric evaluation of the histologic carotid lesions in surgical endarterectomy samples and compared the findings with B-mode ultrasound images.

MATERIAL AND METHODS

The histologic study was carried out on 52 samples of lesions obtained by carotid endarterectomy including the upper section of the common carotid and the section proximal to the bifurcation of the internal carotid. The samples include all the intima thickened by arteriosclerotic plaque (sclerolipocalcific and atheromasic) and the inner third of the media. The quantity of media taken, however, was found to vary considerably. The samples fixed with 10% neutral buffered formalin, decalcified with EDTA (5.8%), were sectioned transversely to give 4-5 mm thick slices which were embedded in paraffin. Of these slices, the one having the greatest stenosis was chosen and transverse serial sections made. One section of 5 µm thickness was taken every 400 µm. The sections were stained with hematoxylin-eosin and observed under an optic microscope. The section having major stenosis was traced using a table microprojector and measured with a computerised semiautomatic image measurer (Videoplan Kontron Zeiss).

Ultrasound analysis was carried out "in vivo" with a high resolution (Biodynamics) system generating a broad pulsed medium frequency ultrasonic band (4 or 8 MHz). The ultrasonic scanning was carried out "in vivo" before surgery longitudinally at 0° (anterior) and at 90° (lateral) to the sagittal plane and, when possible, in posterior position, namely 150-170° to the sagittal plane.

The quantitative parameter calculated was percentage stenosis based on area.

In order to correlate the measurements of the histological sections with the "in vivo" situation, the transverse internal dimension of the lumen, the external dimension and intimal thickening of the endarterectomy samples, determined with the semi-automatic image measurer, were corrected for shrinkage during fixing and embedding.

This was done by multiple linear regression using two independent variables: the amount of calcified atheroma and atheroma. In the model they act together to determine the degree of shrinkage of internal and external dimensions and of intimal thickening.

Each "regression plane" used was obtained from a standardising experiment with a small number of vessels in which the three parameters (external and luminal dimensions and thickening) were measured immediately after surgical removal as well as after fixing and embedding.

The ultrasonic parameter of percentage stenosis was determined from photographs of the ultrasound images using the semi-automatic image measurer. The measurements taken in the points of maximum stenosis in the 3 longitudinal projections were fitted using a mathematical model of interpolation (Newton's Method of Divided Differences) and then successive numerical integration of the function obtained. In the case of only two projections an ellipse having axes equal to the measured values was interpolated. The area percentage of stenosis was thus measured.

Regression linear analysis was applied to obtain the significativity.

The comparison of the qualitative composition of the lesion apparent from the ultrasound image (lesions were classified as "hard", "soft" or "mixed") with the quantitative histologic data (percentage necrotic core, calcification of necrotic core and diffuse, fibrosis) was performed by "Chi square" analysis.

RESULTS AND DISCUSSION

In calculating the shrinkage correction factors for fixing and embedding by regression plane analysis, it was found that calcified plaque shrank the least and fibrous plaque shrank the most. Shrinkage of the vessel was noticeably asymmetric: the shrinkage of the external dimension of the vessel was 10 times greater than that of the luminal dimension. The resulting intimal thickening shrinkage reached values as high as 60%. The presence of calcium or of abundant atheroma lowered this value.

Percentage stenosis from longitudinal ultrasound images reconstructed by mathematical models and the percentage stenosis corrected for shrinkage from histological sections showed a high degree of linear correlation ($y=42.3+0.45.x$; $r=0.45$; $p<0.001$), even if the scattering appears very high (or Pearson's "r" very low).

The ultrasound images obtained through the B-mode devices utilized by the Groups involved in the CNR study "Progression and Regression of Atherosclerotic Lesions" tended to give higher degrees of stenosis: mean histological value = 70.9%; mean echographic value = 74.2% (3 - 9%, cfr. G. Bianciardi et al., 4; G. Weber et al., 7).

This is probably due to the fact that, with the common transducers in clinical use, the "ultrasound intima" does not appear to be constituted only by the intimal lesion but also by a part of the media.

The B-mode over-evaluation should be probably reduced (G. Bond, personal communication) if more sophisticated B-mode devices, specifically aimed at research finalities, would have been used, but we think that the linear correlation found by us both between ultrasound and histologic images making use of the common transducers is maybe even of higher relevance.

The qualitative criteria of evaluation of the ultrasound images as "hard", "soft" or "mixed" compared to the quantitative histological parameters of percentage necrotic core, calcification (of necrotic core and diffuse) and fibrosis was found to correlate significantly in the case of diffuse calcification ($p=0.003$) and, still significantly (even if less so), in the case of necrotic core ($p=0.056$).

We can therefore conclude that ultrasound examination "in vivo" in man of the common carotid and of the carotid bifurcation is valid in estimating the severity of the lesions, even if the high scattering of the regression model obtained by us must be taken on account.

ACKNOWLEDGMENTS

Our thanks to Dr. M.G. Bond, Wake Forest University, Bowman Gray School of Medicine, Winston-Salem, N.C., U.S.A., for his suggestions and helpful criticism.

This study forms part (Grant n° 85.00784.56) of the Italian National Research Council (CNR) Target Project "Preventive Medicine and Rehabilitation", Subproject "Degenerative Diseases", Ob. 44, Coord. by S. Lenzi, Bologna, Italy.

Surgical material and ultrasound images have been kindly given us by Bologna Operative Unit (S. Lenzi: Head, G.C. Descovich, M.S. Benassi, S. Rimondi, Z. Sangiorgi, M. Trianni, F. Zacà) and Perugia Operative Unit (S. Ventura: Head, U. Senin, P.G. Cao, E. Mannarino, L. Moggi, G. Pelliccioli, D. Tazza, E. Signorini, A. Susta).

REFERENCES

1.   Wetzner, SM, Kiser, LC and Bezreh, JS (1984). Duplex ultrasound imaging: vascular applications. Radiology, 150, 507
2.   Inzitari, D, Bianchi, F, Pracucci, G, Albanese, V, Argentino, C, Bono, G, Brambilla, GL, Candelise, L, De Zanche, L, Mariani, F, Passero, S, Prencipe, M and Fieschi, C (1986). The Italian Multicenter Study of reversible cerebral ischemic attacks: IV-Blood pressure components and atherosclerotic lesions. Stroke, 17, 185
3.   Tanganelli, P, Bianciardi, G, Cao, PG, Centi, L, Moggi, L, Novelli, MT, Pelliccioli, G, Senin, U, Signorini, E, Susta, A, Tazza, D and Toti, P (1986) Carotid atherosclerotic lesions: comparative evaluation of echographic, histomorphometric and angiographic data of endoarterectomy samples. In: Ventura, A, Crepaldi, G and Senin U (eds.) "Monographs on Atherosclerosis". Vol. 14, p.189. (Basel: S Karger AG)
4.   Bianciardi, G, Centi, L, Novelli, MT, Tanganelli, P, Toti, P, Weber, G, Senin, U, Susta, A, Mannarino, E,Moggi, L, Cao, PG and Tazza, D (1985) Quantitative and qualitative evaluation of histomorphometric and echografic data on endarterectomy samples. In: "International Congress of angiology". p. 321. (Torino: Ed. Minerva Medica)
5.   Dutreix, JL, Genre, O, Monegier Du Sorbier, Ch, Arbeille, Ph, Lapierre, F, Benhamou, AC, Autret, A and Pourcelot, L (1985) Corrélations ultrasoniques, artériographiques et anatomopathologiques dans 59 cas d'athérosclérose carotidienne. Rev Neurol 141, 128
6.   Weber, G and Tanganelli, P (1985) Valutazione morfometrica pre-operatoria del grado di stenosi carotidea: studio di validazione delle immagini ecografiche. In: Passariello, R and Benedetti Valentini, F (eds.) "Diagnostica per Immagini in Patologia Vascolare". p.349. (Bologna: Monduzzi Editore)
7.   Weber, G, Bianciardi, G, Centi, L, Novelli, MT, Resi, L, Salvi, M, Toti, P and Tanganelli, P (1986) Comparative studies of cerebral atherosclerosis: observations on endarterectomy in man. In: Fidge, NH and Nestel, PJ (eds.) "Atherosclerosis VII". p 593. (Elsevier Science Publisher B.V.)

330

43
Correlative electron microscopy in the study of atherosclerosis

R. Laschi, G. Cenacchi, G. Pasquinelli, P. Preda and
C. Scala

INTRODUCTION

Contributions of E.M. to the study of the arterial wall during atherosclerosis have been significant, by helping in clarifying some of the intricate pathogenetic mechanisms of this disease, particularly on animal models.

But now what has been achieved is no longer enough and new approaches appear to be indispensable: 1) studies on man; 2) all up-to-date morphological facilities (SEM + TEM + IEM + analytical and other new techniques) jointly applied to the same material.

We have undertaken this way, full of difficulties and of many limitations, due particularly to human models always imperfect. Anyway, preliminary results suggest to go on.

Our present observations are devoted on one hand to the cells and extracellular matrix components of apparently unaffected areas near carotid atheromatous plaques, and on the other to the blood cells of atherosclerotic patients. First of all the platelets, whose leading role in the onset and early development of lesions appears very likely. At present we have focused our attention on platelets from type IIa heterozygous hypercholesterolemic patients, a frequent condition in which atherosclerosis develops early.

MATERIALS and METHODS

Arterial wall

Atheromatous carotids taken from patients (n=8) submitted to endo-arteriectomy for atherosclerotic stenosis were studied. All specimens obtained from fibrous plaque and adjacent apparently unaffected areas were treated for:
1) scanning electron microscopy (SEM);
2) transmission electron microscopy, TEM, (on specimens recovered

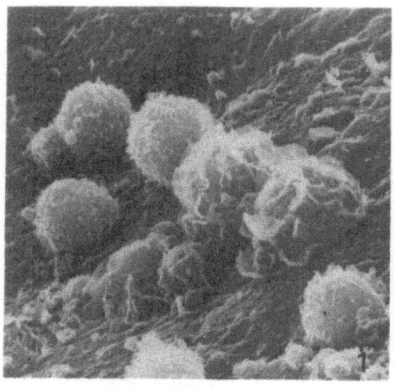 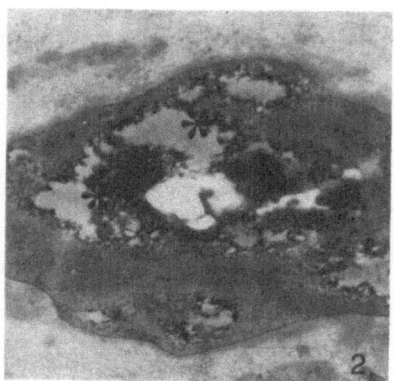

Figure 1. SEM.Focal adhesion of inflammatory cells (monocytes and lymphocytes) to an overtly intact endothelium.   2000 x

Figure 2. TEM. An acid lipase positive SMC: the electron dense granular deposits are localized around phagolysosomes (*).
12,000 x

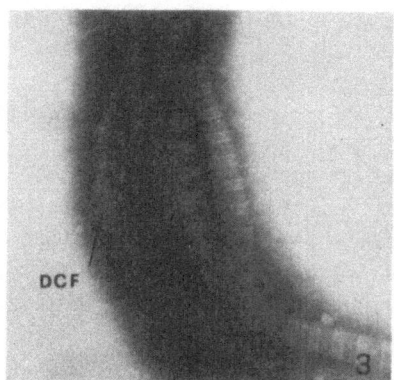 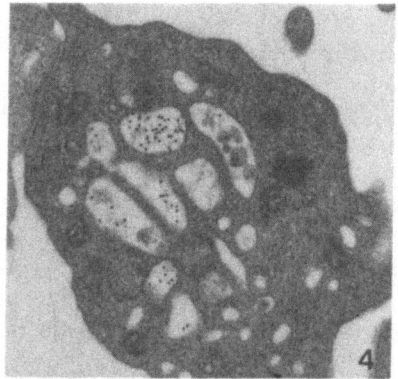

Figure 3. TEM of purified collagen fibrils. A dysplastic collagen fibril, DCF (↑) with poorly packed and frayed appearance.   57,000 x

Figure 4. TEM. Vacuoles in the cytoplasm of a platelet from hypercholesterolemic patient, containing internalized LDL-gold conjugates.   23,000 x

from SEM also), cytochemistry and immunoelectronmicroscopy, IEM, (semithin and thin sections of embedded material).

Purified native collagen fibrils from the same specimens were studied by means of:
1) TEM and IEM (type I and type III collagen fibril labelling with protein A-gold technique);
2) microdensitometric analysis;
3) densitometric gel scans of I, and III collagen extracts.

Platelets

Platelets from patients (n=6) with heterozygous familial hypercholesterolemia (H) have been studied in comparison to normolipidemic controls (n=6). Citrated platelet rich plasma (C-PRP), separated by centrifugation from venous blood, was conventionally processed for SEM and TEM. Aliquots of C-PRP were also frozen in Freon 22 chilled by liquid nitrogen and transferred to the stage of a Balzer's freeze-fracture unit for replicas studies. Internalization of low density lipoproteins (LDL) was carried out on unfixed platelets with LDL conjugated to 20 nm gold particles.

RESULTS

Arterial wall

By SEM, the areas adjacent to the atheromatous plaque seemed to be apparently unaffected. However, in some patients, a focal sticking of blood cells to the endothelium was observed (Fig. 1). Adhesion of these cells occurred both on endothelial cells and on exposed subendothelial matrix where single endothelial cells were degenerating. Platelets were very few. The same specimens, recovered for TEM, allowed to characterize these cells as monocytes and lymphocytes. Moreover the vessel wall, which was apparently unaffected at SEM, showed marked changes: proliferating smooth muscle cells(SMCs), altered extracellular matrix as well as inflammatory cells leading to the formation of fibrous plaque.

Cytochemical demonstration of *acid lipase* in these adjacent areas showed: i) numerous SMCs with a strong positivity mainly around scarce cytoplasmic vacuoles (Fig. 2); ii) myofibroblasts containing the reaction product in the endoplasmic reticulum cisternae and mitochondria, around lipid vacuoles and on the outside of the plasma membrane (small focal deposits); iii) rare macrophage-like cells exhibiting numerous positive lipid-laden phagolysosomes. In the fibrous plaque myofibroblasts and few macrophage-like cells contained some positive lipid vacuoles.

Collagen. At TEM, in both affected (fibrous plaque) and adjacent intima, a generalized and constant lesion consisting of dysplastic collagen fibrils (DCFs, corresponding to the so-called hyperfibres/

hieroglyphic collagen fibrils) has been demonstrated . Ca^{++} ions deposits were seen both along the fibrillar edges of these DCFs and normal collagen fibrils in the adjacent intima. Purified DCFs displayed disordered structure in longitudinal section (Fig. 3). Most fibrils showed a low mean diameter. Preliminary data, obtained by microdensitometric trace of stain distribution on purified fibrils, revealed some alteration in the period range ($\simeq$ 600 Å). IEM study on semithin sections evidenced: i) in the fibrous plaque no significant changes in the ratio between the amount of type I and type III collagen and ii) in the adjacent intima, a type III collagen predominance. Further IEM on thin sections revealed: i) in the fibrous plaque, DCFs were composed of both type I and type III collagen and ii) in the adjacent intima, DCFs were mainly constituted of type III collagen. Sometimes, phagocytized type III collagen fibrils were also seen within the modified smooth muscle cells (myofibroblast-like cells). Antigenic sites evidentiation on 'a' and 'c$_2$' bands of purified collagen fibrils was quite similar to control collagen. Stained gels were scanned at 560 nm in their linear range and chain ratio was computed by an automated system: the analysis of collagen types percentages recovered in the different extracts showed that type III collagen was easier solubilized than type I collagen.

Platelets

SEM was used to estimate the platelet shape and size changes. These parameters, in fact, are both considered to be related to platelet reactivity. Platelets from H patients displayed minimal shape changes, i.e. emission of long , slender pseudopods projecting from the cell periphery. Primary aggregates - clusters of irregularly shaped platelets - were frequently found. The mean platelet diameter showed a statistically significant decrease in the H patients compared with the controls ($p < 0.01$), due to an increased frequency of small platelets.
TEM of platelets from H subjects showed no evident ultrastructural changes. However, an unusual vacuolation of the cytoplasm due to the presence of a large number of membrane complexes of the open canalicular system (OCS) has been observed. Lipid droplets were also evidenced. Freeze-fracture electron microscopy showed, as striking feature of the platelets from H patients, an increased number of the openings of the surface-connected membrane system which were often polarized within focal regions of the fractured plasma membranes. Internalization of LDL in the platelets was investigated by using colloidal gold-LDL conjugates. Our preliminary results showed that internalization of LDL was strongly inhibited in control platelets by preincubation in a medium containing unlabeled LDL,

whereas uptake of LDL seemed to be unaffected by the same preincubation in platelets from H patients (Fig. 4), thus suggesting an altered behavior of LDL receptors.

DISCUSSION

High serum cholesterol levels are associated both to platelet increased reactivity and to their altered prostaglandin metabolism. There is some experimental evidence that hypercholesterolemia could directly affect the platelet production from megakaryocytes at the bone marrow level. Changes in platelet production are supported by: i) the significant presence of circulating small platelets observed in animal models and also in our study and ii) alterations in megakaryocyte membrane development biochemically demonstrated by Schick and Schick (1) and morphologically evidenced by us as an unusual development of the membrane complexes in circulating platelets. This feature could facilitate the exchanges between the external microenvironment and the platelet interior thus rendering platelets hypersensitive to the aggregating stimuli. Moreover the new formed platelets once circulating, could be susceptible to pick up large amount of   cholesterol from the plasma. This is in agreement with our observations on the increased ability of platelets from H patients to accumulate lipoproteins. High platelet cholesterol level can inhibit the expression of specific receptors for PGI_2 and promote TXA_2 synthesis (2). The pathological imbalance between the activities of prostaglandins with opposing effects as well as the hypersensitivity to the external stimuli may lead platelets to adhere to the vessel wall and aggregate.

As for the arterial wall matrix, our findings suggest that DCFs can arise from abnormal collagen fibril aggregation, remodelling or breakdown. IEM, revealing that DCFs in the areas adjacent to fibrous plaques are mainly composed of type III collagen, suggests that DCFs may reflect the effect of the low mechanical resistance of new-abnormally synthetized collagen fibrils against pressure trauma (3).

The cytochemical localization of acid lipase (4, 5) showed that also SMCs are acid lipase-positive and confirmed that: i) very few macrophages are seen both in the adjacent areas and in the fibrous plaque; ii) SMCs are well represented mainly in the adjacent zones; iii) myofibroblasts are much more numerous in the fibrous plaque; iv) macrophage-like cells, SMCs and myofibroblasts are all engaged in hydrolyzing glycerol esters of long-chain fatty acids.

Messages of our work, even though very preliminar, seem to be the following:
1) hypercholesterolemia could affect the platelet reactivity

through alteration in the megakaryocyte metabolism thus suggesting a developmental defect;

2) dedifferentiation of smooth muscle cells during the atheromatous plaque formation produces fibrohystiocytic-like cells able to synthetize as well as phagocytize modified extracellular matrix components and also glycerol esters of long-chain fatty acids, but the new digestive capacity most probably is defective.

3) Ca^{++} ion deposition on collagen fibrils (DCFs as well as normal appearing) also in the carotid areas adjacent to the plaque suggests that these extracellular matrix changes are most likely irreversible.

REFERENCES

1. Schick, BP and Schick, PK (1985). The effect of hypercholesterolemia on guinea pig platelets, erythrocytes and megakaryocytes. Biochem Biophys Acta, 833, 291.

2. Steinberg, D (1983). Lipoproteins and atherosclerosis. Arteriosclerosis, 3, 283.

3. Staubesand, J and Fischer, N (1980). The ultrastructural characteristics of abnormal collagen fibrils in various organs. Connect Tiss Res, 7, 213.

4. Schaffner, TN,Taylor, K, Bartucci, J E, Fischer-Dzoga, K, Beeson, J H, Glagov, S and Wissler, R W (1980). Arterial foam cells with distinctive immunomorphologic and histochemical features of macrophages. Am J Pathol, 100, 57.

5. Davis, H R, Glagov, S and Zarins , C K (1985). Role of acid lipase in cholesteryl ester accumulation during atherogenesis. Atherosclerosis, 55, 205.

44
The role of oxygen free radicals in the ischaemia - reperfusion injury

F. Cuccurullo, A. Mezzetti, A. Arduini, E. Porreca, D. Lapenna and L. Marzio

A potential detrimental effect of reperfusion was first suggested in the late 50's by the work of Jennings and his coworkers (1).

In a detailed study on dog hearts these authors showed that reperfusion of the previously severe ischemic myocardium was not necessarily a beneficial phenomenon.
In fact, their experiments clearly proved that if, on one hand, the reversibly ischemic myocardium was unable to recover with the readmission of an adequate coronary perfusion, on the other hand, the "reperfusion" was capable of inducing a paradoxical derangement of the "blighted" myocardium (1).

Nevertheless, it has recently been suggested that reperfusion may also jeopardize the potentially salvageable myocardium (2,3). More recently, in their work on isolated hearts, reperfused after prolonged periods of normothermic ischemia, Hearse and Nayler pointed out the concept of "reperfusion injury" (2-5).

For a better understanding of this concept, it is

important to outline that the extent of ischemic damage and whether or not reperfusion is beneficial or detrimental to the ischemic myocardium, depends on the degree and the duration of coronary flow reduction (i.e., ischemic period).

In the isolated rat heart (Fig. 1) an abrupt reduction of the coronary flow is always followed by impairment of myocardial function, which results within a few seconds in a significant decline in developed pressure (DP), with a progressive rise in resting tension (RT).

In severely ischemic hearts (Fig. 1) reperfusion does not prevent the derangement of mechanical function and is associated with an irreversible cellular contracture. By contrast, in moderately ischemic hearts (Fig. 1) reperfusion results in a significant lower contracture, which may reverse, with a significant recovery in developed pressure. In all hearts, a peak value of CK release is seen in the early phase of reperfusion and its amount is strictly related to the severity of ischemia.

It is therefore clear that only when the ischemic injury is "severe" (in duration and/or flow reduction) the reperfusion is followed by a paradoxical impairment of mechanical and metabolic heart function.

Probably, there is no single cause for this reperfusion-induced exacerbation of ischemic injury. Instead, it involves a combination of several factors (i.e., ATP depletion, calcium overload, O_2 readmission) (2).
Interestingly, according to other authors, we have found that reperfusion of the ischemic hearts with anoxic medium results in no increase in damage and no significant increase in CK leakage (Fig. 2).

This is axyomatic for O_2 involvement in the reperfusion damage.

Studies in a variety of tissues, including the central nervous system (6), intestine (7) and myocardium (8) suggest that cytosolic oxygen-derived free radicals, O_2 (the superoxide anion), $^{\cdot}OH$ (the hydroxyl radical) and their intermediary, H_2O_2 (hydroperoxide) are generated at an accelerated rate upon reperfusion and contribute critically to ischemia-reperfusion injury.

Several mechanisms for the production of oxygen-derived free radicals have to be taken into account:
1) monovalent reduction of molecular O_2, due to hypoxia-dependent mitochondrial cytochromoxidase inhibition, with

the production of anion superoxide, hydrogen peroxide and hydroxyl radical (9);

2) auto-oxidation of small cytosolic molecules (i.e., catecholamines) (10);

3) formation of free radicals could also occur at the plasma membrane level, via the arachidonic acid enzymatic pathways (11). In this context, phospholipase may be acti-

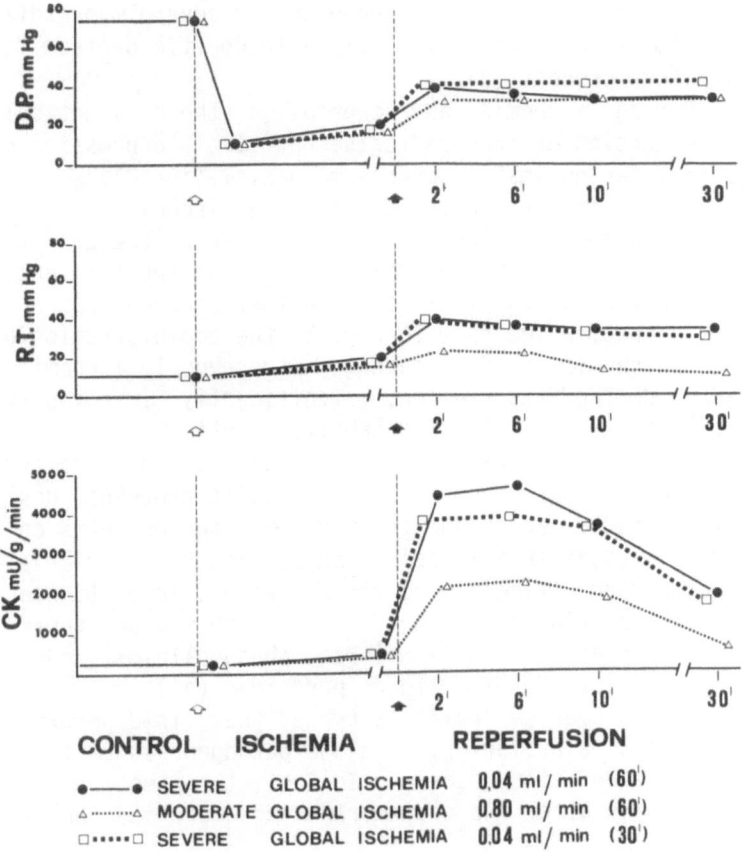

FIGURE 1   The effect of different degrees of ischemia, followed by 30 min reperfusion, on developed pressure (DP), resting tension (RT) and myocardial creatine kinase (CK) release, in the isolated perfused rat heart.

vated by cytosolic-generated free radicals and/or increased availability of Ca^{++} and/or intracellular acidosis (4,12,13);

4) the Ca^{++}-dependent transformation of xanthine dehydrogenase to xanthine oxydase, in the presence of ATP catabolites (i.e., hypoxanthine), evokes the enzymatic production of O_2 and H_2O_2 (14).According to recent studies, this enzymatic pathway has been reported to be localized essentially in the endothelium (15);

5) free radicals may be produced during severe myocardial ischemia (i.e., infarction) via a leukocytic derived inflammatory process (8).

During ischemia and reperfusion, there is not only the production of free radicals, but also a depression of the cellular enzymatic defense mechanism (16-18).

The role of free radicals in myocardial ischemia - reperfusion damage is indirectly suggested by the dramatic protective effect of the administration of specific enzymatic and/or non-enzymatic free radicals scavengers.

In fact, as we show in Fig. 3, the administration of SOD, which is a O_2 scavenger, to severely ischemic hearts during reperfusion, significantly improves the myocardial mechanical and metabolic function.

The reactive free radicals species can oxidize crucial biomolecules, such as DNA, cytosolic proteins, unsaturated fatty acids and the transmembrane proteins containing oxydazable aminoacids, so leading to cellular alteration and ultimately to tissue damage. In particular, the interaction of free radicals with the unsaturated free fatty acids of cell membrane phospholipids, induces the production of toxic lipids peroxides (11).

It has been generally accepted that lipid peroxidation plays a primary role in the pathogenesis of the ischemia-reperfusion damage. In fact, the phenomenon may dramatically alter the biomembrane structure and function (11).

Peroxidation of fatty acids containing three or more double bonds will produce malonildialdehyde (MDA). The presence of this oxydation by-product can be measured with thiobarbituric acid, which, although not a specific or quantitative indication of fatty acid oxydation, correlates with the extent of free radical-induced lipid peroxidation (11,19).

Recently, the possibility of restoring an adequate

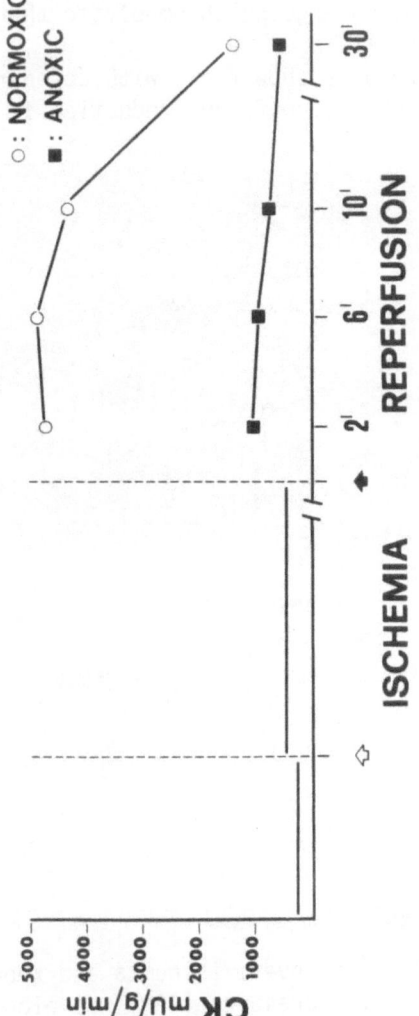

FIGURE 2   The effect of normoxic or anoxic (95% N_2 + 5% CO_2) reperfusion upon
creatine kinase (CCK) leakage in isolated perfused rat heart subjected to
60 min severe ischemia (coronary flow 0.04 ml min^{-1}).

blood supply to the ischemic myocardium, by means of thrombolytic agents or surgical or angioplastic techniques, has emphasized the importance of the reflow injury in human pathology (20).

To test the validity of MDA as an early index of reperfusion and of free radical-induced myocardial damage, we evaluated MDA both in the peripheral and in the coronary sinus plasma of patients suffering from acute myocardial infarction, undergoing thrombolytic therapy with streptokinase.

Our preliminary data show that, with coronary reperfusion (assessed by a significant reduction in S-T seg-

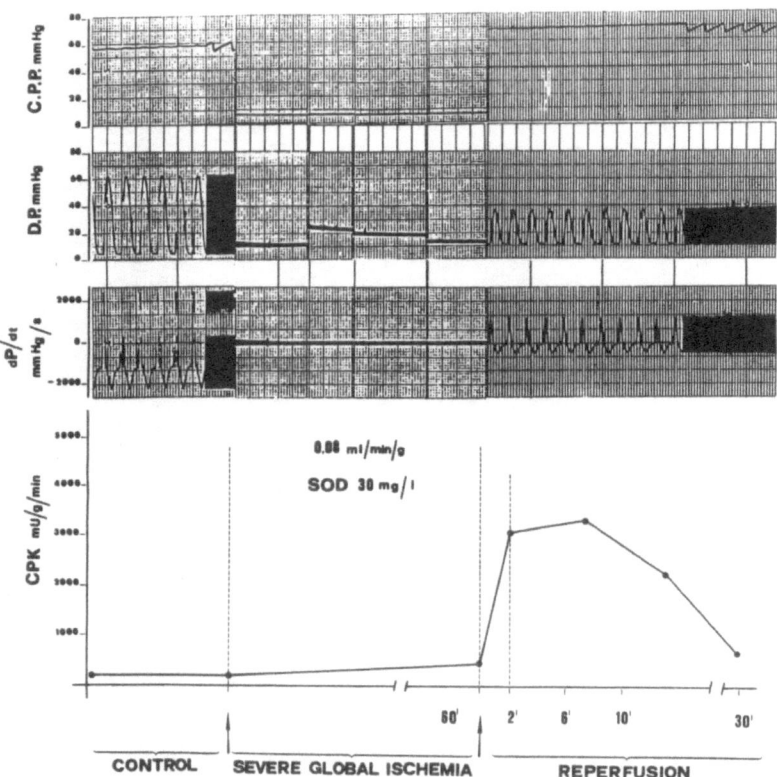

FIGURE 3 The effect of severe ischemia and reperfusion on coronary perfusion pressure (CPP), developed pressure (DP), resting tension (RT), dp/dt and on creatine kinase myocardial release in isolated rat heart,in presence of superoxide dismutase (SOD) 30 mg/l.

ment elevation), plasma MDA level increased rapidly from 4.2 nmol/ml to 5.7 nmol/ml, whereas coronary sinus plasma MDA increased from 7.1 nmol/ml to 9.8 nmol/ml, due to a greater regional MDA concentration. After 30 min reperfusion, MDA levels approached the basal values (Fig. 4).

MDA therefore seems to be a valid and early biochemical index of myocardial reperfusion and could be used in the assessment of reperfusion damage.

Nevertheless, a more extensive and thorough research is needed to confirm these data.

To conclude:
1) myocardial ischemia involves two different types of specific damage: ischemic damage and reperfusion damage;
2) the reperfusion damage depends upon the duration and severeness of ischemia;
3) thrombolytic treatment in acute myocardial infarction emphasizes the need for a new therapeutic approach: the prevention of reperfusion damage.

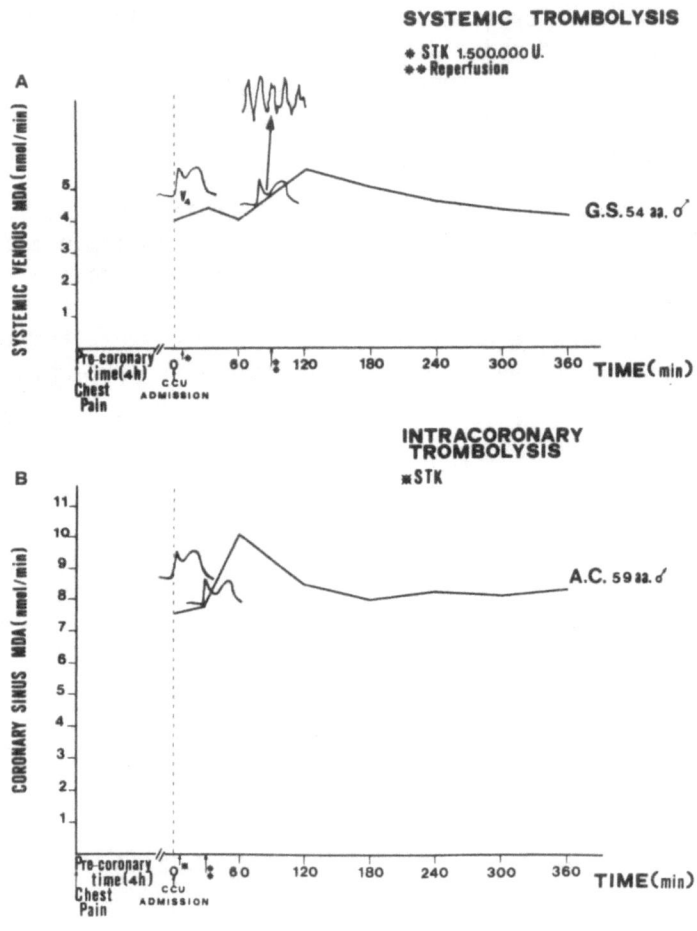

FIGURE 4   Systemic venous and coronary sinus malonildi-
    aldehyde concentration curves from two infarcted
    patients treated with intravenous streptokinase (A)
    or intracoronary streptokinase (B).

References

1.   Jennings, RB, Sommers, HM, Smyth, GA, Flack, HA and Linn H (1960). Myocardial necrosis induced by temporary occlusion of a coronary artery in the dog. Arch Patol, 70, 68
2.   Nayler, WG and Elz, JS (1986). Reperfusion injury: laboratory artifact or clinical dilemma? Circulation, 74, 215
3.   Hearse, DJ (1977). Reperfusion of the ischemic myocardium. J Mol Cell Cardiol, 9, 605
4.   Nayler, WG (1983). Calcium and cell death. Eur Heart J, 4, 33
5.   Nayler, WG, Sturrock, WJ and Panagiotopoulos, S (1985). Calcium and myocardial ischemia. In: Parrott, JR (ed.) "Control and manipulation of calcium movement". p.303. (New York: Raven Press)
6.   Demopoulos, HB, Flamm, ES, Pietronigro, DD,Sezigram, ML (1980). The free radical pathology and the microcirculation in the major central nervous system disorders. Acta Physiol Scand, 492 (suppl.), 91
7.   Parks, DA, Bulkley, GB and Granger, DN (1983). Role of oxygen-derived free radicals in digestive tract disease. Surgery, 94, 415
8.   Werns, SW, Shea, MJ and Lucchesi,BR (1986). Free radicals and myocardial injury: pharmacological implications. Circulation, 74, 1
9.   Fridovich, J (1978). The biology of oxygen radicals. Science, 201, 875
10. Singal, PK, Beamish, RE and Dhalla, NS(1983). Potential oxydative pathway of catecholamines in formation of lipid peroxides and genesis of heart disease. Adv Exp Med Biol, 161, 391
11. Freeman, BA and Crapo, JD (1982). Free radicals and tissue injury. Lab Invest, 47, 412
12. Weiglicki, WB, Dickens, BF and Tong Mak, I (1984). Enhanced lysophospholipid production during free radical injury of lysosomes. Circulation, 70 (Suppl. II), II-80 (Abstr.)
13. Weiglicki, WB, Owens, K, Urschell, CW, Serur, JR and Sonnenblick, EH (1972). Hydrolysis of myocardial lipids during acidosis and ischaemia. In: Dhalla, NS (ed.) "Recent Advances in Studies on Cardiac Structure and Metabolism". p.781. (Baltimore: University Park Press)

14. Chambers, DE, Parks, DA, Patterson, G, Roy, R, Mc Cord, JM, Yoshida, S, Parmley, LF and Dowley, JM (1985). Xanthine oxidase as a source of free radical damage in myocardial ischemia. J Mol Cell Cardiol, 17, 145

15. Schoutsen, D, Keijzer, E and deJong, JW (1986). Heart xanthine Oxidoreductase activity with age; the enzyme is absent from Myocytes. J Mol Cell Cardiol 18 (suppl. 3), 62 (abstr.)

16. Guarnieri, C, Flamigni, F and Caldarera, CM (1980). Role of oxygen in the cellular damage induced by reoxygenation of hypoxic heart. J Mol Cell Cardiol, 12, 797

17. Ferrari, R, Ceconi, C, Curello, S, Guarnieri, C, Caldarera, CM, Albertini, A and Visioli, O (1985).Oxygen-mediated Myocardial damage during ischaemia and reperfusion: role of the cellular defences against oxygen toxicity. J Mol Cell Cardiol, 17, 937

18. Peterson, DA, Asinger, RW, Elsperger, KJ, Homans, DC and Eaton, JW (1985). Reactive oxygen species may cause myocardial reperfusion injury. Biochem Phys Res Comm, 127, 87

19. Satoh, K (1978). Serum lipid peroxide in cerebrovascular disorders determined by a new colorimetric method. Clin Chim Acta, 90, 37

20. Braunwald, E and Kloner, RA (1985).Myocardial reperfusion: A double-edged sword? J Clin Invest, 76, 1713

45
Local and remote effects of acute ischaemic infarction on cerebral glucose metabolism in man

M. Kushner, M. Reivich, C. Fieschi, F. Silver,
J. Chawluk, M. Rosen, A. Burke and A. Alavi

INTRODUCTION

Positron emission tomographic exploration of local cerebral metabolism in acute cerebrovascular diseases have concentrated mostly on the use of 15_O.

Thus, several groups have observed an early increase of oxygen extraction (rOEF), in face of insufficient perfusion (Ackerman (1), Lenzi (2), Baron (3), Wise(4)), while, in subsequent days, the rOEF rapidly drops below the threshold of tissue viability, thus leading to relative or absolute luxury perfusion where blood flow is in excess of the scarce metabolic requirements of the irreparably damaged tissue.

Concurrently, Baron (5) recently demonstrated uncoupling between CMRO and CMRglu, suggesting enhanced glycolysis despite a relative abundance of oxygen, possibly due to local anaerobic conditions.

In addition to local metabolic effects, PET has demonstrated that alterations in the pattern of cerebral metabolism remote from the lesion can be induced by focal cerebral ischemia. Kuhl (6) demonstrated that PET is capable of delineating abnormality earlier than conventional CT and with a wider anatomic distribution. Unanticipated remote metabolic findings have included depression of both metabolism and blood flow in the cerebellum contralateral to supratentorial ischemia (Baron (7), Kushner (8), Pantano (9)). Such findings are not specific but have been reported in conjunction with intracerebral tumors (Patronas, (10)).

MATERIAL AND METHODS

The present study was conducted at the Cerebrovascular Research Center of the University of Pennsylvania and summarizes the clinical, metabolic and anatomic findings in a large series of patients following acute cerebral ischemia.

Imaging of local cerebral glucose metabolism were obtained using 18 F-deoxygluse and positron emission tomography with a modified version of PET V. Data in extenso are reported by Kushner et al (1986).

RESULTS AND DISCUSSION

Thirty-five patients were studied with FDG-PET in the acute phase following focal cerebral ischemia.

One third of patients (12) were studied within three days of the ictus, one third within 4-5 days, one third between 6 days and two weeks. Patients had hemispheric strokes of various severity (4 with complete and 13 with good subsequent recovery of neurological functions), and no patient comatose at the time of the study was included.

In addition to successfully localising the lesion, like CT and MRI, PET was able to define the pattern of cerebral dysfunction, unlike the previous imaging techniques.

The overall sensitivity of PET and CT was similar, but the dimensions of "functional" lesion seen with the metabolic imaging, extended beyond the borders of the CT lesions and were observed also at distance from the ischemic lesions, such as in ipsilateral thalamus in cases of left cortical infarct with aphasia.

A metabolic threshold for irreversible structural changes is hardly defined, due to the limitations of the DG method in acute ischemic tissues.

However, metabolic asymmetries between homologus regions of the affected and unaffected hemisphere allowed to delineate clinical correlations with the severity of the presenting neurological dysfunctions, and with the clinical outcome. Some consistent relationships between clinical

348

outcome and the severity of the metabolic abnormality at presentation were apparent. A normal PET scan or the presence of a mild abnormality (classes I or II) was strongly associated with a good outcome or a complete reversal of the neurological dysfunction (Pearson's R=0.32, p<0.05).

The exceptions to this trend were comprised of 2 cases of lacunar infarction where the course was stable or improvement was only moderate, although the overall degree of clinical disability was mild. Most commonly, a completely normal PET image was found in association with a good recovery. A moderate or severely abnormal PET scan at the outset was also a prognostic indicator.

Patients with moderate or severe metabolic abnormalities (classes III or IV) tended to have a stable disability or only moderate improvement. By examining the reverse situation, it was apparent that patients with poorer outcomes as manifested by only moderate recovery or a stable course tended to have the most severe PET abnormalities.

The prognosic correlates of early metabolic abnormalities suggest future extension of PET studies to objectively monitoring significant effects of treatment in cerebral ischemia.

SUMMARY

Pet studies with 18 F-DG were completed in 35 patients with acute ischemic strokes. Twelve cases were studied within 72 hours, 23 between 4 and 14 days. Results indicate the functional and prognostic significance of early tomographic studies of metabolism, and anticipate possible use of metabolic mapping in the evaluation of treatment.

REFERENCES

1) Ackerman, RH, Correia, JA, Alpert NM, Baron JC, Gouliamos, A, Grotta (1981) Psitron imaging in ischemic stroke disease using compound labeled with oxygen 15. Arch Neurol 38: 537-543

2) Lenzi, GL, Frackowiak, RS and Jones, T (1982) Cerebral

oxygen metabolism and blood flow in human cerebral infarctions. J CBF and Met 2: 321-335.

3) Baron, JC, Rougemont, D, Bouser, MG, Lebrun-Grandie, P, Iba-Zizen, TM (1983) Local CBF, oxygen extraction fraction (OEF) and CMRO2: prognostic value in recent supratentorial infarction in humans. J CBF and Met 3 (suppl): S1-S2

4) Wise, RJS, Bernardi, S, Frackowiak, RSJ, Legg NJ, Jones, T (1983) Serial observations on the pathophysiology of acute stroke. Brain 1983 106: 197-222

5) Baron, JC, Rougemont, D, Soussaline, F, Bustany, P, Crouzel, C, Bousser, MG and Comar D (1984) Local interrelationships of cerebral oxygen consumption and glucose utilization in normal subjects and in ischemic stroke patients: a positron tomography study. J CBF and Met: 140-149

6) Kuhl, DE, Phelps, ME, Kowell, AP (1980) Effect of stroke on local cerebral metabolism and perfusion. Ann Neurol 8:47-60

7) Baron, JC, Bousser, MG, Comar, D et al.(1981): "Crossed cerebellar diaschisis": a remote functional depression secondary to supratentorial infarction in man. J CBF and Met 1 (suppl 1): S500-S501

8) Kushner, MJ, Alavi, A, Reivich, M, Dann, R, Burke, A, Robinson, G (1984) Contralateral cerebellar hypometabolism following cerebral insult. Ann Neurol. 15: 425-434

9) Pantano, P, Baron, JC, Sanson, J, Bousser, MG, Derousne, C, Comar, D (in press) Brain 1986

10) Patronas, NJ, Di Chiro, G, Smith, BH, De La Paz, RL, Brooks, RA, Milan, H, Kornblith, PL, Bairamian, D, Mansi, L (1984) Depressed cerebellar glucose metabolism in supratentorial tumors. Brain Research 291: 93-101

SEROTONIN AND THE CARDIOVASCULAR SYSTEM

46
Serotonin and cardiovascular disease

J.M. Van Nueten, F. De Clerck, W.J. Janssens and
P.A.J. Janssen

INTRODUCTION

The cardiovascular system ensures a continuous suply of nutrients
and oxygen to the cells and a continuous wash-out of waste products
from these cells. If this can no longer be assured, tissue ischemia and dysfunction become unavoidable. The appropriate blood
stream to the tissues is controlled by changes in wall tension and
diameter of the precapillary blood vessels, which helps to determine both peripheral vascular resistance and fluid exchanges at the
capillary level. Active changes in diameter of the blood vessels
are controlled mainly by the sympathetic tone, but can be modulated
by a number of endogenous substances including those formed or released in the vicinity of the vascular smooth muscle cells [1].

One of these substances is serotonin, identified as a gut-
stimulating substance from enterochromaffin cells [2] and as a
vasoconstrictor agent present in serum after blood has clotted [3].
The main sources of serotonin available to the blood vessel wall
are blood platelets, which when they aggregate release serotonin
and other vasoactive substances. The effects of serotonin on the
cardiovascular system are complex and their multiplicity is well
established [3]. Recently, specific serotonergic antagonists such
as ketanserin became available, thus stimulating a revival in fundamental studies on serotonin [4, 5]. Platelet-vessel wall interaction, related in particular to the release of serotonin and other
endogenous substances, may be of crucial significance in the etiology of some cardiovascular diseases [4, 5].

The present review will discuss the experimental and clinical
evidence for a possible role of serotonin in a number of cardiovascular pathological conditions including hypertension and diseases related to impaired tissue perfusion.

PLATELETS

Whereas aggregating platelets are the peripheral source of serotonin, the monoamine itself can induce further aggregation of
platelets in several mammalian species. Although this reaction of
serotonin is comparatively weak in normal human platelets, sero-

tonin strongly augments ("amplifies") the aggregation of human platelets induced by low concentrations of other aggregating substances. Both the direct and amplifying effects of serotonin on platelets are prevented by ketanserin, indicating that S_2-serotonergic receptors are involved (Fig. 1) [6]. The potency of serotonin in respect of amplification is particularly evident when multiple agonists are used to challenge the platelets [7].

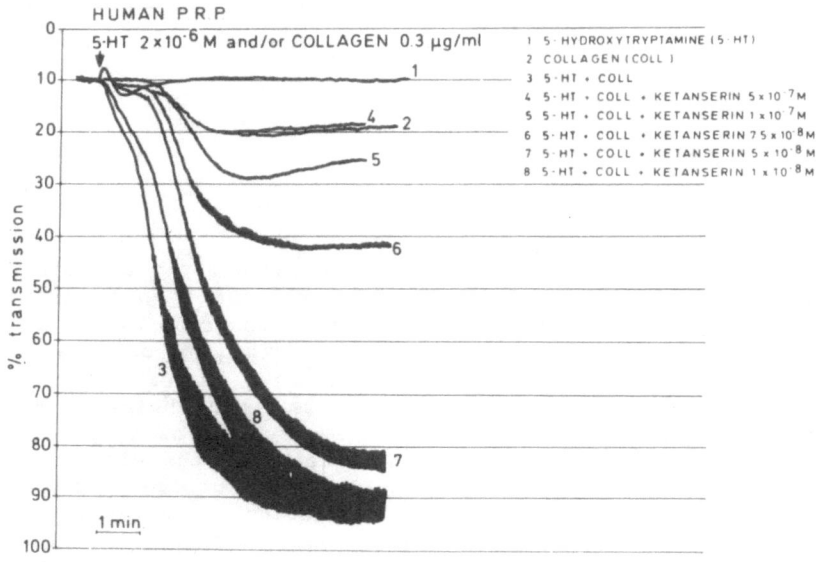

FIGURE 1   Amplification by serotonin (5-HT) and its inhibition by ketanserin of human platelet aggregation induced by a threshold concentration of collagen. (Reproduced from De Clerck et al., 1982, with permission.)

By such mechanisms, serotonin may contribute to the mechanical obstruction of a blood vessel by a platelet thrombus, as observed in experimental conditions. Platelet aggregation and subsequent thrombotic obstruction were observed in canine coronary arteries damaged by mechanically-induced stenosis [8]. The antithrombotic effects of ketanserin in this model substantiate the hypothesis for a contribution of serotonin in this pathological event.

Serotonin is taken up by platelets, where it is stored, and by vascular endothelial cells, where it is inactivated enzymatically, in particular in the pulmonary circulation. Whenever these uptake mechanisms are inhibited and the turnover of platelets is accelerated or when the vascular endothelium becomes dysfunctional or damaged, more serotonin will be presented to the vascular smooth muscle cells. Moreover, since the release of an endothelium-derived relaxing factor will no longer be induced [9], the serotonin-induced vascular contractions come to full expression.

VASCULAR TISSUE

Direct vasoconstrictor effects

Blood vessels - for example cerebral, coronary, pulmonary and um-
bilical arteries, and also collateral arteries of the hindlimb -
contract _in vitro_ when exposed to the monoamine [10, 11]. In most
vascular preparations the contractions evoked with serotonin can be
competitively antagonized by ketanserin, indicating that S_2-seroto-
nergic receptors are involved [10]. In certain blood vessels such
as the basilar and coronary arteries and the saphenous vein of the
dog, another, yet unknown mechanism may also be partly involved,
but even in these blood vessels a substantial contribution to contraction is made by S_2-serotonergic receptors [10]. Aggregating
platelets release serotonin in amounts sufficient to cause contractions of vascular smooth muscle in a variety of isolated blood
vessels. The vasoconstrictor effects of serotonin either exogenous
or released from platelets, are inhibited by ketanserin in a dose-
dependent manner (fig. 2) [12].

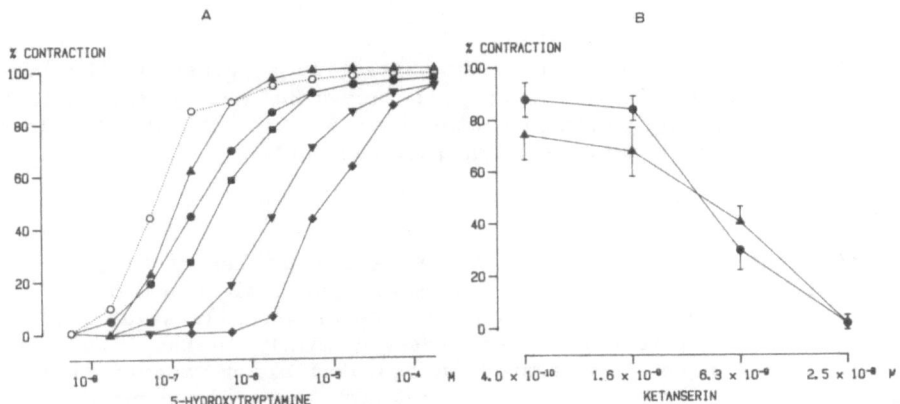

FIGURE 2 A. Effects of ketanserin (30-min incubation) on contractile responses of isolated rabbit pulmonary arteries to
increasing concentrations of serotonin (mean values, n = 5).
Control (o), ketanserin 4.0 x 10^{-10} M (▲), 1.6 x 10^{-9} M (●),
6.3 x 10^{-9} M (■), 2.5 x 10^{-8} M (▼), 1.0 x 10^{-7} M (◆).
B. Contractile responses of isolated rabbit pulmonary arteries
to serotonin (5 x 10^{-7} M) (Δ) or to rat platelets (30,000/μl)
stimulated with thrombin (0.5 U/ml) (o) after incubation (5
min) with increasing concentrations of ketanserin (means ±SEM,
n = 5). (Reproduced from Van Nueten, 1985, with permission.)

Amplifying effects

A threshold concentration of serotonin augments ("amplifies") contractions of isolated blood vessels in response to other agonists.
Thus, the monoamine amplifies the vasoconstrictor response to neurohumoral mediators such as norepinephrine, angiotensin II, hist-

amine, prostaglandin $F_{2\alpha}$ and thromboxane A_2 and to sympathetic stimulation [5]. Such amplification has also been demonstrated when aggregating platelets were used as the source for serotonin (Fig. 3) and was observed in a variety of isolated vascular tissues including human vessels [10, 13]. Amplifying effects have been reported in vivo in various species including man [5]. The amplifying effect of serotonin on the pressor responses to norepinephrine is more pronounced in hypertensive than in normotensive sheep [14].

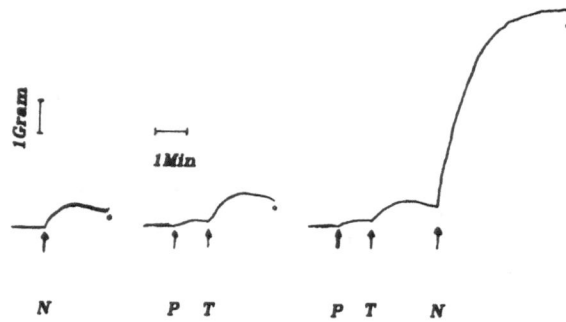

FIGURE 3   Amplification of the contractile response of the isolated rabbit femoral artery to noradrenaline by aggregating rat platelets. N: norepinephrine 5.9 x 10^{-9} M; P: platelets 2500/µl; T: thrombin 0.5 U/ml; •: wash out.

Vasodilator effect

Serotonin has complex actions on the cardiovascular system; it can cause either an increase or a decrease in systemic blood pressure, it can induce peripheral vasoconstriction or vasodilatation [3, 4]. The vasodilator effect has been observed mainly in the intact organism. It can be demonstrated on isolated blood vessels with an elevated tone. In most blood vessels the serotonin-induced vasodilatation is observed when the endothelium is still present. In precontracted coronary arteries serotonin released from aggregating platelets causes opposite, vasodilator or vasoconstrictor responses, depending on the presence or absence of endothelium [15]. In the dog, 2-3 weeks after the superficial femoral artery has been occluded, vasodilatation normally induced by serotonin becomes vasoconstriction, with a reduction in calf blood flow [11].

PATHOLOGY

A variety of vasoactive neurohumoral mediators are continuously released and circulate in the vascular beds at levels too low to induce any effect by itself. In the presence of an amplifying agent (e.g. serotonin released from platelets) such substances may lead to vasoconstriction and even to vasospasm [16]. This will eventually result in pathological conditions due to impairment of regional circulation and deficient tissue perfusion [4, 16]. Am-

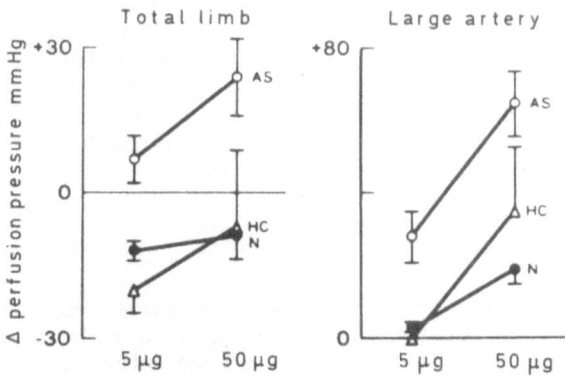

FIGURE 4 Vascular responses to i.a. injections of serotonin in the perfused hindlimb of normal (N), atherosclerotic (AS), and hypercholesterolemic (HC) monkeys. Values are changes in total hindlimb (iliac) perfusion pressure (left) and in the pressure gradient of the large artery segment (iliac perfusion pressure minus dorsal pedal pressure) (right). (Reproduced from Heistad et al., 1984, with permission.)

plifying effects will be of consequence in particular when there is an enhanced release of serotonin from platelets and a concomitant vascular hyperreactivity to serotonin, as observed in a number of cardiovascular diseases, including atherosclerosis and chronic hypertension.

An infusion of serotonin in atherosclerotic monkeys produced a marked decrease in total limb flow, while the opposite effect was observed in normal monkeys; serotonin-induced constriction of large arteries was more pronounced in atherosclerotic monkeys (Fig. 4) [17].

Increased vasoconstriction to serotonin and increased platelet activation has been observed during hypertension in animals and man [4, 18]. The amplifying effect of serotonin on noradrenaline-induced vasoconstrictor or pressor responses is markedly more pronounced in hypertensive than in normotensive animals and in older than in younger animals [14, 19].

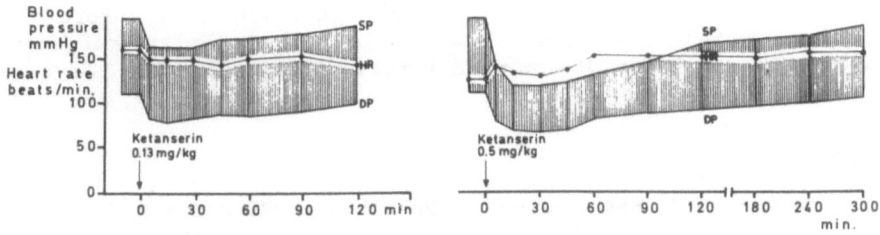

FIGURE 5 Ketanserin (i.v.) dose-dependently decreases systolic (SP) and diastolic (DP) blood pressure in old hypertensive dogs without modifying heart rate (HR) (——) (means; n = 4; data by courtesy of Jageneau, AHM, 1982).

357

This, together with an increased platelet activation during hypertension suggests that serotonin is one of the agents responsible for an increased peripheral vascular resistance. This may, at least partly, explain why the S_2-serotonergic antagonist ketanserin lowers blood pressure not only in hypertensive animals (Fig. 5), but also in hypertensive patients both acutely and chronically, in particular in the elderly [20].

SUMMARY

When activated, platelets release a number of vasoactive substances, including serotonin, resulting in a rise in concentration of the monoamine in the blood. Serotonin induces aggregation of blood platelets and amplifies aggregation induced by other agonists. Platelet-derived serotonin causes vasoconstriction in large arteries, veins and venules and increases vascular permeability. The vasoconstrictor effect can be due to the direct action of serotonin on the vascular smooth muscle or to its potential to amplify the vasoconstrictor response to other endogenous substances. In most blood vessels direct and amplifying vasoconstrictor responses to serotonin released from aggregating platelets are due to activation by S_2-serotonergic receptors since they are inhibited by ketanserin. In some conditions serotonin can cause vasodilatation, in particular at the arteriolar level, by releasing a relaxant factor from the endothelium or by inhibiting sympathetic tone. This vasodilatation is not due to S_2-serotonergic receptor activation since it is not inhibited but enhanced by ketanserin. The net effect of serotonin in a given area of the vascular system is determined by the balance of its vasoconstrictor and vasodilator effects.

The vasoconstrictor effect is more pronounced in a number of chronic pathological conditions such as hypertension, atherosclerosis, cardiopathy, particularly in older individuals and if the endothelium is dysfunctional or absent.

An acceleration of the turnover of platelets, a reduction of the uptake of serotonin by platelets and of its metabolism by the endothelium, and a vascular hyperreactivity to the constrictor response to serotonin have been observed in hypertensive man or animals. These phenomena may lead to an increase in peripheral resistance characteristic of chronic hypertension and suggest a role of serotonin in this disease. This suggestion is reinforced by the observation that the S_2-serotonergic antagonist ketanserin lowers arterial blood pressure in hypertensive patients.

REFERENCES

1. Shepherd, JT and Vanhoutte, PM (1979). "The Human Cardiovascular System. Facts and Concepts". p. 363. (New York: Raven Press)
2. Erspamer, V and Asero, B (1952). Identification of enteramine, the specific hormone of the enterochromaffin cell system, as 5-hydroxytryptamine. Nature, 169, 800
3. Page, IH (1954). Serotonin (5-hydroxytryptamine). Physiol Rev, 34, 563

4. Vanhoutte, PM (1983). 5-Hydroxytryptamine and vascular disease. Fed Proc, 42, 233

5. Van Nueten, JM, Janssens, WJ and Vanhoutte, PM (1985). Serotonin and vascular reactivity. Pharmacol Res Commun, 17, 585

6. De Clerck, F, David, JL and Janssen, PAJ (1982). Inhibition of 5-hydroxytryptamine-induced and -amplified human platelet aggregation by ketanserin (R 41 468), a selective 5-HT$_2$ receptor antagonist. Agents Actions, 12, 388

7. De Clerck, F, Van Nueten, JM, Symoens, J and Janssen, PAJ (1986). Ketanserin in platelet-vessel wall interactions. Agents Actions, in press

8. Bush, LR, Campbell, WB, Kern, K, Tilton, GD, Apprill, P, Buja, LM and Willerson, JT (1984). The effects of alpha$_2$ adrenergic and serotonergic receptor blockade on platelet aggregation in stenosed canine coronary arteries. Circ Res, 55, 642

9. Furchgott, RF (1983). Role of endothelium in responses of vascular smooth muscle. Circ Res, 53, 557

10. Van Nueten, JM, Janssen, PAJ, Van Beek, J, Xhonneux, R, Verbeuren, TJ and Vanhoutte, PM (1981). Vascular effects of ketanserin (R 41 468), a novel antagonist of 5-HT$_2$ serotonergic receptors. J Pharmacol Exp Ther, 218, 217

11. Hollenberg, NK (1985). Segmental vascular responses to serotonin. In: Vanhoutte, PM (ed.) "Serotonin and the Cardiovascular System". p. 165. (New York: Raven Press)

12. Van Nueten, JM (1985). Serotonin and the blood vessel wall. J Cardiovasc Pharmacol, 7, S49

13. De La Lande, IS, Cannel, VA and Waterson, JG (1966). The interaction of serotonin and noradrenaline on the perfused artery. Br J Pharmacol Chemother, 28, 255

14. Myers, JH, Mecca, TE and Webb, RC (1985). Direct and sensitizing effects of serotonin agonists and antagonists in vascular, smooth muscle. J Cardiovasc Pharmacol, 7, S44

15. Cohen, RA, Shepherd, JT and Vanhoutte, PM (1983). Inhibitory role of the endothelium in the response of isolated arteries to platelets. Science, 221, 273

16. Vanhoutte, PM and Houston, DS (1985). Platelets, endothelium, and vasospasm. Circulation, 72, 728

17. Heistad, DD, Armstrong, ML, Marcus, ML, Piegors, DJ and Mark, AL (1984). Augmented responses to vasoconstrictor stimuli in hypercholesterolemic and atherosclerotic monkeys. Circ Res, 54, 711

18. Doyle, AE, Fraser, JRE and Marshall, RJ (1959). Reactivity of forearm vessels to vasoconstrictor substances in hypertensive and normotensive subjects. Clin Sci, 18, 441

19. Janssens, WJ and Van Nueten, JM (1986). The direct and amplifying effects of serotonin are increased with age in the isolated perfused kidney of Wistar and spontaneously hypertensive rats. Naunyn Schmiedebergs Arch Pharmacol, in press

20. De Cree, J, Leempoels, J, De Cock, W, Geukens, H and Verhaegen, H (1981). The antihypertensive effects of a pure and selective serotonin-receptor blocking agent (R 41 468) in elderly patients. Angiology, 32, 137

47
Ketanserin in the treatment of hypertension: clinical review

A. Palermo and A. Libretti

Ketanserin, a selective and specific antagonist for serotoninergic S_2 receptors, has recently been introduced in the pharmacological
management of essential hypertension (1-3). Preliminary results provide strong evidences supporting the hypothesis that serotonin is involved in the etiopathogenesis of this condition (4-5).

So far,Ketanserin has been given approximately to 2000 patients
in different types of controlled studies: in monotherapy, compared to
placebo or other reference drugs, like beta-blockers, diuretics,alpha
methyldopa, or in association. This review is a survey of data-base
made available by Dr.J.Symoens of Janssen Pharmaceutica from world-
wide studies on the effects of chronic treatment with Ketanserin (6).

At first, antihypertensive properties of Ketanserin have been
shown in double-blind, placebo-controlled trials: Ketanserin lowers
either systolic or diastolic blood pressure to a greater degree than
placebo. The dosages currently recommended are 20 or 40 mg twice daily,
higher doses producing an increased incidence of adverse effects and
no added benefit (7). Studies on continous monitoring of blood pressure show that the hypotensive effect is maintained throughout 24 hours
(8).

The fall in blood pressure induced by Ketanserin is progressive:
it begins within two weeks of treatment and keeps on between the 2th
and the 4th week; an additional fall in diastolic blood pressure is
still observed between the 8th and the 12th week. After three months
of monotherapy with Ketanserin (40 mg t.i.d.), systolic and diastolic
blood pressure are reduced by about 10% and 15% respectively (Fig.1).
Neither significant changes in heart rate nor postural hypotension
are observed.

The hypotensive effect of Ketanserin monotherapy is maintained
during long-term treatment over one year, without any effect of tolerance (6) (Fig.2). When the drug is withdrawn, blood pressure rises
back to baseline level over a period of four weeks without any rebound
effect.

361

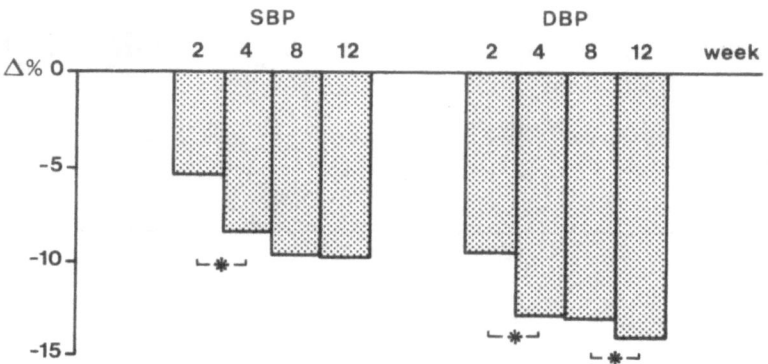

FIGURE 1   Progressive antihypertensive effect of Ketanserin mono –
therapy (40 mg t.i.d.).

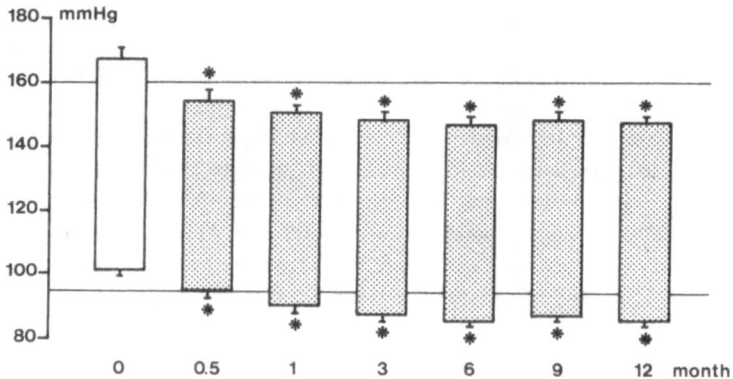

FIGURE 2   Antihypertensive effect of long-term monotherapy with
Ketanserin (from international controlled studies, Ref 6).

The hypotensive effect of Ketanserin depends very much on the
initial blood pressure, so that the fall in blood pressure is greater
in severe rather than in borderline and mild hypertension (Fig.3).
Looking at the response rate as a function of severity of hypertension, blood pressure is normalized, i.e. diastolic blood pressure falls
below 90 mmHg, in about 80% and 70% of patients with borderline and
mild hypertension respectively and in 50% and 30% of patients with
moderate and severe hypertension. Partial responses, defined as a fall
in diastolic blood pressure by 10%, are observed in about 20% and 40%
of patients with moderate and severe hypertension respectively (Fig4)

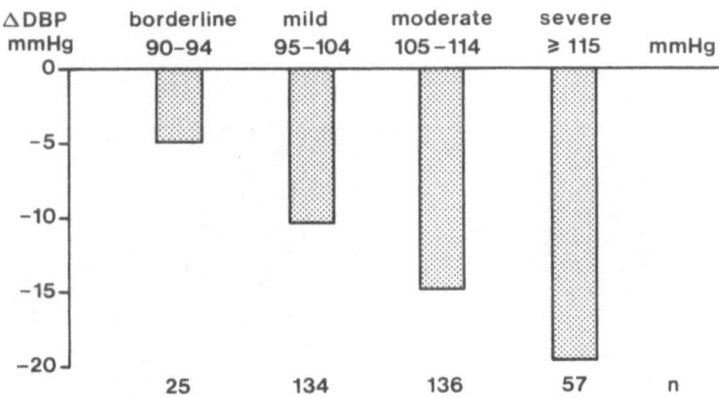

FIGURE 3   Change in diastolic blood pressure at 3 months of mono-
            therapy with Ketanserin at therapeutic doses (40 mg t.i.d.)
            (from international controlled studies, ref. 6)

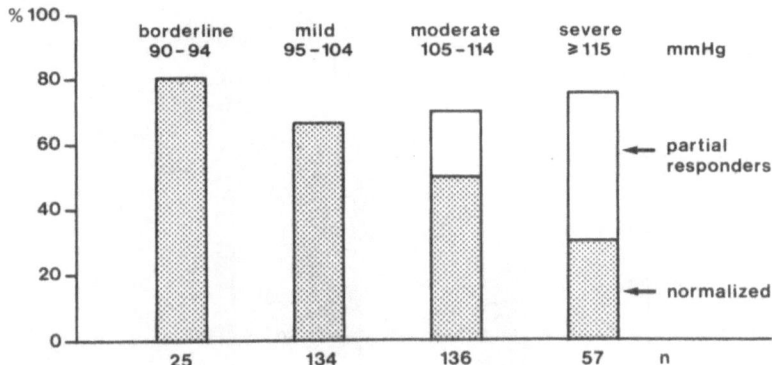

FIGURE 4   Response rate as a function of severity of hypertension
            after 3 months of monotherapy with Ketanserin at thera -
            peutic doses (40 mg t.i.d.) (from international controlled
            studies, Ref. 6).

        Results of international double-blind comparative studies show
that the efficacy and the reponse rate of monotherapy with Ketanserin
(40 mg t.i.d.) or Metoprolol (100 mg t.i.d.) or Hydroclorotiazide
(50 mg) over three months are similar (Fig. 5-6). However, Ketanserin
appears to be particularly more effective in the elderly, unlike the

other drugs (6).

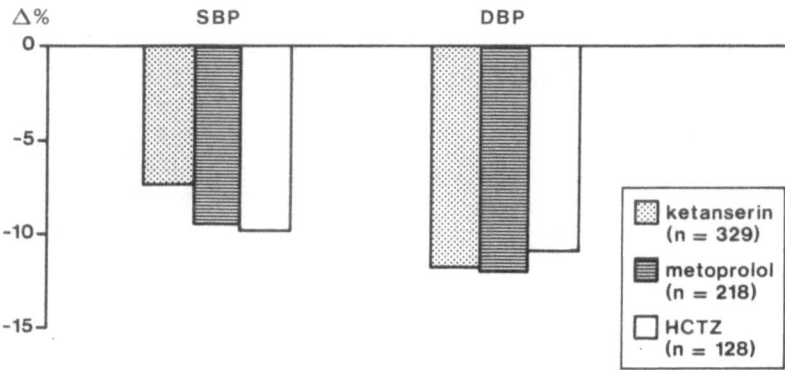

FIGURE 5   Efficacy of monotherapy with Ketanserin, Metoprolol and
            Hydroclorotiazide over 3 months (from international con-
            trolled studies, Ref. 6).

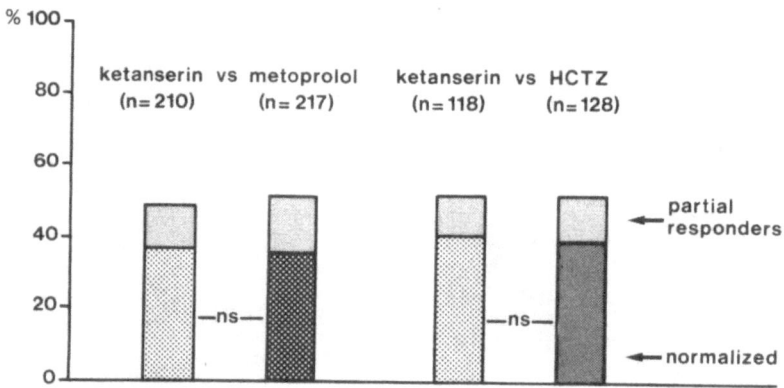

FIGURE 6   Response rate after three months of monotherapy (from
            international controlled studies, Ref. 6).

If monotherapy with Ketanserin fails to normalize blood pressure,
the combination with beta-blockers or diuretics can produce an additional greater effect (fig. 7).
Similarly, an impressive fall in blood pressure is observed giving
Ketanserin to patients unresponsive to previuos therapy with beta -
blockers or diuretics (9).

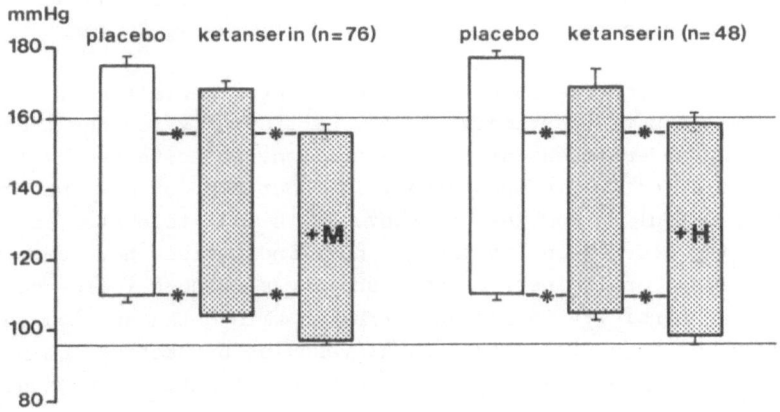

FIGURE 7   Hypotensive effect of association with Metoprolol and
Hydroclorotiazide to Ketanserin in unresponsive patients
(Ref. 6).

Long-term therapy with Ketanserin does not induce any serious adverse reactions. The initial subjective effects (light-headedness,
lack of concentration, drowsiness) are dose-dependent and generally
subside after the initial dose. During chronic treatment the most
frequent adverse reactions are headache, dizziness, fatigue,dispepsia,
dry mouth; however, their incidence is similar to that observed after
placebo (6). The :incidence of drop-out for adverse reactions is very
low, about 5%, at therapeutic doses recommended, but it becomes dramatically higher at doses of 60 mg or more (Fig. 8)

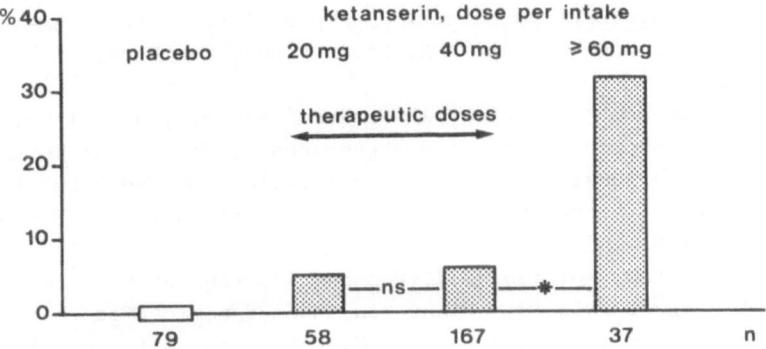

FIGURE 8   Incidence of drop-out for adverse reactions during monotherapy with Ketanserin (Ref. 6).

Long-term therapy does not induce any significant adverse changes in biochemical parameters. A favourable change in the HDL:LDL ratio has been reported (6).

In conclusion, Ketanserin may represent a new alternative in the first-line of antihypertensive drugs, particularly for the treatment of mild and moderate essential hypertension. The data available show that it is effective in monotherapy in about 50% of patients treated and it is useful in combined therapy. It is well tolerated, particularly in the elderly and so far no contraindications have been reported. Moreover, preliminary reports showing a reduced incidence in cardiovascular morbidity in patients treated with Ketanserin suggest that this drug, because of its additional vascular protective action, might be particularly advisable in the treatment of patients with atherosclerosis (6).

REFERENCES

1. Van Neuten JM, Leysen JE, Schnurkes JAJ, Vanhoutte PM: Ketanserin: a selective antagonist of $5HT_2$ serotoninergic receptors. Lancet i: 297-298, 1983.
2. Vanhoutte PM, Van Neuten JM: Ketanserin, a novel antihypertensive drug. J. Pharm. Pharmacol. 35: 339-340, 1983.
3. Schalekamp MADH: Serotonin blockade and hypertension. In "Serotonin and the cardiovascular system" ed. Vanhoutte PM, Raven Press, New York, 1985, 135-145.
4. Symoens J, Vanhoutte PM: Role of serotonin in blood pressure regulation. In "Care of postoperative surgical patient" eds. Smith JAR and Watkins J, Butterworths, London, 1985, 141-164.
5. De Cree J, Leempoels J, Geukens H, De Cock W, Verhaegen H: Are serotoninergic mechanism involved in high blood pressure ? In "5-Hydroxytryptamine in peripheral reactions" Eds. De Clerk F and Vanhoutte PM, Raven Press, New York, 1982, 183-192.
6. Janssen Pharmaceutica, Clinical Research Reports, June 1986.
7. Andren L, Svensson A, Dahlof B, Eggertsen R, Hansson L: Ketanserin in hypertension. Early clinical evaluation and dose finding study of a new $5HT_2$ receptor antagonist. Acta Med.Scand.214: 125-130, 1983.
8. Schalekamp MADH, Woittiez AJJ, Wenting GJ, van den Meiracker AH, Man in 't Veld AJ: Ketanserin: haemodynamic effects and mechanism of action. J. of Hypertension 4 (suppl. 1): S7-S12, 1986.
9. Breckenridge A. : Ketanserin. A new antihypertensive agent. J. of Hypertension 4 (suppl. 1): S13-S16, 1986.

48
Platelets and platelet-related substances in the natural history of atherosclerosis. The role of serotonin

S. Coccheri, G. Biagi and F. Grauso

In the present review some aspects related to plate lets in the pathogenesis and evolution of atherosclerotic and thrombotic vascular disease are discussed.

Platelet-derived materials have been identified in the context of atherosclerotic plaques by means of immunofluorescent techniques at different stages of evolution of the vascular lesion [1] . Thus, Platelet adhesion and interaction with the vascular wall is involved in the origin and evolution of the atherosclerotic plaque also before occurrence of relevant thrombotic complications . Therefore, platelet-endothelial interactions are obviously relevant both in the pathogenesis and in the clinical manifestations of atherosclerosis.

The initial step in platelet-endothelial interac — tions appears to be endothelial damage [2]. The injured endothelium stimulates circulating platelets to adhere to the sub-endothelial structures (as sub-intimal collagen and basal membranes), and to subsequently become activated. Only some of the agents capable of inducing endothelial damage are known, as for instance haemodynamic stress, hypertension, cigarette smoking, hypercholesterolaemia, activated leukocytes, immune complexes, and metabolic products as homocysteine. However, the mechanism of endothelial damage is poorly understood, and occurrence of such event in the human organism cannot be detec — ted and monitored at the present time.

In sites of endothelial lesions platelet adhesion occurs with the contribution of two circulating proteins, Factor VIII von Willebrandt and fibronectin. The following step, platelet activation, is characterized by plate let shape change and emission of contractile pseudopodia, an event predisposing to aggregation. During the activation phase initial release occurs of platelet substances contained in the α granules, as the Platelet Derived Growth Factor. PDGF is a potent stimulator of nuclear and cytoplasmic activities of smooth muscle cells and fibroblasts and seems therefore to be responsible for growth of the atherosclerotic plaque [3]. Other α-granules-derived substances are especially relevant as diagnostic tools for the demonstration of occurring platelet activation, as for instance β-thromboglobulin.

Platelet activation is associated with exposure at the platelet surface of a fibrinogen receptor. In fact, fibrinogen in presence of extracellular Calcium is the main cofactor for platelet aggregation. Intracellular Calcium transfert from microtubuli to free cytoplasma is responsible for the activation of at least three calcium-dependent biochemical pathways capable of inducing different forms of platelet aggregation [4]. These are the following:

a) The cyclic AMP-system. Degradation of CAMP to AMP as catalyzed by calcium-dependent phosphodiesterase enzymes is responsible for reversible platelet aggregation.

b) The Arachidonic Acid pathway. Arachidonic acid, as made available in the platelet membrane by a calcium-dependent phospholipase, undergoes oxidation by means of a cycloxigenase. The final product, thromboxane A_2, is a potent pro-aggregating and vasoconstrictor agent. The same metabolic pathway in endothelial cells leads to synthesis of prostacyclin, a potent physiological antiaggregating and vasodilating substance.

c) The Platelet Activating Factor pathway. In this mechanisms a glycerophospholipid (PAF) with potent pro-aggregating activity is formed, again with a Calcium-dependent mechanism. The pathophysiological role of PAF is however not yet completely understood.

Platelet aggregation is the mechanism by which platelet adhesion becomes amplified and the white thrombus is consolidated, thus offering a solid substrate for localization of blood coagulation and fibrinolytic processes.

Fissuring and ulceration of atherosclerotic plaques occurs as a result of partly unknown haemodynamic and metabolic factors. The subsequent subintimal haemorrhage is a potent stimulus for further platelet aggregation phenomena at the plaque surface. In these conditions, endoluminal thrombosis may develop and coexist with intra or sub-intimal haemorrhage. Platelet embolisation to peripheral districts and growth of intraluminal occlusive thrombosis are therefore closely related events [6] . Sea ling of plaque ulceration by means of endothelial covering and organisation of the intraluminal thrombus and the intraintimal haematoma is the final step of the process giving rise to stable vascular stenosis. Clinico-pa thological correlation have been outlined expecially for coronary heart disease; in this domain, a fissured or ul cerated plaque associated with intraintimal or sub-intimal haemorrhagic and thrombotic material, is linked with clinical events of the type of unstable angina or sudden death. Mural subocclusive or occlusive intraluminal thrombosis correlates with fatal or non-fatal acute miocardial infarction; while sealing, organisation and vascular stenosis correlates with clinical evidence of sta ble angina [7] . Similar clinico-pathological correlations can probably be identified also for other vascular districts.

From the facts and hypotheses outlined, the role of platelet aggregation in atherogenesis and arterial throm bogenesis is very complex. As known, platelet aggregation can be reproduced in vitro by adding different platelet agonists to platelet rich plasma or whole blood under continuous stirring. On the basis of their effects on pla telets, agonists can be divided into weak, moderate and strong. Weak agonists include vasopressin, norepinephrine and serotonin; intermediate are ADP, epinephrine,throm boxane and PAF; the strongest are thrombin and collagen [4]. Besides the strong agonists, it is likely that also the intermediate and weak ones may play a significant pa thophysiological role in vivo, especially by mutual potentiation.

Recent studies have stressed the multiple relationships between serotonin and platelets [4,8,9]. Serotonin is taken up, stored and transported by platelets. Storage occurs in the dense granules from which serotonin can be liberated during the release reaction. Besides storage and transport functions, platelets also react to sero tonin with a weak aggregation response involving only sha pe change and reversible aggregation. However, serotonin is an effective amplifyer of aggregation and release due to other agonists and this property may be even more important in vivo than its direct aggregating effect. Sero tonin may in fact contribute to maintainance of a state of continuous aggregation as for instance occurring in ulcerated or unstable plaques.

Moreover, the release of vasoconstrictive materials, including serotonin from activated platelets may influence collateral circulation and tissue perfusion [10] thus contributing to the modulation of tissue response to vascular occlusion or stenosis [8]. Increased sensitivity of platelets to serotonin observed in a number of patients with vascular diseases may by connected with these phenomena [10]. Both the direct and the amplifying effect of serotonin on platelet aggregation are inhibited [11,12,13,14] by a specific S_2 receptor blocker, ketanserin (table 1, Fig. 1). Preliminary evidence is available on the ability of ketanserin to reduce circulating β - thromboglobulin levels in patients with atherosclerosis and to antagonize hypersensitivity to serotonin of their platelets [15].

On this rationale, a protocol including studies of platelet function has been attached as an auxiliary project to a large international trial on Prevention of Atherosclerotic Complications with Ketanserin (PACK) in patients with claudicatio intermittens, on the basis of previous results [16]. Platelet studies will include the following measurements: β thromboglobulin, platelet factor

Table 1. In vitro effect of ketanserin on platelet aggregation induced by 5-hydroxytriptamine (5-HT). (Mean ± SEM; n = 3) [14]

	Parameters of aggregation	
	Maximum (TU)	Slope (TU/min)
Control	6.0 ± 2.6	11.7 ± 4.7
Ketanserin 1x10^{-8}M	4.9 ± 2.2	8.7 ± 3.4
Ketanserin 2.5x10^{-8}M	2.8 ± 1.2	4.2 ± 2.0
Ketanserin 1x10^{-7}M	0	0

Compound or solvent incubated with PRP 5 min. before the addition of 5x10^{-6} 5-HT. TU = turbidimetric units.

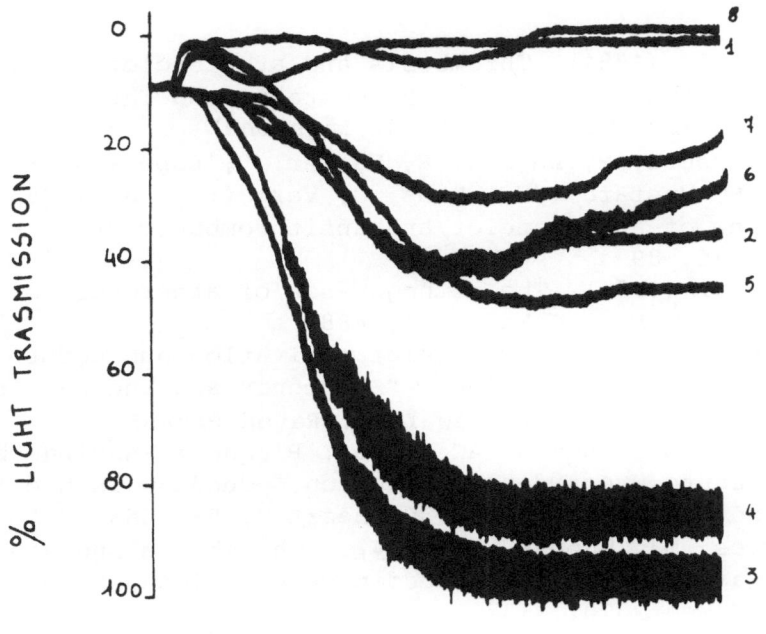

FIGURE 1   In vitro inhibitory effect of ketanserin on
    serotonin amplification of collagen induced plate-
    let aggregation [14]
    1 = Hydroxytriptamine (5-HT)   : 2.5 x 10^{-6}M
    2 = Collagen: 0.5 g/ml
    3 = 5-HY + Collagen
    4 = 5-HY + Collagen+Ketanserin :   1 x 10^{-8}M
    5 =   same   : 2.5 x 10^{-8}M
    6 =   same   :   5 x 10^{-8}M
    7 =   same   :   1 x 10^{-7}M
    8 =   same   :   5 x 10^{-7}M

IV, platelet-bound serotonin, platelet aggregation response to serotonin, ADP and collagen. This trial will pro
bably further elucidate the role of serotonin in the natural history of cardiovascular disease and possibly cla
rify whether specific serotoninergic blockade affects pla
telet function and the clinical evolution in atherosclerosis.

REFERENCES

1.   Woolf, N (1981). Thrombosis and atherosclerosis.In: Bloom Al, Thomas DP, (eds.) "Haemostasis and Thrombosis". p. 527. (Edinburgh: Churchill Livingstone)

2.   Verstraete, M, Dejana, E, Fuster, V, Lapetina, E, Moncada, S, Mustard, JF, Tans, G, Vergaftig, BB (1985). An overview of antiplatelet and antithrombotic drugs.Hae mostasis, 15, 89

3.   Ross, R (1986). The pathogenesis of atherosclerosis An update. New Engl J Med, 314, 488

4.   Holmsen, H (1985). Platelet activation and seroto — nin. In: Vanhoutte, PM, (ed.) "Serotonin and the cardio-vascular system". p.75. (New York: Raven Press)

5.   Davies, MJ, Thomas, AC (1985). Plaque rissuring-the cause of acute myocardial infarction, sudden ischaemic death, and crescendo angina. Br Heart J, 53, 363

6.   Davies, MJ, Thomas, A (1984). Thrombosis and acute coronary-artery lesions in sudden cardiac ischaemic death. New Engl J Med, 310, 1137

7.   De Wood, MA, Spores, J, Notske, R, Mouser, LT, Bur-roughs, R, Golden, MS, Lang, HT (1980). Prevalence of to tal coronary occlusion during the early hours of transmu ral myocardial infarction. New Eng J Med, 303, 897

8.   van Neuten, JM, Janssens, WJ, Vanhoutte, PM (1985). Serotonin and vascular reactivity. Pharm Res Communica — tions, 17, 585

9.   Schaub, RG, Meyers, KM, Sande, RD (1977). Serotonin as a factor in depression of collateral blood flow follo wing experimental arterial thrombosis. J Lab Clin Med , 90, 645

10.   De Clerck, F, Loots, W, Jagenau, A, Nevelsteen, A (1986). Correction by Ketanserin of the platelet-mediat-ed inhibition of peripheral collateral circulation in the cat: measurement of blood flow with radioactive micro — spheres. Drug Development Res, 8, 149

11.   De Cree, J, Leempoels, J, Demoen, B, Roels, V, Ver-haegen, H (1985). The effect of Ketanserin, a 5 HT_2 re-ceptor antagonist, on 5-hydroxytryptamine induced irre-versible platelet aggregation in patients with cardiovas cular diseases. Agents Actions, 16, 313

12.   Vermylen, J, Arnout, J, Deckmyn, H, Xhonneux, B, De Clerck, F (1986). Continuous inhibition of the platelet S_2-serotonergic receptors during the long term adminis-tration of Ketanserin. Thrombosis Research, 42, 721

13. De Clerck, F, David, JL, Janssen, PAJ (1982). Inhibition of 5-hydroxytryptamine and amplified human platelet aggregation by Ketanserin (R41468), a selective $5HT_2$ receptor antagonist. Agents Actions, 12, 388

14. Biagi, G, Grauso, F, Coccheri, S (1986). Unpublished results

15. Verstraete, M (1985). Platelet activation in patients with atherosclerosis of the arteries of the limbs. In: Vanhoutte, PM (ed.) "Serotonin and the cardiovascu — lar system". p.171 (New York: Raven Press)

16. De Cree, J, Leempoels, J, Genkens, H, Verhaegen, H (1984). Placebo-controlled double-blind trial of ketanserin in treatment of intermittent claudication. Lancet ii, 775

49
Prevalence and incidence of leg ischaemia in the general population
J.A. Dormandy

There are countless reports in the literature on the surgical treatment of leg ischaemia. By contrast, relatively little has been published about the incidence and prevalence of intermittent claudication in the general population and the fate of the vast majority of patients who never come to surgery. This review summarises the existing information about the fate of patients presenting with intermittent claudication.

PREVALENCE AND INCIDENCE OF LEG ISCHAEMIA IN THE GENERAL POPULATION

Only a minority of patients with demonstrable atherosclerosis in the legs complain of intermittent claudication. The Basle study showed that two thirds of patients with arteriographically proven occlusion reported no complaint on a questionnaire, and even after a detailed interview, one third were symptom free [1]. Of 14 published studies which looked at a random general population and observed the prevalence of symptoms of intermittent claudication, some relied totally on questionnaires [2-6] while in others the presence of arterial disease was confirmed by an interview and examination [1, 7-12] which in some included non-invasive and invasive vascular tests [1, 8, 11, 12]. Taking these factors into account, it would seem that the prevalence of arterial disease causing intermittent claudication in men below the age of fifty is approximately 1% to 1.5%, rising rapidly with age to over 5% in the older age groups. Using non-invasive tests it has been shown that the prevalence of atheromatous disease in the legs, much of it asymptomatic, is much higher [1, 13]. Unfortunately very little is known of the fate of the asymptomatic subjects with atherosclerosis of the legs.

Only in the Framingham [2] and Basle [11] studies were normal subjects followed over a period of years to determine the incidence of claudication. The 26 years' follow up in the Framingham study probably gives the best indication of the risk of previously asymptomatic subjects developing the symptoms of claudication. The incidence suddenly increases from 0.5% in men aged 50-59 to 3.8% in men aged 60-69 years. In the same population, the incidence of ischaemic strokes was about half and the incidence of ischaemic heart disease about four times that of claudication. In the Basle study [11] the diagnosis was based on careful examination as well as symptoms and the five year incidence of occlusive peripheral arterial disease was 4% for the younger (35-44 years) and 18% for the eldest group (over 65 years). However, only one third of those with detectable arterial disease had symptoms of intermittent claudication.

In most of these studies the ratio of men to women is less than 2, but looking at the disease at a later stage, the ratio of men to women is much higher, ranging from 3 to 13. This would suggest that the prognosis of the local disease in women is much better than in men. In the incidence of the disease, women lag behind men by about 10 years [2].

PROGRESS OF THE LOCAL DISEASE IN PATIENTS PRESENTING WITH INTERMITTENT CLAUDICATION

Traditionally, atheromatous disease of the legs has been regarded as falling in the specialist province of the vascular surgeon. Most reported series have therefore been concerned with the small proportion of claudicants referred to surgical departments. From the study in Oxford [7] only 50% of the patients with claudication had consulted a doctor while in a study of over 18,000 subjects in London the corresponding figure was only 10% [3]. Undoubtedly the vast majority of claudicants are never referred to a specialist centre, possibly because specialists concerned with the non-surgical treatment of leg ischaemia are rare in most countries. Angiologists should be leading the investigation and management of the many patients complaining of intermittent claudication, who are never referred to a vascular surgeon. Looking at studies which are not primarily surgical and therefore give the best approximation to what is likely to happen to the intermittent claudication of the average patient, there is general agreement that in approximately three quarters of the patients the disease will symptomatically stabilize soon after its onset and only about a quarter will significantly deteriorate. Although symptomatically the prognosis is good, the underlying atheromatous disease almost certainly progresses with time, but only between 5% and 15% of those presenting to a doctor will ever require reconstructive arterial surgery. If on the basis of studies by Hughson et al [7] and Reid et al [3] it is assumed that only 10% to 50% of all claudicants consult a doctor then reconstructive surgery is only performed in 1 to 10% of all claudicants. The patient who develops intermittent claudication can be cheered up by the knowledge that he has only a 25% chance of his symptoms continuing to deteriorate and only a 1.5-5% chance of ever requiring a major amputation. Unfortunately, part of the reason for this relatively optimistic outlook for the local disease is that most claudicants will die prematurely of atheromatous disease in another territory.

NON FATAL CARDIAC AND CEREBROVASCULAR EVENTS

The apparent prevalence of coronary artery and cerebrovascular disease in patients presenting with atherosclerotic arterial disease of the legs varies with the nature of the patients studied and the method of screening. Most studies used clinical history and resting ECG and showed a prevalence of 40-60%. In an early non-operative series, relying on clinical history alone for the diagnosis of cerebrovascular disease, the prevalence was only 0.5%, but in a more recent study, looking at a surgical group of patients using Doppler imaging, the prevalence of arterial disease was 52%. Most of these patients will be asymptomatic and it would be important to know what are the chances of a patient presenting with claudication developing symptomatic evidence of serious myocardial or cerebral ischaemia. Unfortunately, there is little data on the incidence of non-fatal myocardial infarction or cerebrovascular accidents in these patients. In the largest study there is simply a general statement that non-fatal coronary and cerebral disease may have developed in at least 20% of claudicants still alive at 5 years [14]. Of the five studies [18-22] with more detailed information on non-fatal myocardial and cerebrovascular events, only the oldest report [18] and the current Northwick Park study [19] distinguished clearly between angina and myocardial infarction; they were also the only studies looking at an unselected group of claudicants. The Framingham study diagnosed claudication solely on history and therefore looked at a relatively benign group of patients [20]. The Basle study considered all patients with evidence of arterial disease in the legs although many did not have symptoms of intermittent claudication [21]. The incidence of non-fatal myocardial infarction seems to be approximately 5% per year, while that of non-fatal cerebrovascular accidents is about 1% to 2%.

MORTALITY OF PATIENTS WITH CHRONIC LEG ISCHAEMIA

There is considerably better information on the incidence of fatal coronary or cerebrovascular events in claudicants. Despite the considerable disparity in patient selection, there is a surprising degree of agreement about the overall mortality. After 5, 10 and 15 years of follow up, the mean mortality from all causes was approximately 30%, 50% and 70% respectively. In the studies where the mortality in claudicants was compared to parallel, age and sex matched, general population, it was over twice that of the general population after 5 years. The analysis of the cause of death is perhaps surprising. In only about half of the cases was death thought to be due to myocardial ischaemia, while the proportion of claudicants dying of cerebrovascular disease was about 10%. In approximately ten percent death was due to vascular events other than stroke or myocardial ischaemia. This group was composed mainly of ruptured aneurysms and visceral infarction.

The importance of recognising the high mortality in claudicants is illustrated in the analysis of one of the largest surgical series, where after the fifth postoperative year, the annual mortality of the patients exceeded the annual rate of graft occlusion [23]. This not only suggests a possible need for revising the indications for surgery but also emphasises the need to concentrate as much on the prevention of the complications of atherosclerosis in other regions as on the prevention of graft occlusion, the traditional preoccupation of the vascular surgeon.

CONCLUSIONS

Our present knowledge of the fate of a patient with intermittent claudications is very incomplete, largely because of the lack of data on the majority of claudicants who never come to the attention of the vascular specialist. Only the following, very tentative conclusions can be drawn from the existing published evidence:

About 1.5% of men under 50 and 5% of men over 50 will develop symptoms of leg ischaemia due to atheromatous disease. The incidence in women is not much lower, but the disease seems to follow a more benign course. In 75% of the men claudication will never become a very serious problem and less than 5% are ever likely to require a major amputation. By contrast, the life expectancy of patients presenting with claudication is very much decreased due to atheromatous disease in other regions of the circulation. Compared to the general population, the claudicants' mortality is twice as high after 5 years.

About 75% of the deaths will be due to atherosclerosis, 50% in the coronaries, 15% in the cerebral region and 10% in the abdomen. There is almost no accurate data on the incidence of non-fatal myocardial infarction or stroke in claudicants. The ongoing multinational study of over 4,000 carefully observed claudicants will go some way towards defining more accurately the fate of the claudicant. This study is aimed at looking at the prevention of atherosclerotic complication by ketanserin (PACK), a serotonin antagonist. It is nevertheless already apparent that patients with claudication, even in the absence of other symptoms, are a very high risk group where active treatment aimed at modifying the progression and complications of atherosclerosis is particularly important.

REFERENCES

1. Widmer LK, Greensher A and Kannel WB: Occlusion of peripheral arteries - A study of 6400 working subjects. Circulation 30: 836-384; 1964.
2. Kannel WB and McGee DL: Update on some epidemiological features of intermittent claudication. J. Amer. Geriatrics Soc. 33:13-18,1985
3. Reid DD, Brett GJ, Hamilton PJS et al: Cardiorespiratory disease and diabetes among middle aged male cival servants. Lancet i: 469-473; 1974.

4.   Bothig S, Metelitsa VI, Barth W et al: Prevalence of ischaemic heart disease, arterial hypertension and intermittent claudication and distribution of risk factors among middle-aged men in Moscow and Berlin. Cor Vasa 18: 104-118; 1976.
5.   DeBacker G, Kornitzer M, Thilly C, Depoorter AM: The Belgian multifactor preventive trial in CVD. Design and methodology. Heart Bulletin 8: 115-124; 1977.
6.   Keys A, Aravanis C, Blackburn H, Buzina R, Djordjevic B S, Dontas A S, Fidanza F, Karvonen M J, Kimura N, Menotti A, Mohacek I, Nedeljkovic S, Puddu V, Punsar S, Taylor H L, Buchmen F S P: A Multivariate Analysis of Death and Coronary Heart Disease.   Seven Countries.   Harvard University Press, 1980, Pages 8-9, 61-62.
7.   Hughson WG, Mann JI and Garrod A: Intermittent claudication: prevalance and risk factors.   Br Med J 1: 1379-1381; 1978.
8.   Isacsson S: Venous occlusion plethysmography in 55 year old men - A population study in Malmo, Sweden.   Acta Med Scand Suppl 537; 8-35 1972.
9.   Reunanen A, Takkunen H and Aromaa A: Prevalence of intermittent claudication and its effect on mortality.   Acta Med Scand 211: 249-256; 1982.
10.   Agner E.   Natural History of Angina Pectoris, Possible Previous Myocardial Infarction and Intermittent Claudication during the Eighth Decade.   Acta Med Scand 210: 271-271, 1981.
11.   Widmer LK, Biland L and Da Silva A: Risk profile and occlusive peripheral artery disease (OPAD).   In: Proceedings of the 13th International Congress of Angiology, Athens 9-14 June, 1985.
12.   Criqui M H, Fronek A, Barrett-Connor E, Klauber M R, Gabriel S, Goodman D.   The prevelance of peripheral arterial disease in a defined population.   Circulation 71, 3: 510-515, 1985.
13.   Criqui M H, Fronek A, Klauber M R, Barrett-Connor E., Gabriel S.   The sensitivity, specificity and predictive value of traditional clinical evaluation of peripheral arterial disease: results form noninvasive testing in a defined population. Circulation 71, 3; 516-522, 1985.
14.   Bloor K: Natural history of arteriosclerosis of the lower extremities.
Ann Roy Coll Surg Engl 28: 36-51; 1961.
15.   Taylor GW and Calo AR: Atherosclerosis of arteries of lower limbs.   Br Med J 1: 507-510; 1962.
16.   LeFevre FA.   Corbacioglu C, Humphries AW and DeWolfe VG: Management of arteriosclerosis obliterans of the extremities. JAMA 170: 656-661; 1959.
17.   Schadt DC, Hines EA, Juergens JL and Barker NW: Chronic atherosclerotic occlusion of the femoral artery.   JAMA 175: 937-940; 1961.
18.   Begg TB and Richards RL: The prognosis of intermittent claudication.   Scot Med J 7 341-352; 1962.
19.   Gilliland E L, Llewellyn C D, Goss D E, Lewis J D.   The morbidity and mortality of stable claudicants - Results of five year follow up.   Presented at 2nd International Vascula Symposium, London, September 1986.
20.   Peabody N C, Kannal W B, McNamara P M.   Intermittent Claudication.   Arch. Surg: 109: 693-697, 1974.

21. De Silva A, Widmer LK, and Muller HR: Cerebrovascular disease and occlusive peripheral artery disease (OPAD). In: Proceedings of the 13th International Congress of Angiology, Athens, 9-14 June 1985.
22. Kallero KS, Bergqvist D, Cederholm C et al: Late mortality and morbidity after arterial reconstruction: The influence of arteriosclerosis in popliteal artery trifurcation. J. Vasc. Surg. 2: 541-546; 1985.
23. Szilagyi DE, Hageman JH, Smith RF et al: Autogenous vein grafting in femoropopliteal atherosclerosis: the limits of its effectivenss. Surgery 86: 836-851; 1979.

ENDOGENOUS OPIOIDS

50
Dynorphin-related peptides in central and peripheral tissues: distribution and possible functions

S. Spampinato and S. Ferri

INTRODUCTION

Dynorphins are a family of opioid peptides deriving, by sequential proteolytic cleavage, from the precursor prodynorphin (1). They include: dynorphin A-(1-32) and the shorter fragments dynorphin A-(1-17) and dynorphin A-(1-8), dynorphin B-29 and dynorphin B. Dynorphins are synthetized throughout the central nervous system in different neural systems (2). Immunoreactive dynorphin perikarya and fibers are particularly concentrated in the hypothalamo-pituitary axis (3). In the anterior pituitary dynorphins occur within gonadotroph cells (4) and within vasopressin neurons in the posterior lobe of the gland (5). These peptides are differentially processed from the precursor in the two pituitary lobes: a) in the adenohypophysis, immunoreactive dynorphin A (ir-dyn A) consists of a high molecular weight form rather than authentic dynorphins; b) in the posterior lobe, dynorphins consist of the small peptides dynorphin A-(1-17), dynorphin A-(1-8) and dynorphin B (6).
Dynorphins are also widely distributed in numerous peripheral tissues including the gastrointestinal tract, the heart and the gonads (6).

1. REGULATION OF PITUITARY DYNORPHINS

We have carried out studies in order to elucidate possible regulatory mechanisms of pituitary dynorphins in the rat.
a) Lesion studies
Discrete lesions of brain areas were achieved as a tool to detect cerebral areas influencing pituitary dynorphins. Particularly, we examined the effect of selective destruction, by radiofrequency lesions, of brain areas known to partecipate in the

regulation of the neuroendocrine system. Ir-dyn A was measured in acetic acid extracts of anterior and neurointermediate lobes by a radioimmunoassay as fully described elsewhere (6) .

As shown in Table 1, selective lesions of the supraoptic and paraventricular nuclei or of the anterior hypothalamic area resulted in a significant decrease of ir-dyn A in the neurointermediate lobe only. On the contrary, ablation of the ventromedial nucleus of the hypothalamus caused a reduction in anterior pituitary ir-dyn A. Lesions placed in the medial preoptic area, in the dorsomedial or in the arcuate nucleus were not associated with any significant modification of pituitary dynorphins.
These data indicate that changes of pituitary dynorphins are associated with the destruction of anatomically and functionally distinct neural systems involved in the regulation of pituitary functions (7).

Table 1. Immunoreactive dynorphin A in the pituitary of rats bearing discrete lesions of brain areas

Experimental group	ir-dyn (fmol/mg protein)	
	Anterior lobe	Neurointermediate lobe
Sham-lesioned	(9) 2068.2 $\pm$ 354.4	10492.6 $\pm$ 1277.4
Supraoptic + paraventricular- -lesioned	(8) 1993.1 $\pm$ 276.1	6952.0 $\pm$ 262.9*
Anterior hypothalamus- -lesioned	(8) 1762.0 $\pm$ 428.5	6718.2 $\pm$ 746.9*
Ventromedial-lesioned	(7) 1484.2 $\pm$ 179.2**	9324.5 $\pm$ 137.6
Medial preoptic area- -lesioned	(10) 2206.8 $\pm$ 176.6	10589.2 $\pm$ 1352.8
Dorsomedial-lesioned	(9) 2195.7 $\pm$ 223.7	11142.6 $\pm$ 973.1
Arcuate-lesioned	(7) 1801.4 $\pm$ 138.5	8196.8 $\pm$ 669.9

* $p < 0.05$; ** $p < 0.01$ VS sham-lesioned rats (ANOVA and Student's t test). Number of rats is shown in parentheses. The values represents the Mean $\pm$ S.E.

b) Endocrine manipulations

Possible effects of endocrine alterations on pituitary dynorphins were investigated. As reported in Table 2, 7 14 and 21 days after ovariectomy a significant increase of ir-dyn A was observed in the anterior pituitary only. This increase was reversed in rats treated with estradiol benzoate (chronically administered from day 14 to day 21 after ovariectomy by silastic tubes implanted subcutaneously). When estradiol benzoate was administered for 7 days to sham-ovariectomized rats, a pronounced decrease of ir-dyn A was observed in the anterior pituitary but not in the neurointermediate lobe (Table 2). These results provide evidence that estrogen may contribute to regulate ir-dyn A in the anterior pituitary. As previously reported, dynorphins in the anterior lobe are contained in gonadotroph cells, thus it is possible that hormonal factors regulating LH and FSH, may influence the levels of these peptides.

Table 2. Effects of ovariectomy (OVX) and estradiol benzoate (EB) (EB) on the pituitary content of a immunoreactive dynorphin A.

Treatment	Days post surgery	ir-dyn (fmol/mg protein)	
		Anterior lobe	Neurointermediate lobe
Sham-OVX	21	553.8 + 38.2	6682.1 + 533.9
OVX	7	987.5 + 102.9*	7067.1 + 704.5
OVX	14	1659.2 + 122.7**	7944.7 + 468.6
OVX	21	1435.9 + 125.9**	6910.3 + 298.9
OVX + EB	21	568.6 + 48.5	6765.4 +1317.8
Sham-OVX + EB	21	252.2 + 41.9	6680.3 + 310.6

* $p < 0.05$; ** $p < 0.01$ sham-OVX group (ANOVA and Student's t test). Each group consisted of 10 rats; the values shown are the Mean + S.E.

2. PRESENCE OF DYNORPHINS IN THE GASTROINTESTINAL TRACT

Particularly significant is the presence of dynorphin-related peptides in the gastrointestinal tract. Ir-dyn A was detected in measurable amounts in acetic acid extracts of rat and human gut specimens (these latter resected for carcinoma and taken at least 8 cm away from the tumor). As shown in Table 3, similar levels of ir-dyn A occur in the stomach, duodenum, jejunum, ileum and colon of both species. The presence of these peptides in the gut is indicative of any physiological role played by dynorphins and still unknown. In addition to enkephalins, dynorphins may be involved in controlling intestinal motility or secretory activity of several digestive glands (8).

Table 3. Levels of immunoreactive dynorphin A in rat and human gastrointestinal tissue.

Tissue	ir-dyn (pmol/g of tissue) Species	
	Human	Rat
Stomach (Fundus)	3.0 ± 0.3 (6)	2.0 ± 0.2 (4)
Duodenum	5.7 ± 0.5 (5)	2.1 ± 0.2 (5)
Jejunum	4.8 ± 2.0 (3)	2.2 ± 0.6 (4)
Ileum	2.3 ± 0.4 (5)	1.3 ± 0.1 (4)
Colon	1.4 ± 0.1 (5)	1.7 ± 0.4 (4)

Number of samples is shown in parentheses. The values represent the Mean ± S.E.

CONCLUSIONS

The present state of knowledge reflects the possible involvement of dynophins in the complex regulation of different biological functions. However, the physiological role is not yet fully established: a challenge for future research.

REFERENCES

1.   Civelli, O, Douglass, J, Goldstein, A and Herbert, E (1985). Sequence and expression of the rat prodynorphin gene. Proc Natl Acad Sci USA, 82, 4291

2.   Khachaturian, H, Lewis, ME, Schafer, MKH and Watson, SJ (1985). Anatomy of the CNS opioid system. Trends Neurosci, 8, 111

3.   Goldstein, A and Ghazarossian, VE (1980). Immunoreactive dynorphin in pituitary and brain. Proc Natl Acad Sci USA, 77, 6207

4.   Khachaturian, H, Sherman, TG, Lloyd, RV, Civelli, O, Douglass, J, Herbert, E, Akil, H and Watson, SJ (1986). Pro-dynorphin is endogenous to the anterior pituitary and is co-localized with LH and FSH in the gonadotrophs. Endocrinol, 119, 1409

5.   Whitnall, MH, Gainer, H, Cox, BM and Molineaux, CJ (1983). Dynorphin-A-(1-8) is contained within vasopressin neurosecretory vesicles in rat pituitary. Science, 222, 1137

6. Spampinato, S and Goldstein, A (1983). Immunoreactive dynorphin in rat tissues and plasma. Neuropeptides, 3, 193

7.   Joseph, SA and Knigge, KM (1978). The endocrine hypothalamus: recent anatomical studies. In: Reichlin, S, Baldessarini, RJ and Martin, JB (eds) "The Hypothalamus". p. 15. (New York: Raven Press)

8.   Ohkawa, H (1985). Dual effects of dynorphin on the non-adrenergic inhibitory potentials and the spontaneous action potentials in the duodenal smooth muscle cells on the guinea-pig. Eur J Pharmacol, 111, 139

51
Aging brain and dementia: change in central opioids and ACTH

G. Nappi, E. Sinforiani, E. Martignoni, C. Pacchetti,
F. Facchinetti and A.R. Genazzani

INTRODUCTION

Alzheimer disease whose symptoms are due to the impairment of
cognitive processes is characterized by a cortical cholinergic
deficit, which seems to originate from dysfunction and/or loss of
neurons of the nucleus basalis of Meynert (1). Recently, the
investigation of neuropeptidergic systems evidenced specific
changes in somatostatin (2) and neuropeptide Y (3) in the brains
of Alzheimer disease patients. Moreover there is agreement in the
literature about reduced B-endorphin (B-EP) (4,5) and B-EP-like
substances (6) in CSF of patients with Alzheimer type dementia
(ATD).
Interestingly, while B-EP levels are reduced only in ATD subjects,
CSF ACTH concentrations have been found to be significantly
reduced both in degenerative and vascular dementia (4). Taking
into account the relationship between ACTH and cholinergic system
(7) and considering the effect of ACTH and its moieties (8) in
learning, memory and behaviour processes, these data seem to
indicate that low CSF levels of ACTH are typical of dementia.
To further investigate the relevance of neuropeptides in cognitive
disorders, we evaluated CSF levels of ACTH, B-EP and B-lipotropin
(B-LPH), which are expressed by the same gene encoding for
proopiomelanocortin (POMC) (9), in various groups of demented
patients including degenerative (Presenile and Senile ATD) and
vascular (MID) forms.

SUBJECTS AND METHODS

Twenty-eight demented inpatients (21 males and 7 females) were
considered for the study. The diagnosis was made on the basis of
detailed history, neurological examination and ancillary
procedures such as CT scan, EEG, blood chemistries and standard
screening for reversible causes of dementia. Scan evaluation was
performed according to the evaluation of Ventricular Index (VI),
Cortical Index (CI) and the dimensions of the 3rd Ventricle (III

389

V) (10,11). The 20 patients fulfilling the clinical criteria for ATD (12) were classified either as suffering from presenile (14 patients; mean age 57.3+5.5) or senile (6 patients; mean age: 77.5+5.9) dementia according to the age (more or less than 65 years) of their initial symptoms (13).
The duration of the disease was similar in both groups: presenile 2.9÷1.9 yr and senile 3.1+ 2.7 yr. The other groups consisted of 8 subjects with MID. The severity of dementia was scored clinically by the Clinical Dementia Rating (CDR) (14) and, as to mental performances, by the Mini Mental State (MMS), whose threshold score for dementia was 24 (15). The Dementia Score (DS) (16) and the Information-Memory-Concentration Test (IMCT) (16) were also applied.
Twelve subjects (mean age: 65.1+11.3) were considered as controls. They were all undergoing investigation for various complaints of possible peripheral or spinal cord origin, but had no evidence of neurological diseases or disc lesion.
The patients' clinical characteristics are shown in Table 1.

Table 1 - Subjects' characteristics

	Controls	ATD	MID
Sex M/F	11/1	15/5	6/2
mean age ± SD (yr)	65.1+11.3	63.5+10.8	68.5÷7.7
range	43-76	46-83	51-76
mean duration ± SD (yr)		3.0+2.1	3.1+3.0
range		1-8	0.2-10
mean CDR score ± SD (16)		2.4+0.5	2.5+0.5
mean MMS score ± SD (17)		11.7+3.6	14.5+2.2
mean DS score ± SD (18)		10.5+4.3	8.7+4.3
mean IMCT score ± SD (18)		13.8+5.2	14.6+5.4

CSF samples were obtained by lumbar puncture after bed rest and overnight fasting between 8 and 9 a.m. in patients free from drugs interfering with CNS neurotransmitters for at least 15 days. Two ml CSF aliquots were freeze-dried and stored under nitrogen until assay. All the patients were characterized by a maintained blood-CSF barrier, evaluated on the basis of the serum-CSF protein gradients and absence of any signs of internal hydrocephalus or

transependymal CSF penetration on computerized tomography.
Sampling and assaying methods to determine CSF B-EP, B-LPH and
ACTH are detailed elsewhere (5).
Statistical analysis was performed by applying one-way ANOVA and
the Student's t test.

RESULTS

Individual concentrations of the three neuropeptides in the
various groups of patients and in controls are reported in Fig. 1.

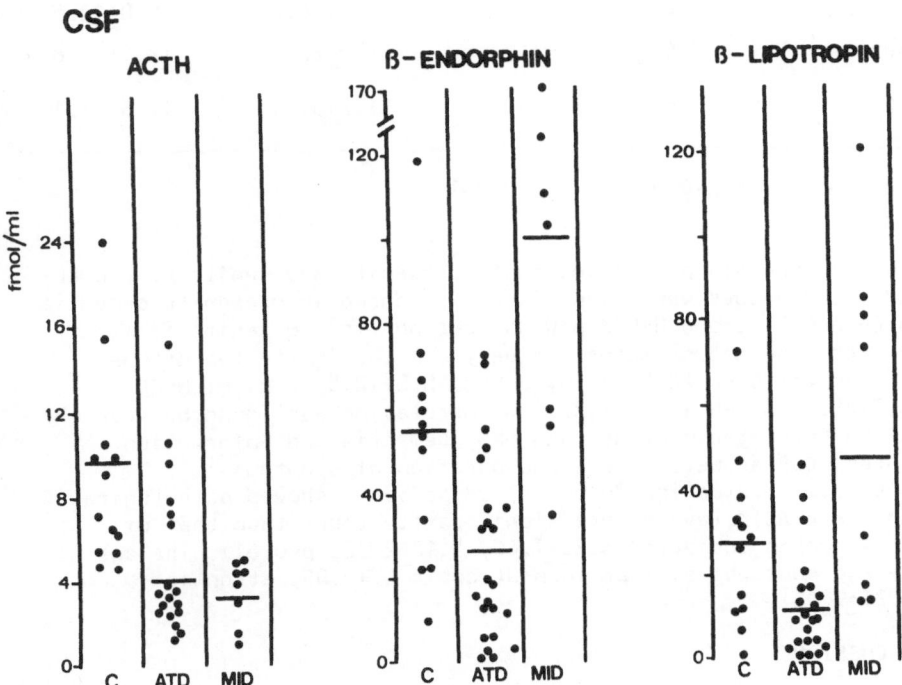

FIGURE 1   Individual levels of CSF ACTH, B-EP and B-LPH in con-
    trols and demented patients.

As mean (+ SD) levels (Table 2), the 28 demented patients showed a
significant decrease in ACTH as compared with controls (F = 8.16,
p<0.01), while B-EP and B-LPH were not different. Considering the
various groups of demented patients, ATD subjects showed
significantly lower values of ACTH (F = 5.22; p<0.05), B-EP
(F = 8.71; p<0.01) and B-LPH (F = 16.33; p<0.001) versus controls.

Table 2.   Mean CSF ACTH, B-EP and B-LPH values in controls and
           demented patients

Subjects	number	ACTH fmol/ml	BEP fmol/ml	BLPH fmol/ml
CONTROLS	12	9.4+5.4*+	53.5+29.2*	23.0+13.5°+
DEMENTED	28	4.6+3.3*	43.4+39.1	22.6+27.6
ATD	20	4.2+3.8+	25.4+21.6*	10.9+11.9°
presenile	14	5.1+4.1	20.5+16.6*	10.0+12.5
senile	6	1.9+1.1	36.9+28.9	12.1+11.8
MID	8	3.6+1.7	81.2+51.1	47.3+41.1

+ p<0.05   * p<0.01   ° p<0.001

Dividing the ATD population in to presenile and senile ATD, B-EP
and B-LPH values were significantly reduced in presenile dementia
(B-EP p<0.01 , and B-LPH p<0.05) but not in the senile form.
However, the actual means are very similar in the two groups
(presenile: B-EP 20.5+ 16.6, B-LPH 10.0+12.5; senile: B-EP
36.9+28.9, B-LPH 12.1+11.8). No correlation was found between the
CSF POMC-related peptides and MMS, Dementia and Information
Scores, CDR as well as age and duration of symptoms.
At CT scan evaluation 20 out of 28 patients showed pathological CI
and their ACTH levels were significantly lower than that of
non-atrophic subjects (3.25+1.40, 5.18+2.32, p<0.01). The age of
the 2 groups was similar (non-atrophic 67+9.05, atrophic
69.25+9.08).

DISCUSSION

Our data indicate that the CSF ACTH levels are reduced in ATD and
MID patients.
It is known that ACTH and its N-terminal fragment, in particular,
show positive effects on different learning and memory tasks.
ACTH 4-9 administered subchronically to elderly patients (17)
improved mood, sociability and ward behaviour. When administered
to ATD patients for 6 months, no improvement was found in memory
functions (17).
Another finding concerns B-EP and B-LPH, which showed levels
inversely related to age in normal subjects (18), while in ATD
patients they were concomitantly and severely reduced. In the
presenile form of ATD, in particular, B-EP appeared severily

reduced (p<0.01 versus controls). Recent data pointed out that
presenile ATD shows peculiar clinical, neuropsychological and
neurobiological peculiar characteristics which are likely to make
it a degenerative neuronal disease in middle age (13). A similar
reduction of CSF B-EP was recently reported by us in patients with
untreated Parkinson's disease, without dementia (19). In contrast
with what has recently been reported by Sulkava et al., MID
patients showed mean CSF B-EP and B-LPH levels similar to
controls. Moreover, we also found increased CSF B-EP and B-LPH
values in subjects who underwent either reversible ischemic
attacks or completed strokes (20).
We do not know which are the mechanisms leading to a reduction of
one or more POMC-related peptides in CSF. In fact we ignore the
organs which contribute to the presence of these peptides in CSF,
except for hypothalanus, whose in vivo secretory ability has been
demonstrated (21). Thus, considering that hypothalamic content of
ACTH, B-EP and B-LPH was found ten times higher in a patient with
presenile ATD (22), it seems likely that a defect of axonal
transport and/or secretion rather than synthesis could account for
the POMC-related peptide abnormalities in CSF.
In conclusion, our data show that the CSF B-EP reduction does not
concern all the dementing processes. Among the 3 POMC-related
peptides we evaluated, the only one that was specifically reduced
in every dementing process, whatever the origin, is ACTH, while
the reduction of B-EP in CSF could be in keeping with a
degenerative process of CNS.

ACKNOWLEDGMENTS

The authors thank Donella Canevari, Laura Delnevo and Anita Diener
for their assistance. This work was partly supported by the
Ministry of Health, Social Medicine Department.

REFERENCES

1. Candy JM, Perry RH, Perry EK et al. (1983) Pathological
   changes in the nucleus of Meynert in Alzheimer's and
   Parkinson's diseases. J Neurol Sci, 59, 277.
2. Rossor MN, Ellison PC, Mountjoy CQ, Roth M, Iversen LL. (1980)
   Reduced amounts of immunoreactive somatostatin in the temporal
   cortex in senile dementia of Alzheimer type. Neurosci Lett,
   20, 373.
3. Allen JM, Ferrier IN, Roberts GW et al. (1984) Elevation of
   neuropeptide Y (NPY) in substantia innominata in Alzheimer's
   type dementia. J Neurol Sci, 64, 325.
4. Facchinetti F, Nappi G, Petraglia F, Martignoni E, Sinforiani
   E, Genazzani AR. (1984) Central ACTH deficit in degenerative
   and vascular dementia. Life Sci. 35, 1691.
5. Sulkava R, Erkinjutti T, Laatikainen T. (1985) CSF B-endorphin
   and B-lipotropin in Alzheimer's disease and multi-infarct
   dementia. Neurology, 35, 1057.

6. Jolkkonen JT, Soininen HS, Riekkinen PJ. (1984) B-endorphin-like immunoreactivity in CSF of patients with Alzheimer's disease. Acta Neurol Scandinav, Suppl 98, 234.

7. Versteeg DHG. (1980) Interaction of peptides related to ACTH, MSH and B-LPH with neurotransmitters in the brain. Pharmac Ther, 11, 535.

8. Wied de D. (1977) Behavioral effects of neuropeptides related to ACTH, MSH and B-LPH. Ann NY Acad Sci, 297, 263.

9. Nakanishi S, Inoue A, Kita T et al. (1979) Nucleotide sequence of cloned cDNA for bovine corticotropin-B-lipotropin precursor. Nature (London), 278, 423.

10. Huckman MS, Fox J, Topel J. (1975) The validity of criteria for the evaluation of cerebral atrophy by CT. Radiology, 116, 85.

11. Hahn FGY, Rim K. (1976) Frontal ventricular dimensions on normal CT. Ann J Roentgend, 186, 593.

12. Diagnostic and Statistical Manual of Mental Disorders, (1980) ed 3. Washington DC, American Psychiatric Association.

13. Seltzer B and Sherwin I (1983). A comparison of clinical features in early and late-onset primary degenerative dementia. One entity or two? Arch Neurol, 40,143.

14. Hughes CP, Berg L, Danziger WL, Coben LA, Martin RL (1982). A new clinical scale for the staging of dementia. Brit J Psychiat, 140, 566.

15. Folstein M, Folstein S, McHugh P. (1975) Mini-Mental State. J Psychiatr Res, 12, 189.

16. Blessed G, Slater E, Roth M. (1968) The association between quantitave measures of dementia and of senile change in the cerebral grey matter of elderly subjects. Br J Psychiatry, 114, 797.

17. Soininen H, Koskinen T, Helkala EL, Pigache R, Riekkinen PJ. (1985) Synthetic ACTH 4-9 (ORG 2766) in treatment of Alzheimer's disease. Neurology, 35, 1348.

18. Facchinetti F, Petraglia F, Nappi G, Martignoni E, Antoni G, Parrini D, Genazzani AR. (1983) Different patterns of central and peripheral B-endorphin, B-lipotropin and ACTH throughout life. Peptides, 4, 744.

19. Nappi G, Petraglia F, Martignoni E, Facchinetti F, Bono G, Genazzani AR. (1985) B-endorphin cerebrospinal fluid decrease in untreated parkinsonian patients. Neurology, 35, 1371.

20. Nappi G, Facchinetti F, Bono G, Petraglia F, Sinforiani E, Genazzani AR. (1985) CSF and plasma levels of pro-opiomelano cortin-related peptides in reversible ischaemic attacks and strokes. J Neurol Neurosurg and Psychiatry, 49, 17.

21. Liotta As, Gildersleeve D, Brownstein MJ, Krieger DT. (1979) Biosynthesis in vitro of immunoreactive 31.000-dalton corticotropin/B-endorphin-like material by bovine hypothalamus. Proc natn Acad Sci (USA), 76, 1448.

22. Facchinetti F, Nappi G, Storchi R, Scelsi M, Sances G, Petraglia F, Genazzani AR. (1985) Abnormal proopiomelanocortin processing in Alzheimer disease. J Neurochem Suppl, 44, 192.

52

Relationship between endogenour opioids and the cardiovascular system: dynorphin measurement in the human heart: ß-endorphin plasmatic levels assay during acute pulmonary oedema

P. Bernardi, F. Fontana, C. Ventura, S. Spampinato,
M. Cavazza, L. Bastagli, N. Spagnolo and S. Lenzi

In recent years a considerable number of informations has been obtained concerning the relationships between the endogenous opioid system (E.O.S.) and the cardiovascular system (1,2).

Opioid receptors have been detected at the level of the cardiovascular system (3).

Both the production sites and the effects of a variety of opioids involved in cardiovascular regulation have been recently characterized. (1, 4)

In the present study we were able to find dynorphin in myocardial atria specimens taken from patients undergoing coronary by pass or valvular surgery. Immuno reactive dynorphin (I_2 - dyn) was measured by the means of a RIA method, by using a higly specific antiserum against the dynorphin ß fragment; the results are shown in table 1.

The cardiac origin of the substance is strongly suggested by the fact that dynorphin is not detectable or is found only in traces in blood circulation.

Dynorphin has yet been found in the atria and ventricles of guinea pig and rat hearts (5). However, to our knowledge, the present data are the first in licterature showing the presence of an endogenous opioid peptide in the human heart.

This finding is of particular interest for the extent of knowledge concerning the role of opioid peptides in the regulation of the heart function. In fact, it is conceivable that opioids, in man, other than by acting through the control nervous system, also directly influence the cardiac function.

The specific dynorphin receptor is the K receptor, wich would explain the slight haemodinamic effects induced by low doses of naloxone (a selective antagonist of the μ opioid receptors) in several diseases exhibiting alterations of the E.O.S.

In our recent study we have shown that morphine, met-enkephalin or leu-enkephalin, reduce the heart rate and the developed tension as well as the coronary resistences in the isolated and perfused rat heart (6). Moreover, these opioids were able to counteract the positive chronotropic and inotropic effects due to isopro - terenol infusion.

In experiments performed in cultured heart cells from chick embrio, opioids reduced the cAMP content and increased cGMP content, thus lowering the cAMP/cGMP ratio.

Such event may partly explain the negative effects induced by the opioids on the mechanical performance of the isolated rat heart. In fact, it is well known that cAMP represents a positive signal for the force of myocardial contraction, whilst, cGMP has been recognized as a mediator of negative inotropic events.

In cardiogenic shock complicating the acute myocardial infarction (AMI), we have found high ß-endorphin plasmatic levels and also we were able to produce a significant increase in the arterial pressure by the intravenous administration of high doses of naloxone. (1)

Naloxone also was able to improve the bradicardia-hypotension syndrome, often occurring in inferior AMI,although in this clinical conditions, no increase in ß - endorphin plasmatic levels was found.In actual part it is possible that other endogenous opioids, i.e. enkephalins or dynorphin are involved in the appearance of the bradycardia-hypotension syndrome.

We have also detected high ß - endorphin plasmatic levels in the course of acute pulmonary oedema (147 $\pm$ 16.5 fmol/ml : mean $\pm$ SEM of 8 patients).It is our opinion that, in this condition, the E.O.S. activation is secondary to ventilation disturbances.

It has been demonstrated that in healthy subjects hypercapnia produced by ventilation of air with high CO_2 levels, causes an increase in plasmatic ß - endorphin. (7),similary in respiratory failure due to bronco-obstructive disease, high endogenous opioid values are frequently found. (8). These agents depress the respiratory centres and increase the respiratory failure. (9). Beneficial effects have been obtained by the use of naloxone in cases with hypercapnia. (8).

Evidence exists for the hypothesis that the activation of the E.O.S., which have been reported in pulmonary oedema, may be a primitive event.

Increased ß - endorphin plasmatic levels during pulmonary oedema of neurogenous origin have been found in sheeps (10) : the pre-treatment with naloxone prevented the onset of pulmonary oedema.

According to the above mentioned studies (11) neurogenous pulmonary oedema depends on : 1) an increased catecholamine release causing higher systemic arterial resistences; 2) a simultaneous release of endorphins responsible for an increased pulmonary capillary permeability.

A disturbance of the vegetative nervous system is often associated with pulmonary oedema wich complicates heart diseases, but the increase in both sympathetic and parasympathetic outflow is able to stimulate the E.O.S.

These consideration strengthen our opinion that morphine may not be the treatment of choice in pulmonary oedema due to a myocardial contractility impairment; the alcaloid, as we have shown in our studies, has negative inotropic effects and can produce myocardial effects, in addition to those elicited by the increased endogenous opioid peptides observed in pulmonary oedema.

Table 1

Immunoreactive dynorphin in human atrial specimens

Diagnosis	Ir-dyn pmol/g
Coronary heart disease	25.3
Coronary heart disease	19.4
Coronary heart disease	21.4
Coronary heart disease	23.0
Coronary heart disease	22.9
Coronary heart disease	36.5
Coronary heart disease	20.7
Coronary heart disease	23.0
Mitral valve disease	20.0
Mitral valve disease	15.5
Mitral valve disease	23.0
Aortic valve disease	24.2
Aortic valve disease	32.5
Aortic valve disease	63.2
Aortic valve disease	24.9
Coronary heart disease + Aortic valve disease	22.0
Coronary heart disease + Aortic valve disease	18.4
Coronary heart disease + Aortic valve disease	20.7
Coronary heart disease + Aortic valve disease	22.5

REFERENCES

1) Bernardi P., Ghezzi F., Grimaldi R., Bastagli L., Minelli C., Cavazza M., Tomassetti V., Fontana F., Ligabue A., Ventura C., Genazzani E. (1986). Variazioni funzionali del sistema degli oppioidi endogeni nell'infarto miocardico acuto. G. Clin. Med. 67, 43.

2) Caffrey J.L., Gangl J.F., Jones C.E. (1985). Local endogenous opiate activity in dog myocardium: receptor blockade with naloxone. Am. J. Physiol. 28, 382.

3) Olson G.A., Olson R.D., Kastin A.J. (1984). Endogenous opiates: 1983. Peptides 5, 975.

4) Lang R.E., Hermann K., Dietz R., Gaida W., Ganten D., Kraft K., Unger Th (1983). Evidence for the presence of eukephalins in the heart. Life Science 32, 399-406.

5) Spampinato S., Golstein A. (1983). Immunoreactive dynorphin in rat tissue and plasma. Neuropeptides 3, 193.

6) Clo C., Muscari C., Tantini B., Pignatti C., Bernardi P., Ventura C. (1985). Reduced mechanical activity of perfused rat heart following morphine or enkephalin peptides administration. Life Science 37, 1327.

7) Weinberger S.E., Steinbrook R.A., Carr D.B., von Gal E.R., Fisher J.E., Leith D.E., Fence V., Rosenblatt M. (1985). Endogenous opioids and ventilatory responses to hypercapnia in normal humans. J. Appl. Physiol. 58, 1415.

8) Santiago T.V., Remolina C., Scoles V., Edelman N.H. (1981). Endorphins and the control of breathing : ability of naloxone to restore flow-resistive load compensation in chronic obstructive pulmonary disease. N. Engl. J. Med. 304, 1190.

9) Weil J.V., Mc Cullough R.E., Kline J.S., Sodal I.E. (1975). Diminished ventilatory response to hypoxia and hypercapnia after morphine in normal man. N. Engl. J. Med. 292, 1103.

10) Peterson B.T., Ross J.C., Brigham K.L. (1983). Effect of naloxone on pulmonary vascular responses to graded levels of intracranial pressure in anesthetized sheep. Am. Rev. Resp. Dis. 128, 1024.

11) Malik A.B. (1985). Mechanisms of neurogenic pulmonary edema. Circulation Research 57, 1.

BEZAFIBRATE, ATHEROSCLEROSIS AND ISCHAEMIC HEART DISEASE

53
Studies on DNA fragment length polymorphism of human apolipoprotein B gene
S. Calandra

INTRODUCTION

Apolipoprotein B (apo B) is the most abundant apolipoprotein of human plasma and plays an important role in
the metabolism of plasma cholesterol and triglyceride.
Apo B is a major constituent of chylomicrons, very low
density lipoprotein (VLDL) and low density lipoprotein
LDL (1, 2). Two types of apo B circulate in human
plasma: apo B-100 and apo B-48; apo B-100 has a MW of
approximately 500,000 daltons, is made in the liver and
is the sole apolipoprotein of human LDL (1, 2). It is
the ligand that mediates LDL clearance by the LDL receptor pathway (3). Apo B-48 has a molecular weight
of approximately 280,000 and is made in the intestine
(1, 2).
    High levels of plasma apo B and LDL are associated
with elevated risk of coronary atherosclerosis, a condi
tion which shows a familial component (4, 5). In addition apo B is elevated in several primary hyperlipoproteinemias which predispose to atherosclerosis (5). In
view of these observations it is reasonable to postula-
te that mutations in the apo B gene locus producing
changes in the synthetic rate and/or in the physico-che
mical properties of apo B lead to elevation of apo B in
plasma thus contributing to the pathogenesis of atherosclerosis.
    The structure and the biosynthesis of apo B-100
and B-48 are not well characterized, in view of the
large size of these molecules their tendency to aggrega
gate and their insolubility in aqueous media after deli
pidation. Great progress in elucidating the structure
of apo B has recently been made through the molecular

cloning of the cDNA for apo B-100. Several apo B-100 cDNA clones which span over a large portion of apo B gene have been characterized (6-13). As expected in view of the putative large size of the apo B gene, several restriction fragment length polymorphisms (RFLPs) have been reported (14-21). In the present comunication we report some RFLPs of the apo B-100 locus in unrelated healthy subjects and in members of a family with low plasma LDL and VLDL cholesterol.

MATERIAL AND METHODS

Subjects
Blood was collected from 7 healthy normolipemic unrelated individuals aged 20-44 years. Four members of a family with low plasma cholesterol were also included in the study. They were healthy subjects which had been identified through a routine blood analysis. The family consisted of: a) two sisters M.R. aged 18 and M.M. aged 14 whose serum cholesterol and triglyceride were 85 and 21 mg/dl (M.R.) and 110 and 29 mg/dl (M.M.) respectively; their HDL-CH was 60 and 50 mg/dl respectively; b) their father (M.P.) aged 46 whose serum cholesterol, triglyceride and HDL-CH were 95, 52 and 45 mg/dl respectively; c) the father's sister (M.B.) aged 47 whose serum cholesterol, triglyceride and HDL-CH were 175, 48 and 50 mg/dl respectively.

Detection of DNA polymorphisms in human leukocyte DNAs
DNA extracted from human leukocytes (22) was digested by various restriction enzymes under the conditions indicated by the supplier (Amersham, England). Complete digestion was ensured by the use of excess enzyme and prolonged incubations. DNA fragments were separated on 1% agarose gel electrophoresis, transferred to nylon membranes (Zeta-Probe) by the method of Southern (23). Pre-hybridization and hybridization of the membranes were performed as specified previously (24). The membranes were blotted dry and exposed to Kodak X-Omat X-ray films at -70°C for 24-72 hours.

Human apo B-100 cDNA probe
The apo B-100 cDNA probe (pB4) was kindly given to us by dr. R. Cortese of the European Molecular Biology Laboratory (EMBL) Heidelberg (West Germany). Details of the clone and the sequence encoding a segment of apo

B-100 have been reported (11). Clone pB4 was labelled by nick-translation (24) and used as hybridization probe for Southern blot analysis of genomic DNA fragments.

Restriction Enzymes

Restriction enzymes used were: Eco RI, Eco RV, Hind III Pst I, Bgl II, Bam HI, Xba I and Pvu II.

Results

Of the 8 enzymes tested in the seven unrelated subjects Eco RI, Eco RV, Xba I and Bam HI gave RFLPs as summarized in table I. These RFLPs appear to be independent of each other.

Table 1.   RFLPs for human apolipoprotein B gene in unrelated normolipemic subjects

Enzymes	Fragment Length (kb)		
Eco RI	15.0	1.1	0.7
	14.0	1.1	0.7
Eco RV	12.0	3.7	3.8
	12.0		3.8
Xba I	8.6	5.0	2.0
		5.0	2.0
	8.6		2.0
Bam HI	8.1	6.9	
	8.1	6.9	6.0

As recently reported by others (21) the most common RFLP was observed with the enzyme Xba I. Fig. 1 outlines the three Xba I phenotypes: X_1X_1 which indicates the homozygosity for the 5.0 and 2.0 kb bands (21), X_2X_2 which indicates the homozygosity for the 8.7 and 2.0 bands and X_1X_2 which indicates the heterozygous condition. Of the seven unrelated subjects, three were heterozygous X_1X_2, two X_2X_2 and two X_1X_1. When the DNA isolated from the four subjects of the family with low serum lipids was analyzed a group of unexpected restriction patterns were observed in DNAs digested with Eco RI, Eco RV, Hind III and Bgl II. Fig. 2 gives an example of these observations by illustrating the RFLP obtained with Eco RV. In the seven unrelated subjects the radioactive probe hybridized two major fragments of 12.0 and 3.8 kb and a minor band of 3.7 kb; in all members of the family with hypocholesterolemia an additional major band of 6.7 kb and other minor bands were observed.

Xbal DIGESTION PATTERN

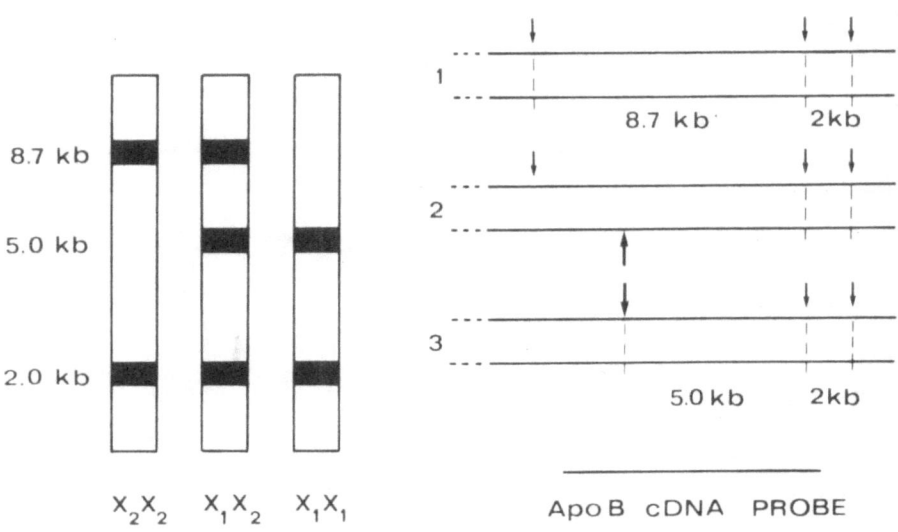

FIGURE 1 Human DNA restriction fragment length polymorphism (RFLP) obtained with the enzyme Xba I. The three phenotypes found in this study are shown on the left. The nomenclature adopted is given in ref. 21

Also in the case of the other enzymes, all members of the family differed from the control subjects but showed identical restriction fragment patterns among themselves. This would suggest that in this family an insertion-deletion event in the apo B-100 gene locus has occurred (25). Studies are in progress to clarify this point.
Finally we confirmed that the Xba I polymorphism is fairly common in the caucasian population. It has been observed that subjects X_1X_1 and X_1X_2 had mean serum triglyceride 36% higher than X_2X_2 subjects and

tend to have higher serum cholesterol (21). Whether the
Xba I   phenotyping   has   a predictive value for assessing   the risk of premature atherosclerotic disease can
only   be established in carefully conducted prospective
studies.

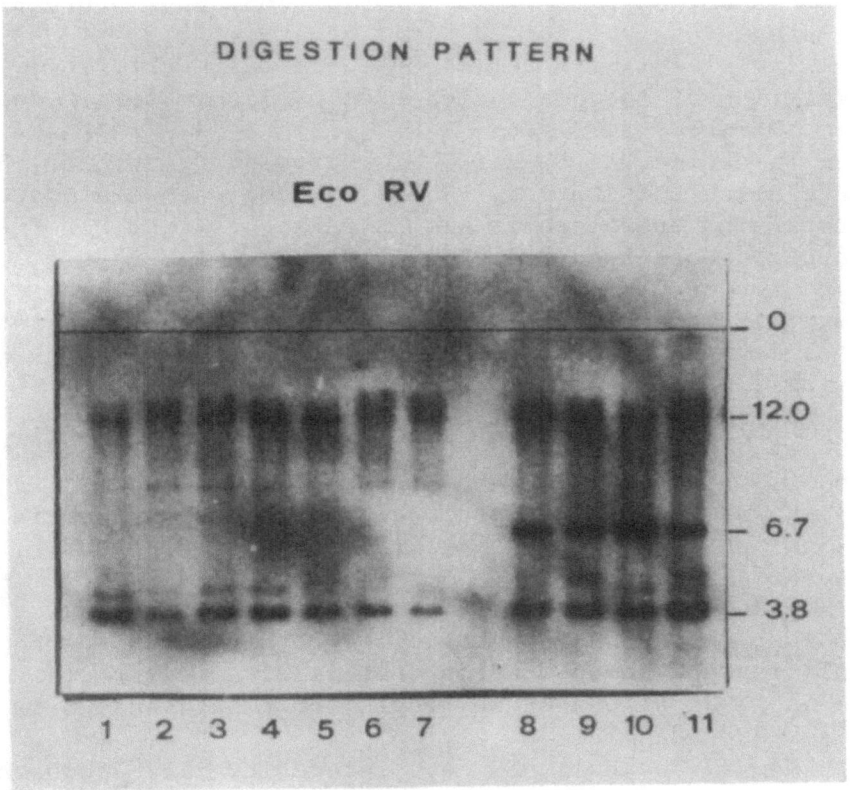

FIGURE 2   Southern   blot analysis   of DNA isolated from
seven unrelated   healthy subjects   (lanes   1-7) and
four   individuals   (lanes 8-11)   of the family with
low VLDL   and LDL cholesterol, after digestion with
Eco RV.   DNA was hybridized   with the 32-P labelled
cDNA apo B probe   (pB4). Numbers   on the right side
indicate the size (in kilobases) of the restriction
fragments. 0 = line of sample application.

REFERENCES

1.   Kane, JP (1983). Apolipoprotein B: structural and metabolic heterogeneity. Ann Rev Physiol, 45, 637
2.   Mahley, RW, Innerarity, TL, Rall, SC Jr. and Weisgraber, KH (1984). Plasma lipoproteins: apolipoprotein structure and function. J Lipid Res, 25, 1277
3.   Brown, MS, Kovanen, PT and Goldstein, JL (1981). Regulation of plasma cholesterol by lipoprotein receptors. Science, 212, 628
4.   Sniderman, A, Shapiro, S, Marpole, D, Skinner, B, Teng, B and Kwiterovich, PO Jr. (1980). Association of coronary atherosclerosis with hyperapobetalipoproteinemia. Proc Natl Acad Sci (USA), 77, 604
5.   Uterman, G (1983). Coronary heart disease. In: Emery, AEH and Rimoin, DL (eds.) "Principles and practi ce of medical genetics ". p. 956. (New York: Churchill Livingstone)
6.   Lusis, AJ, West, R, Mehrabian, M, Reuben, MA, LeBoeuf, RC, Kaptein, JS, Johnson, DF, Schumaker, VN, Yuhasz, MP, Schotz, MC and Elovson, J (1985). Cloning and expression of apolipoprotein B, the major protein of low and very low density lipoproteins. Proc Natl Acad Sci (USA), 82, 4597
7.   Huang, LS, Clark Bock, S, Feinstein, SI and Breslow, JL (1985). Human apolipoprotein B cDNA clone isolation and demonstration that liver apolipoprotein B mRNA is 22 kilobases in length. Proc Natl Acad Sci (USA), 82, 6825
8.   Knott, TJ, Rall, SC Jr., Innerarity, TL, Jacobson, SF, Urdea, MS, Levy-Wilson, B, Powell, LM, Pease, RJ, Eddy, R, Nakai, H, Byers, M, Priestley, LM, Robertson, E, Rall, LB, Betsholtz, C, Shows, TB, Mahley, RW and Scott, J (1985). Human apolipoprotein B: structure of carboxyl-terminal domains, sites of gene expression, and chromosomal localization. Science, 230, 37
9.   Wei, CF, Chen, SH, Yang, CY, Marcel, YL, Milne, RW, Li, WH, Sparrow, JT, Gotto, AM, Jr. and Chan, L (1985). Molecular cloning and expression of partial cDNAs and deduced amino acid sequence of a carboxyl-terminal fragment of human apolipoprotein B-100. Proc Natl Acad Sci (USA), 82, 7265
10. Law, SW, Lackner, KJ, Hospattankar, AV, Anchors, JM, Sakaguchi, AY, Naylor, SL and Brewer, BH Jr. (1985) Human apolipoprotein B-100: cloning, analysis of liver mRNA, and assignment of the gene to chromosome 2. Proc

Natl Acad Sci (USA), 82, 8340

11. Shoulders, CC, Myant, NB, Sidoli, A, Rodriguez, JC, Cortese, C, Baralle, FE and Cortese, R (1985). Molecular cloning of human LDL apolipoprotein B cDNA. Athero sclerosis, 58, 277

12. Protter, AA, Hardman, DA, Schilling, JW, Miller, J, Appleby, V, Chen, GC, Kirsher, SW, McEnroe, G and Kane JP (1986). Isolation of a cDNA clone encoding the amino terminal region of human apolipoprotein B. Proc Natl Acad Sci (USA), 83, 1467

13. Protter, AA, Hardman, DA, Sato, KY, Schilling, JW, Yamanaka, M, Hort, YJ, Hjerrild, KA, Chen GC and Kane, JP (1986). Analysis of cDNA clones encoding the entire B-26 region of human apolipoprotein B. Proc Natl Acad Sci (USA), 83, 5678

14. Chan, L, VanTuinen, P, Ledbetter, DH, Daiger, SP, Gotto, AM, Jr. and Chen, SH (1985). The human apolipoprotein B-100 gene: a highly polymorphic gene that maps to the short arm of chromosome 2. Biochem Biophys Res Commun, 133, 248

15. Priestley, L, Knott T, Wallis, S, Powell, L, Pease, R, Simon, A and Scott, J (1985). RFLP for the human apo lipoprotein B gene: I; Bam HI. Nucl Acids Res, 13, 6789

16. Priestley, L, Knott, T, Wallis, S, Pease, R and Scott, J (1985). RFLP for the human apolipoprotein B gene: II; Eco RI. Nucl Acids Res, 13, 6790

17. Priestley, L, Knott, T, Wallis, S, Powell, L, Pease, R and Scott, J (1985). RFLP for the human apolipoprotein B gene: III; Eco RV. Nucl Acids Res, 13, 6791

18. Priestley, L, Knott T, Wallis, S, Powell, L, Pease, R and Scott, J (1985). RFLP for the human apolipoprotein B gene: IV; MspI. Nucl Acids Res, 13, 6792

19. Priestly, L, Knott, T, Wallis, S, Powell, L, Pease, R, Brunt, H and Scott, J (1985). RFLP for the human apo lipoprotein B gene: V; Xba I. Nucl Acids Res, 13, 6793

20. Frossard, PM, Gonzalez, PA, Protter, AA, Coleman, RT, Funke, H and Assmann, G (1986). Pvu II RFLP in the 5' of the human apolipoprotein B gene. Nucl Acids Res, 14, 4373

21. Law, A, Wallis, SC, Powell, LM, Pease, RJ, Brunt, H, Priestley, LM, Knott, TJ, Scott, J, Altman, DG, Miller, GJ, Rajput, J and Miller, NE (1986). Common DNA polymorphism within coding sequence of apolipoprotein B gene associated with altered lipid levels. Lancet, i, 1301

22. Kunkel, LM, Smith, KD, Boyer, SH, Borgaonkar, DS,

Wachtel, SS, Miller, OJ, Breg, WR, Jones, HW Jr. and Rary, JM (1977). Analysis of human Y-chromosome-specific reiterated DNA in chromosome variants. Proc Natl Acad Sci (USA), 74, 1245
23. Southern, EM (1975). Detection of specific sequences among DNA fragments separated by electrophoresis. J Mol Biol, 98, 503
24. Tarugi, P, Calandra, S and Chan, L (1986). Changes in apolipoprotein A-I mRNA level in the liver of rats with experimental nephrotic syndrome. Biochim Biophys Acta, 868, 51
25. Gusella, JF (1986). Recombinant DNA techniques in the diagnosis of inherited disorders. J Clin Invest, 77 1723

Acknowledgement

This study was supported by the Progetto Finalizzato Inge gneria genetica e Basi Molecolari delle Malattie Ereditarie of the Italian Research Council (CNR). The authors wish to thank dr. G. Bittolo-Bon who allowed them to study his patients.

54
Porphyrins, tumors and atherosclerosis

A. Pagnan, G. Jori, P. Pauletto, G. Scannapieco,
S. Biffanti and C. Dal Palù

Several porphyrins are accumulated in significant amounts and
retained for relatively long periods of time (up to 4 weeks) by
solid tumors and other rapidly growing tissues, including embryonic
and traumatized tissues, atheromatous plaques, and psoriatic cells.
This property, associated with the ability of porphyrins of acting
as photosensitizing agents after irrediation with visible light,
represents a new therapeutic modality, termed photodynamic therapy
(PDT). This technique is attracting the interest of clinicians,
especially for the treatment of cancer; at the same time, there is a
burst of basic studies aimed at lucidating the photobiological,
pharmacological and toxicological properties of porphyrins in vitro
and in vivo. This is emphasized by the numerous books and reviews on
the subject published in the last few years (1-7).

The affinity for tumors appears to be maximal for those
porphyrins which display a relatively high degree of hydrophobicity
(octanol/water partition coefficient in the 3-12 range). This
finding is probably due to the fact that hydrophobic porphyrins in
the serum interact preferentially with lipoproteins. One component
of the lipoprotein class, namely the LDL fraction, is responsible
for the delivery of a large fraction of the injected porphyrins to
hyperproliferating tissues through a specific receptor-mediated
process. On the other hand, other lipoproteins (HDL) and albumin act
as carriers of porphyrins mainly to skin districts and constituents
of the reticuloendothelial system, such as liver and spleen. The
clearance of porphyrins from normal tissues is usually complete
within 48 hours after administration of the drug; however, skin
exhibits an anomalous behavior and detectable amounts of porphyrins
are often recovered from this tissue up to 15 days after injection.
Neoplastic tissues release the accumulated porphyrins at a much
slower rate than healthy tissues. The latter property has been
ascribed to a combination of several factors, including the lower pH
tumor components, the poor efficiency of the lymphatic drainage and
the presence of lipid-rich clusters which incorporate porphyrins and

make them inaccessible to serum proteins.

Actually, pharmacodynamic studies have shown that tumor-bound porphyrins are preferentially located in the cytoplasmic and endothelial cells. A significant amount of porphyrins is also present in the connective tissue and, to a minor extent, in the macrophages. The heterogeneous endotissutal distribution of porphyrins is somewhat dependent on the complex composition of Photofrin II (often called DHE), i.e. the porphyrin most frequently used in clinical PDT; Photofrin II contains a covalent dimer of hematoporphyrin (60-70%) in the form of several different isomers, as well as variable amounts of other porphyrins of different chemical structure and aggregation state. Good tumor-localizing properties have also been found for monomeric hematoporphyrin (Hp), as well as for some water-insoluble derivatives of Hp. Since the latter compounds are characterized by a greater degree of purity than DHE, it is possible that their biodistribution is more selective.

In any case, all of the above mentioned porphyrins possess an absorption band in the 620-630 nm region. These light wavelengths are suitable for clinical PDT, since they are endoved with a relatively deep penetration into biological tissues and are not competitively absorbed by the endogenous chromophores typical of mammalian tissues : as a result, tissue volumes with diameters as large as 1 cm can be often illuminated with no concomitant photodamage of the normal tissues where the tumor grows. This circumstance minimizes the risks of undesired side effects of PDT and allows the repetition of the phototreatment.

As regards the mechanism of the tumor damage after porfhirin photosensitization, two independent processes have been observed: i) direct lysis of neoplastic cells, which is the consequence of the photoinduced peroxidation of steroids and lipids and cross-linking of membrane proteins; ii) vascular damage, mainly arising from photodestruction of endothelial cells. Both events require the presence of oxygen in the microenvironment of the photoexcited porphyrin molecule. Oxigen acts by two parallel reaction pathways:

i) Reaction with radical intermediates formed during the primary electron transfer between the photoexcited porphyrin (P*) and selected substrates (Sub):

$$P^* + Sub \longrightarrow P^{+\cdot} Sub^{-\cdot}$$
$$Sub^{-\cdot} + O_2 \longrightarrow Sub_{ox}$$

ii) Electronic energy acceptor from the photoexcited porphyrin with generation of a cytotoxic and highly reactive oxygen species, namely singlet oxygen ($^1O_2$):

$$P^* + O_2 \longrightarrow P + {}^1O_2$$
$$^1O_2 + Sub \longrightarrow Sub_{ox}$$

In both cases, owing to the short lifetime of the reactive transients (P*, Sub$\overline{\cdot}$, $^1O_2$), the whole photoprocess occurs within a limited spatial range; thus, only the tissue area surrounding the photoexcited porphyrin molecule is subjected to the photodamage.

On the basis of the outlined mechanisms, the most common PDT protocol for the treatment of tumors involves the intravenous injection of Photofrin II (or Hp) at a dose of 2-5 mg/Kg body weight of the patient. After about 48 hours, the tumor area is irradiated with light wavelength(s) in the 620-630 nm interval; the total light dose delivered to the tumor ranges between 100 and 600 J/cm^2 depending on the size of the neoplastic area and the optical features of the tumor (e.g., the degree of pigmentation). The dose-rate must be kept below a threshold value of 300 mW/cm^2 to avoid the onset of hyperthermic effects which would overlap and possibily mask the photochemical process. The red light is usually obtained from a cw Argon-dye laser or a pulsed gold-vapor laser. For external tumors or located in directly accessible cavities, the laser emission is focused on to the neoplasia by means of optical fibers coupled with the light source; in the case of deep-sited or large tumors, the optical fibers are either included in an endoscope or inserted into a needle, which is then infixed into the tumor mass (intestinal PDT). Thus, a sufficient light fluence is driven to the site to be irradiated independently of the size or depth of the latter.

PDT is now in a controlled (phase III) clinical trial for the treatment of bladder and endobronchial tumors. Moreover, PDT is being considered as a valuable therapeutic option either as a primary treatment, for palliation or as on adjuvant therapy. In general, PDT is most effective toward malignant tumors which are thin and localized. Thus, carcinoma-in-situ and early invasive carcinoma of the skin, oral and vaginal mucosa, bronchial mucosa and bladder often give satisfactory responses. Moreover, PDT is utilized for palliation of inoperable or obstructive cancers or cancers recurring after conventional therapeutic modalities. There is now a general agreement that the previous application of chemo- or radio-therapy does not influence the efficacy of PDT. Thus, it appears ethically acceptable to use PDT with those tumors which are unresponsive to standard therapies, since the mechanism of PDT action on cells and tissues is different from those typical of cytotoxic chemicals and ionizing radiations.

In analogy with tumors, recently it has been shown that porphyrins are also retained in atherosclerotic plaques of rabbit and monkey aortas (8, 9).
Studies from our group have demonstrated that hematoporphyrin (Hp) also accumulate in the atherosclerotic lesions (fig. 1) of another animal species represented by the Broad Breasted White Turkey (BBWT)

411

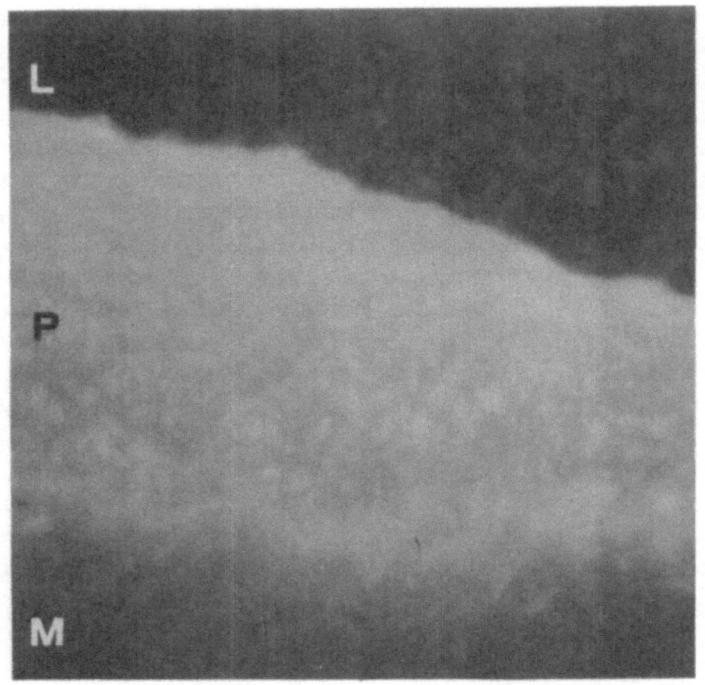

Figure 1 Histological section taken from abdominal aorta of BBWT 24 hours after i.v. injection of 10 mg/Kg hematoporphyrin. The specimen was photographed under fluorescence microscope. The atherosclerotic plaque shows an intense fluorescence, which progessively decreases towards the underlying media.
L = lumen; P = plaque; M = media

The interest for this experimental model relates to the fact that BBWT is spontaneously hypertensive and atherosclerotic; the atherosclerotic process is confined to the abdominal aorta, while the thoracic tract is free from any lesion and exhibits a marked medial hypertrophy, due to the chronic hypertension (10). In this animal species we have observed after Hp injection a significant accumulation of the dye also in the media of the thoracic tract which is free from atherosclerotic lesions (fig. 2).

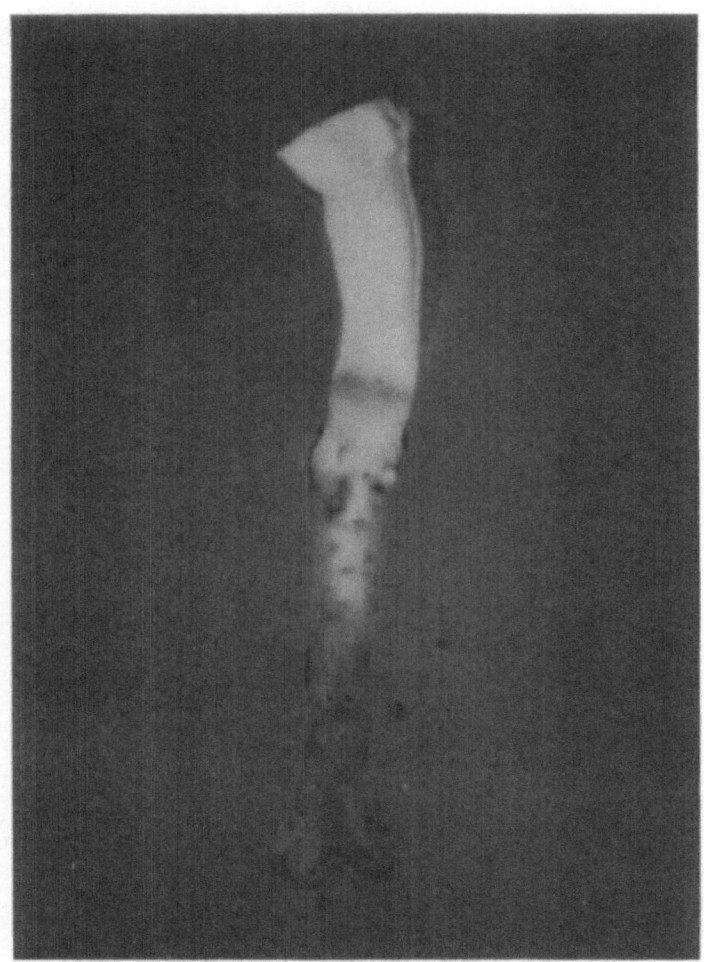

Figure 2 Aorta taken 24 hours after i.v. injection of 10 mg/Kg hematoporphyrin, observed under UV light. The entire luminal surface of the abdominal tract shows an intense fluorescence; no fluorescence is observed in the thoracic tract.

This finding suggests that other substrates than atherosclerotic lesions are able to take up Hp. It is however important to outline that the thoracic aorta releases the bound Hp more rapidly than the abdominal tract. Based on the above observations, we postulated that the cellular basis for the specific Hp uptake by the arterial wall

413

could be represented by the vascular smooth muscle cells. To test this hypothesis we set up secondary cultures of smooth muscle cells in vitro, obtained by explants of aortic wall. We could demonstrate that smooth muscle cells from the thoracic aorta bind higher Hp quantities than the smooth muscle cells from the abdominal tract. Even more interesting, the cellular binding of aqueous Hp is significantly lower than that observed for the LDL-Hp complex, suggesting the esistence of a specific receptor-mediated mechanism.

REFERENCES

1. Doiron, D and Gomers, CJ (1984). Porphyrin localization and treatment of tumors. Alain R Liss, New York.
2. Kessel, D (1984). Photochem Photobiol, 39, 851
3. Andreoni, A and Cubeddu, R (1984). Porphyrins in tumor phototherapy,. Plenum Press, New York.
4. Jori, G and Perria, CA (1985). Photodynamic therapy of tumors and other diseases. Libreria Progetto, Padova.
5. Dougherty, TJ (1985). Clin Chest Med, 6, 219.
6. Moan, J (1986). Lasers Med Sci, 1, 5.
7. Van Den Bergh, H (1986). Chem Britain, 22, 5.
8. Spears, JR Serur, J Shropshire, D Paulin, S (1983). J Clin Invest 71, 395.
9. Litvack, F Grundfest, WS Forrester, JS et al. (1985). Am J Cardiol, 56, 667.
10. Pagnan, A Thiene, G Pessina,AC Dal Palù, C (1980). Artery, 6, 320

55
Influence of physical exercise on plasma lipoprotein pattern in healthy subjects

P. Oriente, G. Di Fraia, A. Spanó, L. Postiglione,
G. Casaburo, A. Pepe and F. Murru

INTRODUCTION

A growing body of experience has demonstrated that physical activity may be protective against C.H.D.[1].

Various hypotheses on the possible pathogenic processes through which physical activity may operate have been proposed, but it has been generally accepted that physical activity may exert its effect reducing some of the known coronary risk factors[2].

The influence of physical exercise on plasma lipids and lipoproteins, which have been widely accepted to be among some of the major coronary risk factors, has gained increasing scientific attention in recent years[3,4].

The "typical" lipoprotein pattern in well-trained subjects, shows a low VLDL fraction, normal or low LDL (relatively poor in triglycerides) and a cholesterol rich triglycerides poor HDL fraction associated with a high level of Apo A_1. This pattern is associated with a low risk for the development of atherosclerosis.

Despite extensive cross-sectional and longitudinal research on a population with different levels of physical activity, i.e. sedentary subjects, on active subjects and athletes on a regular and different physical exercise program, there is still a lack of consensus on the type, the intensity and duration of physical exercise able to affect the lipoprotein pattern as well as on a possible threshold value of physical exercise above which antiatherogenic lipoprotein changes may occur.

In order to shed more light on these problems we evaluated some possible changes of the lipoprotein pattern in correlation with different types and intensity of exercise in both sedentary and active subjects (agonist or not) by four different investigations carried out in the last decade.

In the first the effect of a regular and mild physical exercise program with respect to sedentary control was defined[5,6].

In the second we evaluated the effect of the different kinds of physical activity in athletes well trained for competition, in subjects with mild physical activity and in a sedentary control group[7].

In the third an intensive short program of a particular type of physical training (aerobic exercise maxime represented) in three professional basket-ball teams was studied[8].

In the fourth study we evaluated the effects of a program of aerobic physical activity conducted in a moderate way and for a long period in sedentary subjects[9].

METHODS

325 subjects (242 men and 83 women) were examined in the four studies. The investigation included medical history, clinical examination, ECG and several chemical analyses. The same clinical instrumental and laboratory procedures were used.

Clinical examination consisted of anthropometric measurements: body weight (determined with a standard beam scale), height (determined with a fixed ruler attached to the scale) and thickness of four skinfolds: biceps, triceps, subscapular and subcostal (determined with the Harpender caliper), and Body Mass Index (weight $kg/height^2$) and Body Fat percent (sum of the four skinfolds).

Blood pressure and heart rate were taken according to the WHO advised methods. Blood analyses were performed on venous blood drawn from subjects fasting from 12-14 hours.

Cholesterol and triglycerides in serum and in lipoprotein fractions were evaluated by enzymatic colorimetric methods (CHOD-PAP and GPO-PAP*)[10,11,12].

Lipoprotein fractions were obtained be preparative ultracentrifugation at three different densities (1.006 g/ml for VLDL, 1.063 g/ml for LDL and 1.210 g/ml for HDL)[13].

HDL was also evaluated by the phosphotungstate Mg^{++} precipitation method[14,15].

LDL was calculated using the indirect method.

Apoprotein A, A and B were evaluated by simple radial immunodiffusion (RID**)[16,17,18].

VO_2 max (maximal oxygen consumption) measurement were obtained with the Ostrand procedure[19].

---

* Boehringer Biochemica Mannheim
** M-Partigen, Istituto Boehring-Scoppito (AQ)

RESULTS

In the first study 150 subjects (75 males and 75 females) aged from 18 to 26 years have been examined.

They were attending the Faculty of Physical Education (ISEF) and had 12 hours of physical training four times a week. Physical Training included swimming, gymnastics, rhythmic gymnastics (women only), basket-ball, volley-ball and fencing (men only).

In Table 1 data on plasma and lipoproteins lipid concentrations of ISEF students compared with data of a population sample of inactive subjects of the same area are reported (Olivetti study).

Total cholesterol has been found significantly lower in active men with respect to the controls while VLDL, LDL and HDL - cholesterol concentrations have been found to be very similar in the two groups; men and women alike (when these values were corrected for different methods used).

Total triglycerides concentration is lower in active men (ISEF) as compared to the sedentary group (Olivetti).

Data on the lipoprotein profile of this group of young active subjects compared with a working population with low physical activity led to the conclusion that only prolonged and heavy exercise both in men and women can increase HDL-cholesterol concentration, whereas lighter physical activity might not significantly affect this lipoprotein fraction but may affect plasma cholesterol and triglycerides concentration in men.

In the second study 98 male subjects, 42 athletes (15 judokas, 14 sprinters and 14 marathon runners) well-trained for competition, 25 students from ISEF and 30 inactive subjects have been considered.

Type, duration and intensity of physical exercise was as follows: A) hard way: judokas (12 hrs/weekly, 5 times a week), sprinters (16 hrs/weekly, 6 times a week), marathon runners (16 hrs/weekly, 6 times a week); B) moderate (12 hrs/weekly, 4 times a week).

The mean values of plasma and lipoprotein lipids, apoprotein A and B and VO_2 max of the three groups of athletes, on active (ISEF) and control groups are reported in Table 3. Total and VLDL and LDL cholesterol concentration have been found significantly lower in the active group with respect to the control group.

HDL-cholesterol concentration has been found significantly higher in the marathon group as compared to the other ones: the values being very similar between sedentary and other active groups.

Total and VLDL, LDL and HDL triglycerides have been found significantly lower in all active groups.

Apoprotein B concentration has been found, similarly to cholesterol concentration, lower in active groups than in the sedentary controls.

417

On the contrary apoprotein A, according to HDL cholesterol concentration trend, is significantly higher in marathon runners.

The VO_2 max value, as expected, is significantly higher in the marathon group with respect to the other ones.

The results indicate that cholesterol and triglycerides concentration are lower in all active subjects than in sedentary controls.

Moreover the most favorable lipoprotein pattern has been found in the group of athletes in which aerobic metabolism is maximally utilized for the energy request. In the marathon group, in fact, the VO_2 max values have been found higher than the other groups in which higher values of HDL-cholesterol and apoprotein A have been reported.

In the third study 27 basket-ball players (18 males and 9 females) have been studied before and after an exercise training program designed to increase the capacity and the aerobic power metabolism (4 hrs daily, 6 times a week).

In Table 2 we report the mean values and S.D. of plasma cholesterol and triglycerides, HDL-cholesterol and apoprotein A, A_1 and B concentration in basket-ball players of both sexes before and after a month of training.

A significant decrease of the total cholesterol concentration has been demonstrated only in men, whereas HDL-cholesterol concentration and apo A_1 have been found to be increased in both sexes.

Minor changes have been found for triglycerides concentration.

After training this value decreased slightly in men probably due to the major intake of carbohydrates during training.

The results showed that this type of physical intensive exercise, mainly through the increased aerobic capacity, was able to significantly determine the increase of HDL-cholesterol as well as apoprotein A_1 concentration.

In the fourth study 50 sedentary life-style middle-aged men undergoing a program of moderate physical exercise consisting of a 10 km run 3 times weekly for 6 months have been studied.

In Table 4 lipids lipoprotein and apoprotein concentrations and VO_2 max values are reported. Total cholesterol, LDL cholesterol and total triglycerides concentrations have been found significantly decreased after one month with respect to the baseline values. The lowest values have been reached in the fourth month.

HDL-cholesterol starts to increase only during the second month while APO A and Apo A_1 only show an increase during the first month reaching the highest values in the fourth month.

VO_2 max progressively increased during the program reaching a significant value in the third month.

Table 1 Cholesterol and triglycerides of plasma and lipoprotein fractions concentrations (mg/dl) in ISEF students and in Olivetti population sample

| | ISEF | | OLIVETTI | |
	MEN n=75	WOMEN n=75	MEN n=40	WOMEN n=26
Age (yrs)	22 ± 2.0	21 ± 2.0	25 ± 2.0	25 ± 2.0
Tot.-Chol.	152 ± 13.5	164 ± 11.6	170 ± 30.5	165 ± 27.4
VLDL "	8 ± 3.5	6 ± 2.7	13.1*	7.7*
LDL "	103 ± 20.3	111 ± 23.9	96 ± 28.9	100 ± 22.4
HDL "	41 ± 6.3	48 ± 6.9	41°	50°
Tot.-Tg	88 ± 15.6	96 ± 20.3	92*	73*
VLDL "	54 ± 9.7	43 ± 10.6	48*	37*
LDL "	22 ± 7.9	26 ± 6.2	17 ± 6.2	17 ± 3.5
HDL "	12 ± 3.5	26 ± 3.5	9 ± 3.5	17 ± 3.5

$\bar{x}$ ± S.D.

* Geometric mean

° Values corrected for different methods

Table 2 Plasma lipids, HDL-cholesterol and A, A_1 and B apoprotein concentrations (mg/dl) in basket-ball players before and after one month of training

| | MEN(n=18) | | WOMEN(n=9) | |
	BASELINE		BASELINE	
Age (yrs)	24 ± 6.0		24 ± 6.0	
BMI	23 ± 1.7	23 ± 2.1	22 ± 1.8	23 ± 1.0
Tot-Chol.	151 ± 15.0	138 ± 12.0*	134 ± 10.0	121 ± 15.0
HDL-Chol.	49 ± 14.0	60 ± 13.0**	51 ± 18.0	61 ± 15.0**
Tot-Tg	68 ± 5.0	87 ± 9.0	57 ± 5.0	47 ± 5.3
Apo A	157 ± 16.6	170 ± 14.3	159 ± 15.0	174 ± 25.2
Apo A_1	98 ± 5.6	137 ± 5.6**	122 ± 10.6	135 ± 10.3**
Apo B	65 ± 6.7	56 ± 8.7	85 ± 10.0	81 ± 7.8

$\bar{x}$ ± S.D.; BMI = Body Mass Index

*p 0.01   **p 0.05 (Student's t-test)

419

Table 3 Cholesterol and triglycerides of plasma and lipoprotein fractions, apoproteins A and B concentrations (mg/dl), VO_2 Max values in three groups of athletes in active (ISEF) and control group

N.	Control group (30)	ISEF Students (25)	Judokas (15)	Sprinters (14)	Marathon runners (14)
Age (yrs)	23 ± 2.0	23 ± 1.0	22 ± 2.0	20 ± 2.0	21 ± 2.0
BMI	24 ± 2.1	23 ± 1.4	25 ± 2.6	22 ± 1.3	21 ± 1.4
Tot.-Chol	174 ± 25.9	152 ± 31.2*	152 ± 31.2*	144 ± 22.2*	147 ± 20.6*
VLDL "	11 ± 5.3	7 ± 2.1*	5 ± 2.9*	5 ± 2.2*	6 ± 1.9*
LDL "	125 ± 22.1	106 ± 23.4	107 ± 28.6	99 ± 19.9*	90 ± 17.4*
HDL "	40 ± 6.1	39 ± 4.9	39 ± 5.2	40 ± 5.9	52 ± 6.5*
Tot.-Tg	97 ± 33.2	73 ± 25.4	51 ± 12.7*	61 ± 15.7*	64 ± 20.35*
VLDL "	56 ± 25.6	38 ± 15.5	24 ± 8.9*	29 ± 14.8*	25 ± 11.1*
LDL "	28 ± 11.5	22 ± 11.5	19 ± 6.9*	24 ± 6.8	32 ± 19.1
HDL "	12 ± 5.4	10 ± 3.5	8 ± 3.7	8 ± 4.0	8 ± 2.6
Apo A	214 ± 30.2	212 ± 22.1	205 ± 19.9	218 ± 29.1	235 ± 30.7*
Apo B	96 ± 22.8	83 ± 21.9	85 ± 21.9	82 ± 20.6	83 ± 13.8
VO_2 Max	48 ± 9.8	47 ± 7.4	45 ± 10.8	51 ± 14.2	62 ± 12.0*

$\bar{x}$ ± S.D.; BMI = Body Mass Index; VO_2 Max (ml/min/kg BW); * p 0.05   Analysis of variance (F) in the four groups versus control group.

Table 4 Cholesterol and triglycerides of plasma and lipoprotein fractions, apoproteins A, A_1 and B concentrations (mg/dl), VO_2 Max values in 50 male subjects during 5 months of the training

	BASELINE	I	II	MONTHS III	IV	V
Age(yrs)	24 ± 1.9			31 ± 3.0		
BMI		23 ± 1.0	23 ± 1.8	23 ± 1.1	23 ± 1.6	23 ± 1.3
Tot.-Chol.	180 ± 9.1	162 ± 9.8**	155 ± 20.2**	152 ± 20.1**	149 ± 19.8**	145 ± 18.4**
VLDL "	11 ± 3.4	10 ± 5.8	8 ± 3.9	9 ± 4.3	8 ± 3.8	8 ± 3.9
LDL "	124 ± 31.4	108 ± 28.5**	103 ± 25.9**	97 ± 25.6**	94 ± 24.2**	93 ± 26.3**
HDL "	40 ± 6.1	40 ± 4.6	45 ± 4.1*	49 ± 4.8**	52 ± 4.0**	52 ± 4.7**
Tot.-Tg	96 ± 23.9	75 ± 20.7**	73 ± 18.4*	71 ± 18.4*	65 ± 19.9*	62 ± 20.3*
VLDL "	54 ± 16.9	41 ± 15.7*	39 ± 14.5*	38 ± 12.2*	35 ± 12.4*	37 ± 14.7*
LDL "	24 ± 8.9	21 ± 6.3	21 ± 7.0	19 ± 8.1	17 ± 8.2	17 ± 7.3
HDL "	10 ± 2.3	10 ± 2.3	11 ± 20.4	11 ± 3.6	12 ± 2.7	11 ± 3.7
APO A	133 ± 36.6	150 ± 17.1*	152 ± 16.6*	154 ± 15.7*	157 ± 16.5*	159 ± 16.1*
APO A_1	113 ± 12.6	119 ± 9.9	130 ± 10.5*	135 ± 9.13**	134 ± 23.3**	136 ± 15.5**
APO B	83 ± 16.7	82 ± 14.4	79 ± 14.1	77 ± 14.1	74 ± 12.9	75 ± 13.2
VO_2 Max	45 ± 10.1	48 ± 9.5	52 ± 10.2*	54 ± 14.2**	55 ± 9.8**	55 ± 8.9**

$\bar{x}$ ± S.D.; BMI = Body Mass Index; VO_2 Max (ml/min/kg BW); * p 0.05   ** p 0.01 (analysis of variance (F) versus baseline values).

421

CONCLUSION

The results obtained in the four studies according to the data in the literature support the thesis that in clinically healthy people physical exercise affects the plasma lipoprotein pattern. The relationship between physical activity and lipids is not unequivocal but remains to be interpreted with respect to the biological and life style variability in the practicing subjects as well as the physical exercise characterized by type, intensity, duration, time and frequency of practice.

At present it seems well documented that physical exercise, mild and intensive, is able to lower plasma cholesterol and triglycerides concentration, while only physical exercise in which aerobic capacity is stimulated (in an intensive way for a short period and/or for a long period in a moderate way) is able to increase HDL-cholesterol and Apo A_1 concentration.

REFERENCES

1. Froelicher, V.F., Oberman,A. (1972). Analysis of epidemiological studies of physical inactivity as risk factor for coronary artery disease. Prog. Vardiovasc. Dis., 15, 41.
2. Kannel, W.B., Sorlie, P. (1979). Some health benefits of physical activity. The Framingham Study. Arch. Inter. Med., 139, 857.
3. Lewis, C.L., Bonow, R., Schaefer, E., Bruwer, M.B., Lindgeren, F.T. (1980). Effect of exercise conditioning on plasma high density lipoproteins and other lipoproteins. Atheroclerosis, 37, 529.
4. Wood, P.D., Haskell, W.L. (1979). The effect of exercise on plasma high density lipoproteins lipids, 14, 417.
5. Oriente, P., Farinaro, E., Spanò, A., Di Fraia, G., Coraggio, S., Postiglione, L. (1981). Lipoprotein profile in a group of young people on regular physical activity (ISEF study). Atheroscl. Clin. Evaluat. and Therapy. MTP Press Ltd, 367, 372.
6. Farinaro, E., Oriente, P., Paggi, E., Panico, S., Mancini, M. (1979). L'indagine di Pozzuoli "Olivetti". Rapporto conoscitivo sullo stato delle Indagini Epidemiologiche in Italia nel Campo dell'Arteriosclerosi. Vol.II, 177-201. CNR Progetto Finalizzato Medicina Preventiva, Subprogetto ATS-RF$_2$ (Roma: Consiglio Nazionale delle Ricerche).
7. Oriente, P., Spanò, A., Di Fraia, G., Postiglione, L., Cimmino, F., Murru, F., Pepe, A. (1983). Concentrazioni dei lipidi e delle lipoproteine in giovani adulti praticanti attività fisica moderata ed in atleti impegnati in differenti sports a

livello agonistico. Med. dello Sport, Vol.36, n. 6, 557-62.

8. Di Fraia, G., Spanò, A., Pepe, A., Cimmino, F., Murru, F., Postiglione, L., Oriente, P. (1984). Valutazione dei lipidi, lipoproteine ad alta densità ed apoproteine A, A_1 e B del siero in atleti prima e dopo un programma di allenamento preagonistico. Atherosclerosis and Cardiovascular Diseases. Ed. Compositori, Bologna.

9. Oriente, P., Postiglione, L., Fi Fraia, G., Spanò, A., Pepe, A., Murru, F. (1986). Modificazioni dei lipidi e delle frazioni lipoproteiche indotte dall'esercizio fisico in soggetti adulti dell'area napoletana. Prog. Fin. Med. Prev., C.N.R. Roma, (Italy).

10. Match, F.T., Lees, R.W. (1968). Practical methods for plasma lipoprotein analysis. Adv. Lipid Res., 6, 1.

11. Klosa, S., Hagen, A., Gruf, H. (1975). Méthode de dosage colorimétrique du cholesterol par voie entièrement enzymatique adaptée à tous les types d'autoanalyseurs. Organization del Laboratoires Biologie Prospective. III Colloque de Punt-à Mousson, l'Expansion Scientifique Française, Paris, 505.

12. Buccolo, G., Davis, M. (1973). Quantitative determination of serum triglycerides by use of enzyme. Clin. Chem., 19, 475.

13. Carloson, K. (1973). Lipoprotein fractionation. J. Clin. Path., Suppl. 5, 26.

14. Burstein, M., Sholnich, M.R., Morfin, R. (1970). Rapid method for the isolation of lipoproteins from human serum by precipitation with polyanions. J. Lipid Res., 11, 583.

15. Kostner, G.M. (1976). Enzymatic determination of cholesterol in high density lipoprotein fractions preparated by polyanion action. Clin. Chem., 22, 625.

16. Bradby, G.V.H., Valente, A.J., Welton, K.W. (1978). Lancet, 2, 1271.

17. Schonfield, G. (1978). Lipids, 13, 951.

18. Reman, F.C., Vermond, A. (1978). The quantitative determination of apolipoprotein A_1 in human serum by radial immunodiffusion assay (RID). Clin. Chem., Acta, 87, 387.

19. Shephard, R.J., Allen, C., Benale, A.J.S., Davies, C.T.M., Di Prampero, P.E., Medman, R., Merriman, J.E., Myhre, K., Simmons, R. (1968). The maximum oxygen intake: an international reference standard of cardiorespiratory fitness. Bull. WHO, 38, 757.

56
Long-term experience with bezafibrate in different types of hyperlipidemia

D. Sommariva, A. Branchi, M. Tirrito, D. Bonfiglioli,
L. Bellintani, C. Ottomano and A. Fasoli

INTRODUCTION

Bezafibrate has been shown in several studies to have effective hypocholesterolemic and hypotriglyceridemic activity |1-6|. Thus the drug may be of benefit in primary and secondary prevention of atherosclerosis. From this point of view, two aspects seem to be of particular interest. The first one is the effect of the drug on lipoprotein subfractions that are believed to play different roles in atherogenesis. The second one is the long-term effectiveness and safety of bezafibrate therapy since the hypolipidemic treatment must be continued for years or decades.

In this paper we report the modifications of the lipoprotein pattern induced by bezafibrate in different types of hyper-lipoproteinemia during 8 month treatment.

MATERIAL AND METHODS

The study was carried out on 108 patients known to have primary hyperlipoproteinemia. Their ages ranged from 19 to 84 years (mean of 50.4 ± 1.04).Sixty one were males and 47 females. According to the WHO criteria, 49 patients were classified as type IIa, 37 as type IIb and 22 as type IV. All the patients were on low fat low cholesterol diet since more than 2 months before entering the study.

Serum samples were taken after an overnight fast at the beginning of the study and 1 month later. Then the patients were put on bezafibrate 200 mg t.i.d. therapy.

Total and lipoprotein cholesterol (C) was determined by the CHOD-PAP method and total and lipoprotein triglycerides (TG) by the DHBS-color method (Ames-Miles Italiana S.p.A., Cavenago Brianza). Serum lipoproteins were fractionated by a mixed ultracentrifugation

(d. 1.006 and 1.125) and precipitation (phosphotungstate/Mg++)
procedure as previously described |6|.

Table 1. Serum lipids and HDL-cholesterol in 106 hyperlipoproteinemic
patients before and after 1 month of treatment with bezafibrate

	-30 days	basal	+30 days	P (+30 vs b)
Type IIa N=47				
Serum cholesterol	310.1±12.19	317.2±10.67	253.7±9.16	<0.001
Serum triglycerides	116.5±5.94	115.7±6.46	~ 38.6±5.36	<0.001
HDL cholesterol	57.0±2.28	57.8±2.04	62.1±2.26	<0.01
Type IIb N=37				
Serum cholesterol	300.1±5.63	298.4±5.91	241.2±6.68	<0.001
Serum triglycerides	224.1±10.37	242.3±12.22	120.1±8.64	<0.001
HDL cholesterol	50.4±1.84	47.4±1.81	57.8±2.87	<0.001
Type IV N=22				
Serum cholesterol	249.6±14.51	248.0±15.15	229.3±12.03	<0.05
Serum triglycerides	556.8±53.21	533.9±65.47	270.9±35.94	<0.005
HDL cholesterol	38.0±2.74	36.4±2.79	44.0±2.69	<0.05

RESULTS

During the first month of follow-up, before the start of
bezafibrate therapy, no significant changes in serum lipids occurred
in the 3 groups of patients. After 1 month of bezafibrate in 47 type
IIa serum C decreased on the average by 20%, serum TG by 23% and
HDL-C increased by 7%. In type IIb patients serum C fell by 19%,
serum TG by 50% and HDL-C rose by 22%. In type IV patients serum
C decreased by 8%, serum TG by 49% and HDL-C increased by 21%
(table 1).

In 68 patients the lipid distribution in lipoprotein fractions
was studied before and after 1 month of bezafibrate therapy. As it
can be seen in table 2, the change in serum C level of type IIa
patients was mostly accounted for by the decrease in LDL-C (-54.8
mg/dl). Both C and TG in VLDL fraction significantly decreased and
HDL-C rose owing to the increase in C of the HDL_3 subfraction. In
Type IIb patients (table 3) the fall of serum C concentration was
due to a decrease of C content in both VLDL and LDL while C in HDL_2
and HDL_3 subfractions significantly increased. TG decreased in all
the 3 main lipoprotein fractions; the fall in VLDL-TG accounting
for 80% of the diminution of serum total TG. In type IV patients

Table 2. Lipoprotein cholesterol and triglycerides in 33 type IIa patients before and after 1 month of therapy with bezafibrate

	basal	30 days	P
VLDL cholesterol	20.3±3.20	12.7±2.12	< 0.05
VLDL triglycerides	55.4±6.67	33.5±4.76	< 0.001
LDL cholesterol	237.8±13.70	183.0±12.58	< 0.001
LDL triglycerides	41.8±2.02	37.2±2.37	< 0.05
HDL$_2$ cholesterol	29.5±2.47	30.2±2.18	N.S.
HDL$_3$ cholesterol	29.4±1.30	33.0±0.97	< 0.005

(table 4), major variations concerned VLDL lipids. VLDL-C decreased on the average by 58% and VLDL-TG by 59%. LDL-C as well as HDL-C significantly increased (21%). The change of HDL-C level was due to the raise of C of the HDL$_2$ (33%) and HDL$_3$ (14%) subfractions, though this latter variation did not reach the statistical significance.

Twenty seven type IIa, 21 type IIb and 16 type IV patients continued the treatment for 8 months. As it can be seen in figure 1, no further significant changes, beyond the ones recorded at the first month, occurred in serum C, HDL-C and serum TG levels during the following 7 months of treatment.

DISCUSSION

Results of this study confirm the effectiveness and safety of bezafibrate in the treatment of the commonest types of hyper-lipoproteinemia. As shown in previous studies |5| bezafibrate besides having a lowering effect on elevated lipoprotein lipids, increases C content of HDL$_2$ and HDL$_3$ subfractions. While the increase of HDL$_3$-C is present in all the 3 groups of patients, though in type IV patients the change do not reach the statistical significance (possibly due to the small series of patients), the increase in HDL$_2$-C can be observed in type IIb and in type IV but not in type IIa patients.

The fact that HDL$_2$-C increases only in patients with elevated serum VLDL concentration and the presence of an inverse correlation between the decrease in VLDL-C and TG and the increase in HDL$_2$-C (r=-0.38 and -0.43 respectively) strongly suggest that both changes are due, at least in part, to a stimulatory effect by the drug on lipoprotein lipase |7|. Such an effect may explain also the increase

Table 3. Lipoprotein cholesterol and triglycerides in 25 type IIb patients before and after 1 month of therapy with bezafibrate

	basal	30 days	P
VLDL cholesterol	53.8±4.40	15.3±2.57	< 0.001
VLDL triglycerides	170.1±10.93	67.7±9.11	< 0.001
LDL cholesterol	199.6±7.27	172.8±8.54	< 0.005
LDL triglycerides	60.8±5.82	43.2±3.51	< 0.05
HDL$_2$ cholesterol	19.5±1.87	29.7±2.86	< 0.001
HDL$_3$ cholesterol	29.3±1.29	33.1±1.24	< 0.001

in LDL-C serum concentration in type IV patients after bezafibrate. In fact, in presence of high VLDL level an excess of VLDL are converted into LDL through the activation of lipoprotein lipase |8| and this may overwhelm the increased ability of LDL uptake and degradation produced by bezafibrate by enhancing the production of specific receptors for LDL |9|. Many effects of bezafibrate on lipoprotein pattern seem then to be largely dependent on the amount of VLDL catabolized.

The hypolipidemic effect of bezafibrate remained constant throughout the period of the study. In no case safety laboratory parameters showed pathological changes. Three patients complained of heartburn, 1 of diarrhea and 1 of skin rash during the treatment.

In conclusion the changes in lipoprotein pattern produced by bezafibrate are consistent with a reduction of cardiovascular risk. The drug is then suitable for long-term use in primary and secondary prevention of atherosclerosis.

Table 4. Lipoprotein cholesterol and triglycerides in 10 type IV patients before and after 1 month of therapy with bezafibrate

	basal	30 days	P
VLDL cholesterol	86.0±11.98	36.3±11.28	< 0.001
VLDL triglycerides	338.0±59.40	139.8±32.59	< 0.02
LDL cholesterol	114.1±11.76	137.6±8.89	< 0.05
LDL triglycerides	56.2±7.26	46.5±5.27	N.S.
HDL$_2$ cholesterol	14.2±1.76	18.9±2.48	< 0.05
HDL$_3$ cholesterol	24.1±1.61	27.4±1.82	N.S.

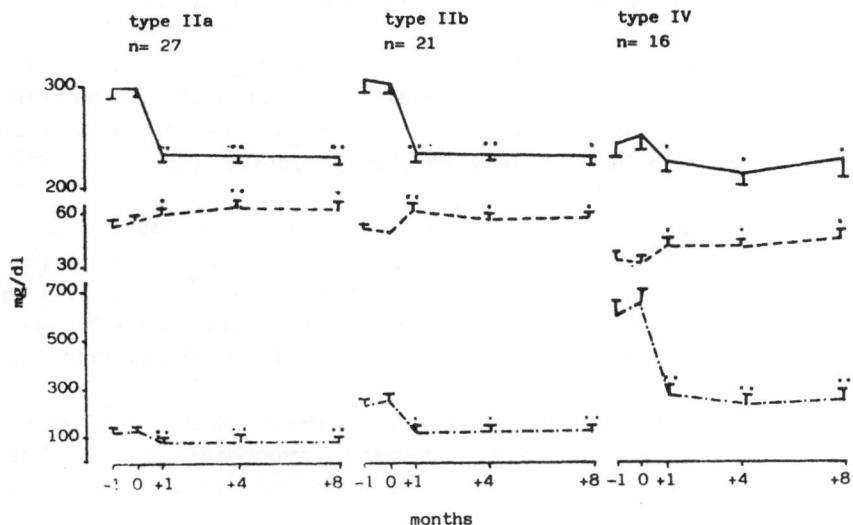

FIGURE 1 Mean changes in total (−) and HDL cholesterol (− −) and in
serum triglycerides (−·−) during 8 month treatment with
bezafibrate (°P < 0.05   °°P < 0.001 vs time 0 level)

REFERENCES

1.   Olsson, AG, Rossner, S, Walldius, G, Carlson,LA, Lang,PD(1977).
Effect of BM 15075 on lipoprotein concentrations in different types
of hyperlipoproteinemia. Atherosclerosis, 27, 279

2.   Oster, P, Schlierf, G, Lang, PD, Andreas, J, Muhlbeyer, W,
Schellenberg, B, Vollmar, J (1980). Effect of bezafibrate and
clofibrate on diurnal lipid and lipoprotein profiles in healthy
volunteers and patients with hypertriglyceridemia. In: Greten, H,
Lang, PD, Schettler, G (eds.) "Lipoproteins and Coronary Heart
Disease". p.145. (New York, Baden-Baden, Cologne: Gerhard Witzstrock
Publ. House)

3.   Fellin, R, Martini, S, Crepaldi, G, Senin, U, Mannarino, E,
Avellone, G, Notarbartolo, A, Capurso, A, D'Agostino, C, Montaguti,
U, Celin, D, Descovich, GC, Mantovani E (1981). Multicenter trial
with bezafibrate in primary hyperlipidemias. Curr Therap Res, 29,657

4.   Olsson, AG, Lang, PD, Vollmar, J (1985). Effect of bezafibrate

during 4.5 years of treatment of hyperlipoproteinemia. Atherosclerosis 55, 195

5. Sommariva, D, Tirrito, M, Bonfiglioli, D, Pogliaghi, I, Branchi, A, Ottomano, C, Bellintani, L (1985). Changes in serum lipoprotein pattern following bezafibrate. Differential effects in type IIa and in type IIb hyperlipoproteinemic patients. Pharmacol Res Comm, 17, 1181

6. Sommariva, D, Tirrito, M, Bonfiglioli, D, Pogliaghi,I, Branchi, A, Cabrini, E (1986). Long-term effects of bezafibrate and of a bezafibrate and cholestyramine combination on lipids and lipoprotein lipids in type IIa hypercholesterolemic patients. Int J Clin Pharm Res, 3, 249

7. Klose, G, Behrendt, J, Vollmar, J, Greten, H (1981). Effect of bezafibrate on the activity of lipoprotein lipase and hepatic triglyceride hydrolase in healthy volunteers. In: Greten, H, Lang, PD, Schettler, G (eds.) "Lipoproteins and Coronary Heart Disease". p.182. (New York, Baden-Baden, Cologne: Gerhard Witzstrock Publ. House)

8. Sigurdsson, G, Nicoll, A, Lewis, B (1975). Convertion of very low density lipoprotein to low density lipoprotein. A metabolic study of apolipoprotein B kinetics in human subjects. J Clin Invest 56, 1481

9. Stewart, JM, Packard, CJ, Lorimer, AR, Boag, D, Shepherd, J (1982). Effects of bezafibrate on receptor mediated and receptor independent catabolism in type II hyperlipoproteinemic subjects. Atherosclerosis, 44, 355

57
Role of fibrinogen in atherosclerosis: therapeutic effects of bezafibrate in short-term treatment
G. Pagano, G. Niort, P. Nuccio and A. Bulgarelli

INTRODUCTION

Fibrinogen has been recognized as a primary risk factor for the development of acute cardiovascular disease |1,2| if not of atherosclerosis itself |3| by enhancing red cell and platelet aggregation |4,5|, increasing rheologic stasis |6| and amplifying the coagulative cascade when in higher concentrations. In this view it seems of interest to lower chronically enhanced fibrinogen down to normal in a stable way. A drug which specifically lowers plasma fibrinogen being at the same time maneageable, long-acting, orally administerable and showing negligible side effects should be chosen for this purpose. Bezafibrate is an antilipaemic drug which could fit these features |7|. In order to elucidate the extent and the quality of this effect we undertook the following study.

MATERIALS AND METHODS

We studied 56 hospitalized patients affected by chronic atherosclerotic vasculopathy and hyperfibrinogenemia (638 $\pm$ 23 S.E.M. mg/dl) without intercurrent acute pathologies in the last three months, not taking any drug which could significatively affect the haemorheologic pattern from at least 15 days and no clinical or laboratory evidence of renal disfunction.

These subjects were divided into two groups which followed different treatments: they were randomly assigned to each study and to the drug or to the placebo treatment as well.

The first group (group A) was composed of 32 patients, aged 56 $\pm$ 7 S.E.M. years, range 43-72: 10 of these subjects were treated with bezafibrate 200 mg twice a day, 6 of them 200 three times a day, while 16 underwent placebo treatment. Fibrinogen values (Behring NOP-Partigen immunodiffusion slabs) were checked three times during a period of observation which lasted between 35 and 40 days. Moreover, in this group we considered plasma fibrinogen in 6 patients who, by chance, had suspended the therapy (bezafibrate 400 mg/day) later on because of incoming clinical factors: the values refer to subsequent controls and the time past from the interruption was chosen at random for each case.

Twenty-four subjects, aged 57 $\pm$ 4 S.E.M. ys, range 40-73, composed group B: they were treated alternatively with bezafibrate 400 mg/day or placebo. This time some more haemorheological parameters were studied before and after a 15 days-treatment: blood filterability |8| as a whole measure of blood viscosity, BTG (Amersham RIA-kit), PF4 (Abbot RIA-kit) and platelet aggregating threshold for ADP (Sigma) and collagen (Semmelweiss) as indexes of platelet activation and release |9,10,11| and those haematological values which could affect by themselves these measures (WBC count, hematocrit, lipids and blood glucose) |12,13,14|.

Results are expressed as mean $\pm$ S.E.M.

As platelet aggregating thresholds we considered the lowest ADP concentration able to provoke a second wave aggregation (in a population of young healthy normals, in our experience, it is $\sim$ 2μM) and the percentage of aggregation at the collagen concentration which is half of that sufficient to provoke a 100% aggregation in the same population (5μg/ml).

Statistical analysis was performed by Student's t test for paired samples.

RESULTS

GROUP A. A progressive dose-dependent decrease of fibrinogen plasma concentrations was recorded in treated patients (653 $\pm$ 27.1 vs 356 $\pm$ 22.4 mg/dl p $<$ 0.001) unlike the placebo group (585 $\pm$ 2 vs 577 $\pm$ 26 mg/dl N.S.).From figure 1, the decrease appears prompt and reaches its maximum effect in 10-15 days: the higher daily dose of bezafibrate obtains a quickier and more incisive effect. Anyway, the decrease is permanent and the final effect, independently from the dose used on fibrinogenemia reaches a mean decrease of 45% at the end of the first month.

In the six patients which discontinued the treatment,fibrinogen values rose progressively: the increase in absolute value correlates well with the number of days after the suspension (r = 0.91 p $<$ 0.001, y=30.89+8.91x) (fig.2).

GROUP B. In the shorter study, treated patients fibrinogen plasma levels decreased significatively (652.7 $\pm$ 41 vs 348.3 $\pm$ 18.2 mg/dl, p $<$ 0.001) compared to the placebo group (664.1$\pm$ 25.52 vs 652.9 $\pm$ 24.86 mg/dl, N.S.) (fig.3). Blood filterability at 0.5 and 1 ml, platelet aggregating thresholds for ADP and

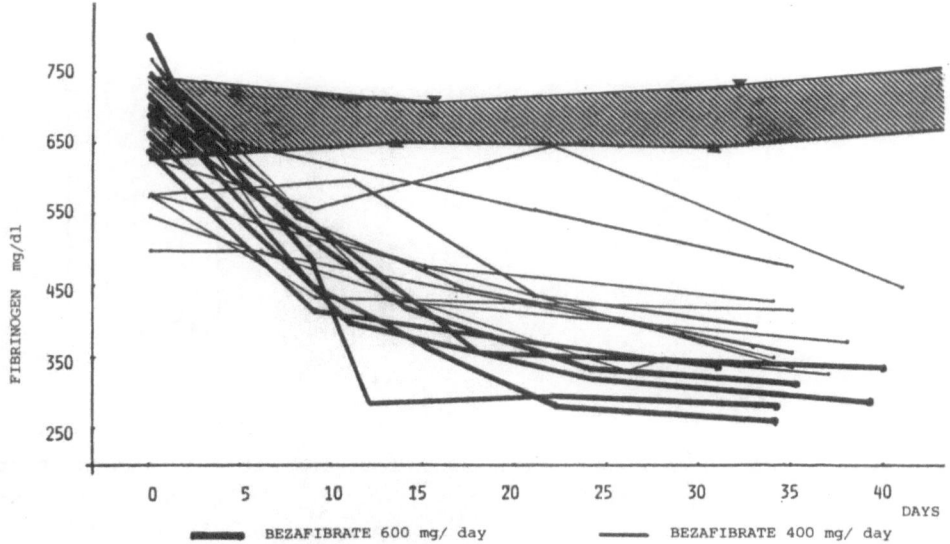

FIGURE 1   Fibrinogen concentrations in 16 placebo (shaded area) and
16 bezafibrate-treated (thin lines 400 mg/day, bold lines 600 mg/
day) group A patients during the observation period.

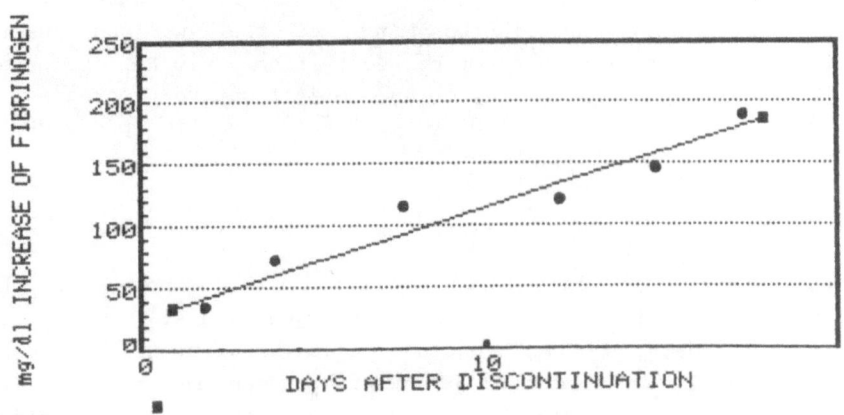

FIGURE 2.   Regression curve between days after suspension of bezafibrate treatment (x) and absolute value increase of plasma
fibrinogen (y) in 6 patients of group A ($y = 30.89 + 8.91x$,
$r = 0.91$, $p < 0.001$)

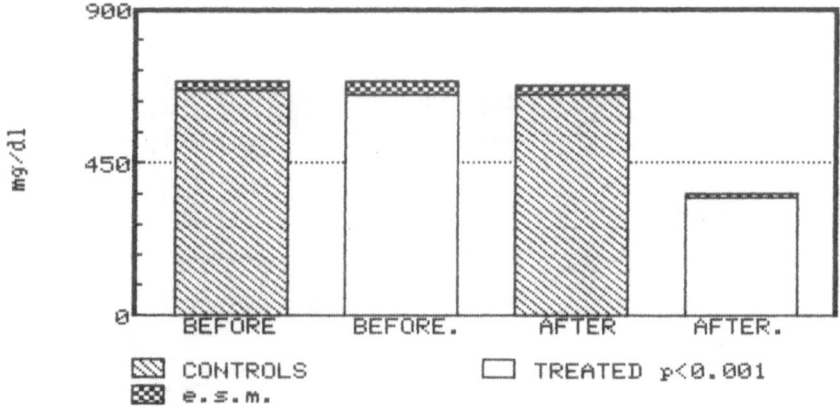

FIGURE 3 Fibrinogen concentrations before and after a 15 days short-term treatment with bezafibrate 400 mg/day in 12 hyperfibrinogenemic subjects compared to a placebo group (n=12), $p < 0.001$.

collagen and PF4 have all returned into the normal range after bezafibrate treatment, even if near the upper limits, while BTG doesn't reach normal values during the period of time observed (15 days), but decreases significatively so that it can be presumed at the moment, that it would probably happen like for the other values, in a longer period of therapy (Table 1).

No significative variations in the haematologic variables cheked were observed after and before the treatment both in the treated patients and the placebo group, so that we can assert that the results obtained are not biased by them. Only HDL-cholesterol plasma levels show a rapid and significative increase in the treated patients (36.6 ± 1.07 vs 48.1 ± 1.1 mg/dl, $p < 0.005$), as reported by others |15| (Table 2).

CONCLUSIONS

Bezafibrate is an antilipaemic drug which has shown, in the past, the ability of lowering plasma fibrinogen values.

From our data, we can conclude that bezafibrate treatment (400,600 mg/day) can normalize plasma fibrinogen in 15 days with no further variation when the therapy is mantained and patient clinical conditions are unchanged. Its effect is rapid, dose-dependent and the discontinuation of it is followed by a rebound increase of fibrinogen values.

At the same time, the haemorheological values tested are specifically reduced. In particular, a reduction of platelet reactivity to aggregants (ADP and collagen) and spontaneous peri-

TABLE 1. Group B haemorheological parameters in bezafibrate-treated and placebo patients before and after treatment.

TREATMENT :	PLACEBO n=12		BEZAFIBRATE n=12	
	before	after	before	after
Blood filterability sec/ml				
1.00 ml	27.7 + 1.6	26.6 + 1.1	26.9 + 0.9	17.5 + 1.2 **
0.50 ml	12.64+ 0.7	12.6 + 0.4	12.8 + 0.31	9.7 + 0.4 **
BTG ng/ml	97.7 + 7.4	100.9 + 8.9	89.9 + 8	52.6 + 1.8 *
PF4 ng/ml	47.4 + 1.8	43.8 + 1.5	49.4 + 1.4	7.8 + 1.1 **
ADP (uM) (2nd wave)	1.32+ 0.3	1.50 + 0.2	1.3 + 0.2	2.4 + 0.4 **
collagen (%) (5ug/ml)	70.3 + 0.9	75.2 + 1.1	74.5 + 4.8	49.1 + 4.7 **

* $p < 0.02$
** $p < 0.001$

TABLE 2. Group B haematological variables cheked during the tests

	BEFORE		AFTER		
PLACEBO (n=12)					
CHOLESTEROL	155.3 + 5.3		146.5 + 5.7	mg/dl	N.S.
TRIGLYCERIDES	131.6 + 8.9		127.1 + 9.4	mg/dl	N.S.
HDL-CHOLESTEROL	37.3 + 0.66		37.4 + 0.6	mg/dl	N.S.
BLOOD GLUCOSE	80.8 + 2.1		78.6 + 1.8	mg/dl	N.S.
HT	39 + 0.79		39.9 + 0.4	%	N.S.
WBC	7660 + 643		7600 + 391	/ml	N.S.
BEZAFIBRATE (n=12)					
CHOLESTEROL	178 + 7.0		168 + 6.1	mg/dl	N.S.
TRIGLYCERIDES	87 + 6.5		78 + 6.7	mg/dl	N.S.
HDL-CHOLESTEROL	36.6 + 1.07		48.2 + 1.05	mg/dl	$p < 0.005$
BLOOD GLUCOSE	76.6 + 3.9		81 + 6.8	mg/dl	N.S.
HT	38.1 + 0.9		40 + 0.9	%	N.S.
WBC	6765 + 552		6805 + 415	/ml	N.S.

pheral activation (measured as BTG and PF4) is evident, probably consequent to lowered plasma fibrinogen: this, together with a decrease of intrinsic plasma viscosity, due to fibrinogen itself, results in a normal blood filterability, i.e. an increased blood fluidity, which is certainly favourable to a vascular flow amelioration, especially in peripheral districts. The prompt and significative increase of HDL-cholesterol together with the return almost to normal of the haemorheological parameters tested help in this sense and in the view of preventing the acute complications of atherosclerosis. A possible positive effect on the instauration of the disease may also be proposed according to the theory of R.Ross |16|.

Bezafibrate seems to be of value in chronic treatment of hyperfibrinogenemia in atherosclerotic patients by selectively reducing fibrinogen plasma concentrations so ameliorating the haemorheological pattern in these subjects. The low side-effects and the good maneageability of the drug support this indication.

AKNOWLEDGEMENTS

This work was partially supported by a grant from the "Consiglio Nazionale delle Ricerche" n°85.00695.56 - progetto finalizzato "Medicina Preventiva e Riabilitativa".

REFERENCES

1.   Wilhelmsen,L, Svardsudd,K, Korsan-Bengsten,K, Larsson,B, Welin,L and Tibblin,G (1984). Fibrinogen as a risk factor for stroke and myocardial infarction. New Engl J Med, 311,501.

2.   Meade,TW, Chakrabarti,R, Haines,AP, North,KRS, Stirling,I, Thompson,GSG and Brozovic,MB (1980). Haemostatic function and cardiovascular death. Early results of a prospective study. Lancet, 1, 1050.

3.   Sadoshima,S and Tanaka,K (1979). Fibrinogen and LDL in the development of cerebral atherosclerosis. Atherosclerosis,34,93.

4. Schmidt-Schönbein,H, Gallash,G, Gosen,vJ, Volger,E and Klose,HJ (1976). Red cell aggregation in blood flow.II. Effect on apparent viscosity of blood. Klin Wochenschr, 54, 159.

5.   Di Minno,G, Thiagarajan,P, Perussi,B, Martinez,J, Shapiro,S, Trinchieri,G and Murphy,S (1983). Exposure of platelet fibrinogen-binding sites by collagen, arachidonic acid and ADP: inhibition by a monoclonal antibody to glycoprotein IIb-IIIa complex. Blood, 61, 140.

6.   Dormandy,JA (1983). L'influenza dell'emoreologia sulla pratica della medicina clinica. La Ricerca Clin Lab, 13 (Suppl.3),7.

7.   Lowe,GDO (1984). Evaluation of rheological therapy by orally administered drugs. Clin Haemorheol, 4, 159.

8.   Reid,HL, Barnes,AJ, Lock,PJ, Dormandy,JA and Dormandy,TL (1977). A simple method for measuring erythrocyte deformability. J Clin Pathol, 29, 855.

9.   Wu,KK and Hoak,JC (1976). Spontaneous platelet aggregation in arterial insufficiency. Mechanisms and implications. Thromb Haemost, 35, 702.

10.   Files,JC, Malpass,TW, Yee,EK, Ritchie,JL and Harker,LA(1981). Studies of human platelet alfa-granule release in vivo. Blood,58,363

11.   Kubisz,P, Parizek,M, Seghier,F, Holan,J and Cronenberg,S(1985). Relationship between platelet aggregation and plasma BTG levels

in arteriovascular and renal diseases. Atherosclerosis, 55, 363.

12.   Chien,S, Schmalzer,EA, Lee,MML, Impelluso,T and Skalar,R(1983). Role of white blood cells in filtration of blood cell suspensions. Biorheology, 20, 11.

13.   Burrows,AW (1981). BTG in diabetes: relation with blood glucose and FpA. H Metab Res, 11 (Suppl), 22.

14.   Muggeo,M, Calabrò,A, Businaro,V, Moghetti,P, Padovan,D and Crepaldi,G (1983). Correlazione tra parametri metabolici ed emoreologici nel diabete mellito e nelle iperlipidemie. La Ricerca Clin Lab, 13 (Suppl 3), 165.

15.   Schwandt,P and Weisweiler,P (1980). Effect of bezafibrate on the high-density lipoprotein subfractions HDL2- and HDL3 in primary hyperlipoproteinemia type IV. Artery, 7, 464.

16.   Ross,R (1986). The pathogenesis of atherosclerosis - An update. New Engl J Med, 20, 448.

NICOTINIC ACID DERIVATIVES, ATHEROSCLEROSIS AND ISCHAEMIC HEART DISEASE

58
Effects of Acipimox on in vivo insulin sensitivity in obese subjects and NID diabetics

P. Cavallo-Perin, E. Pisu, A. Bruno, C. Baggiore,
S. Marena, L. Boine and G. Pagano

ABSTRACT

The increase of plasma FFA could be implicated in the mechanism
of insulin resistance at post-receptorial level. To evaluate
the effects of an inhibitor of lipolisis (acipimox) on in vivo
insulin sensitivity, we performed a 3H-glucose i.v. infusion
and an euglycemic hyperinsulinemic clamp, with plasma FFA determination in 6 non-diabetic obese patients and in 6 non-obese NID
diabetics. Fasting plasma triglycerides were also measured. The
tests were performed in both groups after acipimox (750 mg/day
for 6 weeks) and after placebo, in random sequence. The values
of plasma FFA, glucose production and glucose utilisation, in
both groups, were not significantly different after acipimox
and placebo. After acipimox, plasma triglycerides levels were
significantly ($p<0.001$) lower in both groups, while fasting plasma
glucose levels were significantly ($p<0.025$) lower in NIDD patients.
These results indicate that, although acipimox at the dose employed
does not reduce plasma FFA and insulin resistance, it is able
to reduce plasma triglycerides in both groups and to ameliorate
fasting plasma glucose levels in NID diabetics.

INTRODUCTION

Obesity and non insulin-dependent diabetes mellitus are considered
insulin resistant states, according to Yalow an Berson [1]. High
plasma FFA levels have been implicated in the mechanism of insulin
resistance at the post-receptor site [2]. An in vivo anti-lipolytic
activity of acipimox has been reported [3]. The aims of the present
study are: 1) to evaluate whether the anti-lipolytic action of
acipimox is also present in obese subjects and NID diabetic patients;
2) to study the effects of the drug on insulin resistance; 3) to pro-

pose an explanation of the insulin resistance mechanism in these two conditions on the basis of the hypothetical reduction of plasma FFA levels.

MATERIAL AND METHODS

Six non-diabetics obese patients with impaired glucose tolerance [4], BMI 35.2+4.9, age 46+8 yr, and no family hystory of diabetes and six non-obese non-insulin dependent diabetics (NIDD), BMI 24.4+2.1; age 60+6 yr, were studied.

Both groups have normal renal function as assessed by creatinine clearance. The only ongoing treatment was glibenclamide 10-15 mg/day in the diabetic group. Each patient was treated with acipimox (750 mg/day for 6 weeks) and placebo in random sequence. The usual diet and physical activity were maintained constant in each subiect during the study. A continuous i.v. infusion of D-6-3H-glucose (Amersham, U.K.) (0.2μCi/min for 240 min, with a priming dose of 25μCi) was commenced at 8 a.m. after an overnight fast. The euglycemic glucose clamp [5] was done by infusing 40 mU/m2/min of biosynthetic human insulin (Normal Humulin, Eli Lilly Co. Ltd, USA) using artificial pancreas (Biostator Ames, USA). Plasma glycerol and FFA were measured (enzymatic methods) fasting and every 40 min during clamp. Plasma triglycerides were also measured (Worthington-Cooper Biomedical-Freehold-NJ) on fasting state. The tests were performed at the end of each treatment. All patients gave their informed consent. Blood glucose levels automatically measured by the Biostator were also checked on plasma every 5 min. with a Beckman II Glucose Analyzer. Reproducibility was good (less than 5% variation). Plasma glucose values were used for calculation of all indices. Glucose metabolic clearance rate (ml/kg/min) was calculated as previously reported by us [6]. Endogenous glucose production (mg/kg/min) was calculated using the formula: [(3H-glucose infusion/s.a.)-(pVC/s.a.)(dt/ds.a.)] where s.a.= specific activity, p= 0.65, V= plasma volume, C= glucose concentration, negative values being regarded as 0.

Specific plasma radioactivity during 3H-glucose infusion was determined according to Issekutz at al. [7]. Insulin was measured by solid-phase antibody radioimmunoassay (Kornig Kit, Metfield, Ma).

All values were expressed as mean + 1 S.E.M. Student's t test by paired data was used for statistical evaluation of the differences between values recorded after acipimox and placebo.

RESULTS

Mean values of plasma glucose, insulin and triglycerides on fasting state and during clamp and mean values of glucose production and utilisation are reported in Tab.1. After acipimox plasma triglycerides levels were significantly lower in both groups, while fasting plasma glucose values were significantly lower in NIDD patients only.

Table 1.

	ACIPIMOX	PLACEBO	Significance
OBESE PATIENTS			
FASTING PLASMA GLUCOSE (mg/dl)	94.7±2.7	88.7±2.8	n.s.
FASTING PLASMA INSULIN (uU/ml)	20.8±1.4	19.5±1.7	n.s.
PLASMA TRIGLYCERIDES (mg/dl)	97.0±9.4	148.5±12.7	p<0.001
GLUCOSE PRODUCTION (mg/kg/min)	1.6±0.2	2.0±0.1	n.s.
GLUCOSE UTILISATION(mg/kg/min)	2.6±0.3	3.1±0.3	n.s.
NON INSULIN-DEPENDENT DIABETICS			
FASTING PLASMA GLUCOSE (mg/dl)	133.2±11.1	160.0±17.9	p<0.025
FASTING PLASMA INSULIN (uU/ml)	10.7±1.2	13.5±0.7	n.s.
PLASMA TRIGLYCERIDES (mg/dl)	128.6±10.1	169.8±11.5	p<0.001
GLUCOSE PRODUCTION (mg/kg/min)	2.9±0.4	3.2±0.7	n.s.
GLUCOSE UTILISATION(mg/kg/min)	5.4±0.6	4.4±0.1	n.s.

Plasma FFA and glycerol levels on fasting state and during clamp are reported in Fig.1 and 2. The differences between placebo and acipimox are not statistically significant both in obese and NIDD patients.

Body weight values were not significantly changed during the study both in obese and NIDD patients.

Fig. 1　　　　　　　　　OBESE

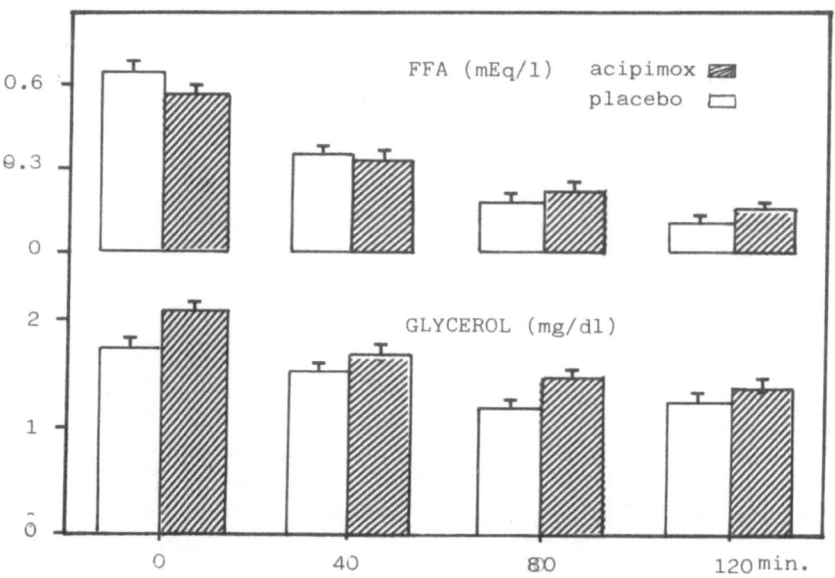

Fig. 2　　　　NON INSULIN-DEPENDENT DIABETICS

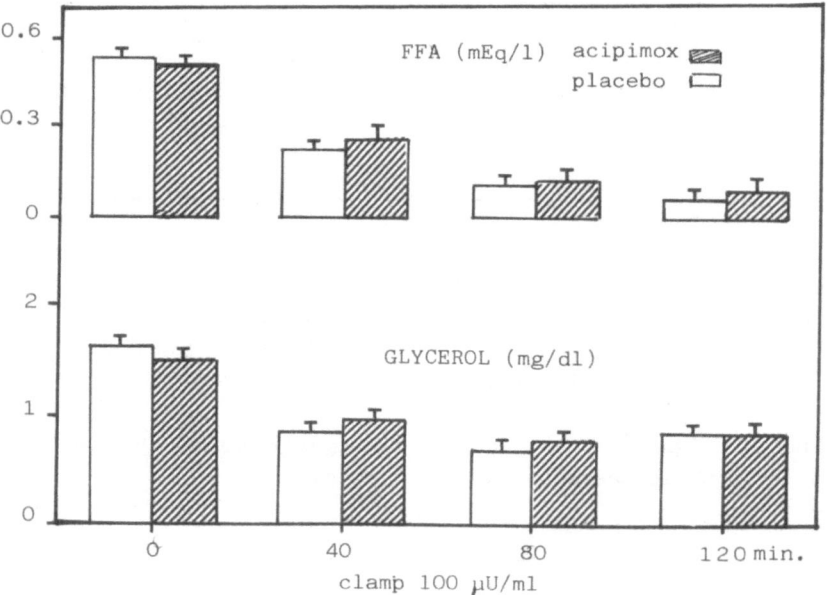

DISCUSSION

Several mechanisms have been proposed to explain insulin resistance in obesity and NIDD [8]. Among them, a possible interpherence by FFA on insulin action at the postreceptor level has been postulated [2]. A reduction of lipolysis has been reported after the administration of acipimox [3]. Acipimox is usually employed in man in the therapy of hypertriglyceridemia [9]. The present study was performed to evaluate whether the treatment with acipimox (750 mg/day) for 6 weeks is able to reduce plasma FFA levels in obese and NIDD patients and whether this effect produces an amelioration of insulin sensitivity in these patients.

Our results indicate that the anti-lipolytic effect of acipimox, evaluated by plasma FFA and glycerol levels, is not evident both in fasting state and during hyperinsulinemic steady-state. The lack of reduction of plasma FFA levels after acipimox did not give the opportunity to evaluate their implication in the mechanism of insulin resistance of these patients. Furthermore, our study indicates that acipimox, in the regimen employed, does not affect insulin resistance in any other different way. Nevertheless, acipimox produced a significant reduction of plasma triglycerides levels both in obese and NIDD patients and a significant reduction in fasting plasma glucose in NIDD patients only. The first result is consistent with the well established anti-hypertriglyceridemic effect of the drug [9] and suggests its efficacy also in presence of plasma triglycerides levels in the normal range. This result, obtained without a significant decrease of glycerol and FFA levels, support the hypothesis that acipimox may exert different mechanisms of triglycerides control other than the proposed anti-lipolytic action. Since the reduction of fasting plasma glucose took place without a reduction in body weight, no explanation of this metabolic effect of acipimox can be derived from the present study.

In conclusion, even though acipimox did not ameliorate insulin sensitivity, it produced a favourable metabolic effect in reducing plasma glucose and triglycerides in the patients studied.

AKNOWLEDGEMENTS

This work was partially supported by a grant from the "Consiglio Nazionale delle Ricerche" No. 85.00695.56 Progetto Finalizzato "Medicina Preventiva e Riabilitativa" Sottoprogetto SP4 "Malattie Degenerative" and No. 85.00788.04. We are grateful to the Eli Lilly Co. Ltd., U.S.A., for supplying the biosynthetic human insulin used in the study.

445

REFERENCES

1.   Yalow , RS and Berson, SA (1970). Insulin resistance. In:
Ellemberg, M and Pifkin, H (eds) "Diabetes Mellitus:Theory and
Pratical". p.389-402.(McGraw-Hill Book Co. Inc. New York)

2.   Kolterman, OG, Scarlett, JA and Olefsky, JM (1982). Insulin
resistance in non insulin-dependent, type II diabetes mellitus.
Clin Endocrinol Metab, 11, 363-385

3.   Fuccella, LM, Goldaniga, G, Lovisolo, P, Maggi, E, Musatti,
L, Mandelli, V and Sirtori, CR (1980). Inhibition of lipolysis
by nicotinic acid and by acipimox. Clin Pharmacol Ther, 28,
790-795

4.   National Diabetes Data Group (1979). Classification and
diagnosis of diabetes mellitus and other categories of glucose
intolerance. Diabetes, 28, 1039-1057

5.   De Fronzo, RA, Tobin, JD and Andres, R (1979). Glucose clamp
technique: a method for quantifying insulin secretion and resistance,
Am J Physiol, 237(3),E214-E222

6.   Cavallo-Perin, P, Cassader, M, Bozzo, C, Bruno, A, Nuccio, P,
Dall'Omo, AM, Marucci, M,and Pagano, G (1985). On the mechanism of
insulin resistance in human liver cirrhosis: evidence of a combined
receptorial and postreceptor defect. J Clin Invest, 75, 1659-
1665

7.   Issekutz , BJ, Allen, M and Borkow, I (1972). Estimation
of glucose turnover in the dog with glucose-2-T and glucose-U-
14C. Am J Physiol, 222, 710-712

8.   Kahn, C (1978). Insulin resistance, insulin insensitivity, and
insulin unresponsiveness: a necessary distinction. Metabolism,
27, 1893-1908

9.   Sirtori, CR, Gianfranceschi, G, Sirtori, M, Bernini, F, Descovich, G, Montaguti, U, Fuccella, LM and Musatti, L (1981). Reduced
triglyceridemia and increased high density lipoprotein cholesterol
levels after treatment with acipimox, a new inhibitor of lipolysis.
Atherosclerosis, 38, 267-271

59
The lipid-lowering effect of the acipimox: comparison with tiadenol and probucol

S. Bertolini, N. Elicio, S. Valice, G. Pistocchi,
S. Cuzzolaro, G. Montagna, A. Serafini and
R. Balestreri

INTRODUCTION

Acipimox (5-methylpyrazine carboxylic acid 4-oxide) is a nico-tinic acid derivative which mainly exerts its hypolipidaemic effect by reducing lipolysis in adipose tissue and free fatty acid (FFA) flux to the liver, leading to a smaller precursor pool for Very-Low-Density Lipoproteins (VLDL) and Low-Density Lipoproteins (LDL) synthesis (1). In comparison to nicotinic acid, Acipimox has been shown to be more effective in decreasing plasma FFA with a longer duration of activity and a lesser rebound following drug withdrawal (2). Here we first give the results obtained during a double blind comparative study between the effects of Acipimox and Tiadenol in type IIb and IV patients, and then the results of an open study in subjects with familial hypercholesterolemia treated with Cholestyramine alone, and with Cholestyramine plus Probucol or Acipimox.

PATIENTS AND METHODS

Double blind trial (Acipimox vs. Tiadenol)

Forty-four patients with primary hyperlipoproteinemia (22 IIb and 22 IV) were typed according to WHO criteria (3). After 1 month period of stabilization on prudent isocaloric diet (50% carbohydrate, 30% fat, 20% protein, cholesterol $\leq$ 300 mg/day, alcohol proscribed) and Placebo, the patients were stratified for hyperlipidemia type and allocated at random into two treatment groups, according to a predetermined schedule based on a table of random numbers. Group A (11 type IIb and 11 type IV; 12 males and 10 females; mean age 52.8, from 37 to 67 years; 25.0+0.7 Body Mass Index) was treated with Aci-pimox 150 mg t.i.d. during the 1st month and with 250 mg t.i.d. du-ring the 2nd and 3rd month. Group T (11 type IIb and 11 type IV; 17

Table 1. Effect of Acipimox (A) and Tiadenol (T) on body weight (Kg), plasma lipids (mmol/l) and apoproteins (mg/dl) in hyperlipoproteinaemic patients type IIb.

months		Baseline	Placebo	A(150mgtid) T(400mgtid)	A(250mgtid) T(800mgtid)	
		-1	0	1	2	3
b.wt.	A	64.7±2.3	64.7±2.5	64.0±2.6	64.4±2.6	64.4±2.6
	T	69.3±2.9	69.1±3.0	69.1±3.0	68.7±3.0	69.3±3.0
Tc	A	7.47±0.26	7.47±0.28	6.93±0.34^a	6.76±0.27^b	6.41±0.20^b
	T	7.44±0.28	7.57±0.25	6.84±0.20^a	6.15±0.22^c	6.30±0.21^b
LDLc	A	4.96±0.31	4.99±0.31	4.59±0.34	4.41±0.29^a	4.03±0.20^b
	T	5.04±0.26	5.24±0.26	4.71±0.17	4.08±0.19^c	4.14±0.19^b
HDLc	A	1.35±0.08	1.32±0.08	1.40±0.07	1.50±0.08^b	1.54±0.07^c
	T	1.16±0.07	1.20±0.05	1.20±0.06	1.21±0.07	1.21±0.08
HDL2c	A	0.40±0.05	0.39±0.05	0.42±0.03	0.53±0.04^c	0.54±0.04^c
	T	0.31±0.03	0.32±0.03	0.30±0.03	0.29±0.02	0.30±0.04
HDL3c	A	0.94±0.04	0.92±0.03	0.99±0.05	0.97±0.04	1.00±0.03^b
	T	0.86±0.04	0.89±0.03	0.90±0.03	0.92±0.05	0.92±0.05
TG	A	3.05±0.32	3.08±0.45	2.48±0.26	2.22±0.19^a	2.19±0.20^a
	T	3.26±0.25	2.95±0.20	2.43±0.15^a	2.27±0.16^a	2.52±0.25
apoAI	A	131.6±7.6	136.0±6.8	146.6±6.2^b	152.5±6.6^c	160.6±6.6^c
	T	121.2±6.8	129.2±6.8	127.6±8.0	131.4±9.8	135.5±9.3
apoB	A	163.4±7.6	162.2±6.4	156.5±8.1	143.7±5.1^b	144.6±5.8^a
	T	176.6±5.8	172.7±5.5	156.1±4.7^a	146.1±6.5^b	155.7±3.3^a

Mean±SEM; N= 11/11 (lipids), N= 8/8 (apoproteins)
^{a}P<0.05, ^{b}P<0.01, ^{c}P<0.001: significance of differences with respect to placebo period (Student's t test for paired data).

males and 5 females; mean age 52.9, from 38 to 67 years; 26.3±0.7 Body Mass Index) assumed Tiadenol 400 mg t.i.d. during the 1st month, and 800 mg t.i.d. during the 2nd and 3rd month. The clinical and bio chemical evaluations of the patients were done in basal conditions, at the end of the placebo period and every month during the pharmaco logical treatment. Plasma samples were collected at each visit to de termine cholesterol (Tc), LDL cholesterol (LDLc), HDL cholesterol (HDLc) and its fractions (HDL2c, HDL3c), triglycerides (TG) and apoproteins AI and B (apo AI, apo B). Blood was drawn after a 12-14 h overnight fast using evacuated tubes (Terumo VT050 Na) containing EDTA -Na$_2$ (final conc. 1.5 mg/ml of blood). Cells were removed within 20 minutes by low-speed centrifugation (1500 x g for 30 minutes at 4°C). All lipid assays were made within 4 hours of blood sampling, plasma samples being stored under refrigeration until assayed. Apo-

Table 2. Effect of Acipimox (A) and Tiadenol (T) on body weight (Kg), plasma lipids (mmol/l) and apoproteins (mg/dl) in hyperlipoproteinaemic patients type IV.

		Baseline	Placebo	A(150mgtid) T(400mgtid)	A(250mgtid) T(800mgtid)	
months		-1	0	1	2	3
b.wt	A	73.1+3.1	73.0+3.2	72.8+3.3	72.7+3.3	73.2+3.4
	T	75.4+2.9	74.9+2.8	74.8+3.0	74.9+3.0	74.9+3.0
Tc	A	6.29+0.4	6.21+0.33	6.09+0.26	5.98+0.17	6.16+0.27
	T	5.57+0.28	5.60+0.29	5.41+0.24	5.51+0.33	5.30+0.23
LDLc	A	3.33+0.24	3.39+0.18	3.62+0.16	3.68+0.15	3.90+0.29
	T	3.31+0.34	3.45+0.33	3.57+0.26	3.63+0.28	3.48+0.25
HDLc	A	1.19+0.06	1.17+0.06	1.26+0.06	1.27+0.04	1.27+0.06
	T	1.06+0.08	1.05+0.08	1.08+0.08	1.11+0.08	1.08+0.09
HDL2c	A	0.29+0.05	0.28+0.04	0.37+0.05[a]	0.41+0.06[b]	0.39+0.06[a]
	T	0.25+0.03	0.22+0.03	0.23+0.04	0.23+0.04	0.21+0.03
HDL3c	A	0.89+0.02	0.88+0.03	0.89+0.03	0.86+0.05	0.89+0.04
	T	0.85+0.06	0.84+0.06	0.86+0.06	0.89+0.04	0.89+0.05
TG	A	5.17+1.12	5.26+1.56	3.56+0.92[a]	3.28+0.70[a]	3.22+0.68[a]
	T	5.71+1.05	5.43+1.04	3.83+0.57[a]	3.54+0.38[a]	2.99+0.26[a]
apoAI	A	112.7+7.0	119.5+5.3	129.7+6.0[a]	130.9+4.6[b]	134.2+4.4[b]
	T	108.2+7.5	114.3+7.5	114.7+7.3	118.3+7.0	118.3+7.1
apoB	A	136.8+12	136.5+13	138.2+14	128.9+12	134.1+14
	T	115.9+14	123.7+13	110.4+11[a]	115.1+12	108.0+11[a]

Mean+SEM; N= 11/11 (Tc,TG), N= 8/8 (LDLc, HDLc, HDL2c, HDL3c), N= 10/10 (apoproteins). [a]$p<0.05$, [b]$p<0.01$: significance of differences with respect to placebo period (Student's t test for paired data).

lipoproteins were assayed within 1 month in plasma aliquots kept at -30°C until analysis. Cholesterol and triglycerides in whole plasma, and cholesterol in HDL and HDL3 fractions, were measured with enzymatic methods (4,5). HDL cholesterol was determined in the supernatant after precipitation of the apo B-containing lipoproteins (VLDL, LDL) by heparin and manganese chloride (final conc. 184 UI/ml, 92 mmol/l respectively); HDL2 and HDL3 cholesterol subfractions were obtained according to Gidez et al. (6). LDL cholesterol concentrations were calculated as suggested by Wilson et al. (7): LDLc = Tc - HDLc - (0.166 x TG). Apolipoproteins AI and B were measured in whole plasma by rocket immunoelectrophoresis according to Curry et al. (8,9) using monospecific antisera (sheep anti-apo AI, Boehringer Mannheim; rabbit anti-apo B, Behringwerke); standard sera for apo AI

Table 3. Mean percent changes after 3 months of treatment with Acipimox (A) and Tiadenol (T).

type		Tc	LDLc	HDLc	HDL2c	HDL3c	TG	apoAI	apoB
IIb	A	-14	-19	+17	+38	+ 8	-29	+18	-11
	T	-17	-21	NS	NS	NS	-15(NS)	NS	-10
IV	A	NS	+15(NS)	+ 8(NS)	+39	NS	-39	+12	NS
	T	NS	NS	NS	NS	NS	-45	NS	-13

Table 4. ANCOVA for repeated measures: group A (IIb + IV) vs. group T (IIb + IV) and their mean percent changes after 3 months.

variable	nA/nT	mean change(%) after 3 months		between treatments(adj)	between periods	interaction
		A	T	P	P	P
Tc	22/22	- 8	-12	<0.05	NS	NS
HDLc	19/19	+14	+ 1	<0.005	<0.05	NS
HDL2c	19/19	+37	0	<0.001	<0.01	<0.01
HDL3c	19/19	+ 6	+ 5	NS	NS	NS
TG	22/22	-35	-34	NS	NS	NS
apoAI	18/18	+15	+ 4	<0.005	<0.001	NS
apoB	18/18	- 6	-11	NS	NS	NS

and apo B were obtained from Immuno Diagnostika and from Behringwerke respectively. Quality assurance of the test systems resulted in the following: the day-to-day coefficients of variation were 3.3% for Tc, 4.2% for TG, 30% for apo AI and 4.8% for apo B; the within-day coefficients of variation were 2.2% for HDLc and 3.2% for HDL3c. The statistical significance of differences between treatment values and placebo values was checked for each group and each type by Student's t test for paired data. Significance of differences between the effects of Acipimox and Tiadenol was evaluated by factorial analysis of covariance for repeated measures in order to correct any difference between the groups in pre-treatment values (10).

Open trial (combined drug therapy for familial hypercholesterolemia)

Eight patients with heterozygous familial hypercholesterolemia (5 males and 3 females; mean age 45.0, from 25 to 59 years; 23.4+2.1 Body Mass Index; 3 with previous myocardial infarction), after a 2

Table 5. Plasma lipid changes induced by cholestyramine (C), Chole-styramine plus Probucol (C+P) and Cholestyramine plus Acipimox (C+A) in 8 patients with heterozygous familial hypercholesterolemia.

	DIET	TREATMENT (% change from diet)			
		C	C+P	C	C+A
weeks	0	6	12	18	24
Tc (mmol/l)	9.85+0.95	-18	-26	-19	-22
LDLc "	7.75+0.93	-22	-28	-22	-26
HDLc "	1.35+0.25	- 5(NS)	-23	- 7(NS)	+ 4(NS)
HDL2c "	0.42+0.15	-10(NS)	-37	-11(NS)	+10(NS)
HDL3c "	0.94+0.09	- 3(NS)	-16	- 5(NS)	0
LDLc/HDLc	5.97+1.99	-17	- 6(NS)	-17	-29[a]
TG (mmol/l)	1.63+0.54	+ 3(NS)	-11(NS)	- 7(NS)	-28
b.wt.(Kg)	64.5+8.3	NS	NS	NS	NS

[a]Significantly different from C (P<0.05) and C+P (P<0.01) periods (analysis of variance and Newman-keuls test).

months period of stabilization on low cholesterol ($\leq$ 200 mg/day) diet containing less than 10% of calories as saturated fat, were sequentially treated with: diet and Cholestyramine 12 g/day; diet and Cholestyramine 12 g/day and Probucol 500 mg b.i.d.; diet and Cholestyramine 12 g/day; diet and Cholestyramine 12 g/day and Acipimox 250 mg t.i.d.. Each treatment lasted 6 weeks. After the diet alone, and at the end of each period of treatment, plasma concentrations of Tc, LDLc, HDLc, HDL2c, HDL3c and TG were determined as previously descri bed. The statistical evaluation of the results was per formed by the analysis of variance and by Newman-Keuls test for multiple comparisons.

RESULTS AND COMMENTS

Double blind trial

The results are shown in table 1-4. Both Acipimox and Tiadenol decreased to the same extent Tc, LDLc and apo B in type IIb, TG in type IV and TG in type IIb and IV considered together; in type IV Acipimox induced a not significant increase of LDLc level. HDLc and apo AI rose in patients treated with Acipimox, where only HDL2 subfraction contributed to HDLc increase. In the Tiadenol group, HDLc, its subfractions and apo AI did not change. The unlike mechanisms of action of the two drugs may explain the different effects observed. Acipimox, inhibiting lipolysis and FFA flux to the liver, reduces triglycerides and VLDL synthesis (2); it also improves VLDL removal probably trought increasing lipoprotein lipase activity in the adipose tissue, like nicotinic acid (11). This suggestion seems to be supported by the tendency of LDLc to increase, coupled with HDL2c enhancement, in type IV. Moreover, HDL2c increase may be due to the decrease of hepatic lipase activity found in type III and IV patients during Acipimox treatment (12); this enzyme, indeed, is well known to be involved in HDL2 catabolism (13). Finally, the increase of apo AI might depend on a decrease in the apoprotein catabolism as found during treatment with nicotinic acid (14). Tiadenol inhibits VLDL synthesis in the liver, reducing the VLDL-LDL pool in the plasma (15). No other mechanisms of action of this drug have been demonstrated and therefore its lack of effect on the HDL system was to be expected. With both Acipimox and Tiadenol, no significant changes in the routine laboratory tests (blood cells counts, haemoglobin, BUN, creatinine, bilirubin, SGOT, SGPT, alkaline phosphatase, blood sugar and uric acid) were observed. Three patients complained of gastrointestinal disturbances and flushing during Acipimox, but these side effects were moderate and interruption of the treatment was not necessary.

Open trial

Combined drug therapy gives the best result in familial hypercholesterolemia, and improves compliance allowing a reduction of the daily dose of the bile sequestrant resin, which is badly tolerated in most patients. Several reports have shown remarkable reductions of LDL cholesterol level using cholestyramine associated to Probucol; moreover, the recent finding that Probucol prevents oxidative modification of LDL particles (16) allows us to presume that this drug may prevent the progression of atherosclerosis. Nevertheless, the decrease of HDLc and apo AI, induced by Probucol, remains the "black hole" of this kind of treatment. In this connexion, the Cholestyramine-Acipimox combined therapy (table 5) seems to give a better result, leading to a consistent LDLc reduction, as Cholestyramine-Probucol does, and unchanging or increasing HDLc level.

REFERENCES

1. Stirling, C, Mc Aleer, M, Reckless, JPD, Campbell, RR, Mundy, D, Betteridge, DJ and Foster, K (1985). Effects of acipimox, a nicotinic acid derivative, on lipolysis in human adipose tissue and on

cholesterol synthesis in human jejunal mucosa. Clinical Science, 68, 83

2.   Fuccella, LM, Goldaniga, G, Lovisolo, PP, Maggi, E, Musatti, L, Mandelli, V and Sirtori, CR (1980). Inhibition of lipolysis in man by nicotinic acid and by acipimox, a new anti-lipolytic agent. Clin Pharmacol Ther, 28, 790

3.   Beaumont, JL, Carlson, LA, Cooper, GR, Fejfar, Z, Fredrickson, DS and Strasser, T (1970). Classification of hyperlipidemias and hyperlipoproteinemias. WHO Bull, 43, 891

4.   Siedel, J, Schlumberger, H, Klose, S, Ziegenhorn, J and Wahle-feld, AW (1981). Improved reagent for the enzymatic determination of serum cholesterol. J Clin Chem Clin Biochem, 19, 838

5.   Wahlefeld, AW (1974). Triglycerides determination after enzy-matic hydrolysis. In: Bergmeyer, HU (ed.) "Methods of Enzymatic Ana lysis". P.1831. (New York and London: Verlag Chemie Weinheim Aca-demic Press)

6.   Gidez, LI, Miller, GJ, Burstein, M, Slagle, S and Eder, HA (1982). Separation and quantitation of subclasses of human plasma high density lipoproteins by a simple precipitation procedure. J Lipid Res, 23, 1206

7.   Wilson, PWF, Zech, LA, Gregg. RE, Schaefer, EJ, Hoeg, JM, Sprecher. DL and Brewer, HB Jr. (1985). Estimation of VLDL choleste rol in hyperlipidemia. Clin Chim Acta, 151, 285

8.   Curry, MD, Alaupovic, P and Suenram, CA (1976). Determination of apolipoprotein A and its constitutive AI and AII polipeptides by separate electroimmunoassays. Clin Chem, 22, 315

9.   Curry, MD, Gustafson, A, Alaupovic, P and Mc Conathy, WJ (1978). Electroimmunoassay, radioimmunoassay and radial immunodiffusion assay evaluated for quantification of human apolipoprotein B. Clin Chem, 24, 280

10.   Winer, BJ (1971). Statistical principles in experimental design (New York: Mc Graw-Hill)

11.   Nikkila, EA and Pykalisto, O (1968). Induction of adipose tis-sue lipoprotein lipase by nicotinic acid. Biochim Biophys Acta, 152, 421

12.   Stuyt, PMJ, Stalenhoef, AFH, Demacker, PNM and Van't Laar, A (1985). A comparative study of the effects of Acipimox and Clofibra-te in type III and type IV hyperlipoproteinemia. Atherosclerosis, 55, 51

13.   Eisenberg, S (1984). High density lipoprotein metabolism. J Lipid Res, 25, 1017

14.   Packard, CJ, Stewart, JM, Third, JLHC, Morgan, HG, Lawrie, TDV and Shepherd, J (1980). Effects of nicotinic acid therapy on high-density lipoprotein metabolism in type II and in type IV hyperlipo-proteinaemia. Biochim Biophys Acta, 618, 53

15.   Franceschini, G, Poli, A, Catapano, AL, Gatti, E, Sirtori, M Gianfranceschi, G and Sirtori, CR (1981). Pharmacological studies on Tiadenol in type IV patients. Evidence for a mechanism of action different from other lipid-lowering drugs. Atherosclerosis, 40, 245
16.   Parthasarathy, S, Young, SG, Witzum, JL, Pittman, RC and Stein berg, D (1986). Probucol inhibits oxidative modification of low density lipoprotein. J Clin Invest, 77, 641

60
A controlled trial on the hypolipidemic effect of Acipimox in type IIA and IIB hyperlipoproteinemia

M.A. Averna, A. Stanzial, F. Bonafanti, G. Di Fede,
G. Montalto, M. Muggeo and A. Notarbartolo

INTRODUCTION

Nicotinic acid (NA) is one of the most potent lipid lowering agents, but the long-term use of this drug in patients at risk is problematical because of the seriousness of side effects[1,2,3].

Acipimox (A), a NA strongly-related compound, was found to be 20 times more active, with longer-lasting antilipolytic action and no rebound effect on plasma FFAs[4]; furthermore, A can be given in doses about five times lower than NA.

The aim of this study was to evaluate in a controlled trial the hypolipidemic action and side effects of A in a daily dose of 750 mg in type IIA and type IIB hyperlipoproteinemic (HLP) patients as compared to Fenofibrate (F), a well-tested lipid-lowering drug[5,6,7,8].

MATERIALS AND METHODS

Forty type II HLP patients, previously informed about the aim of the research, were randomized in two equal groups for study on either A or F treatment. The HLP patients underwent a one month wash-out period with placebo and isocaloric diet; four patients interrupted the trial during this period and were not replaced. In group A there were 10 IIA and 8 IIB patients - 9 males and 9 females - mean age 54 years, age range 33 to 72; mean body weight (b.w.) 68.3 ± 2.50, and in group F 11 IIA and 7 IIB patients - 7 males and 11 females - mean age 55 years, age range 19 to 73, mean b.w. 64.8 ± 2.92. Admission criteria were defined according to the following basal values: IIA total cholesterol (TC) > 250 mg/dl, total triglycerides (TG) < 200 mg/dl; IIB TC > 250 mg/dl; TG > 200 mg/dl; LDL-C $\geq$ 180 mg/dl. Patients with secondary hyper-lipoproteinemia, diabetes, hepatic or renal failure, malignancy, al-coholism, pregnancy, peptic ulcer, gut malabsorption, hypersen-sitivity to drugs and NA especially, or administered within the preceding 3 months with hypolipidemic drugs were excluded.

Patients on isocaloric diet were given A 750 mg t.i.d. after meals for 3 months; assessments of therapy were made at the start of the trial (t_{-1}), after one month on diet and placebo period (t_0), and after one, two, three months of drug treatment plus isocaloric diet (t_1, t_2, t_3). In each period the levels of TC, TG, HDL-C were measured; at t_{-1}, t_0, and t_3 periods, the levels of VLDL-C and LDL-C were measured too. Blood samples were taken after twelve hours fast in the morning; blood count, urea, creatinine, SGOT, alkaline phosphatase, uric acid, glycemia were also evaluated. Side effects of the drugs, heart rate, blood pressure, b.w. were re-corded every month. TG, TC, VLDL, LDL, HDL cholesterol were determined by the enzymatic methods (Boehringer) (9); lipoproteins were isolated by a preparative ultracentrifuge Beckman L_2-65.

Statistical evaluation of the differences at t_{-1}, t_0 and t_3 were carried out by Student's t test for paired data; the statistical com-parison between A and F treatments was performed by the covariance analysis.

RESULTS

Throughout the study no changes in b.w. were noted either during A or F treatment (Figure 1). The plasma lipid and lipoprotein con-centrations and (VLDL-C+LDL-C)/(HDL-C) ratio values found in HLP patients are given in Table 1 (A) and in Table 2 (F). After one month placebo period, lipid and lipoprotein values were similar to the start of trial values, but TG which decreased by 20% in the IIB A group and by 12% in the IIB F group; these differences were not statistically significant. TC decreased during A intake (Table 1) by about 12% in IIA and 17% in IIB patients (p < 0.01); in IIB the TG and VLDL-C fell respectively by about 34% and 28% (p < 0.01); LDL-C decreased by 17% in IIA (p < 0.01) and in IIB patients al-though in the latter the differences was statistically not significant; HDL-C increased, but not significantly, by 11% in IIA and 7% in

IIB. The (VLDL-C + LDL-C)/(HDL-C) ratio values were reduced significantly from 6.30 to 4.57 in IIA (p < 0.05), and from 9.11 to 6.31 in IIB, although this decrease was not significant because of the great variability of the data.

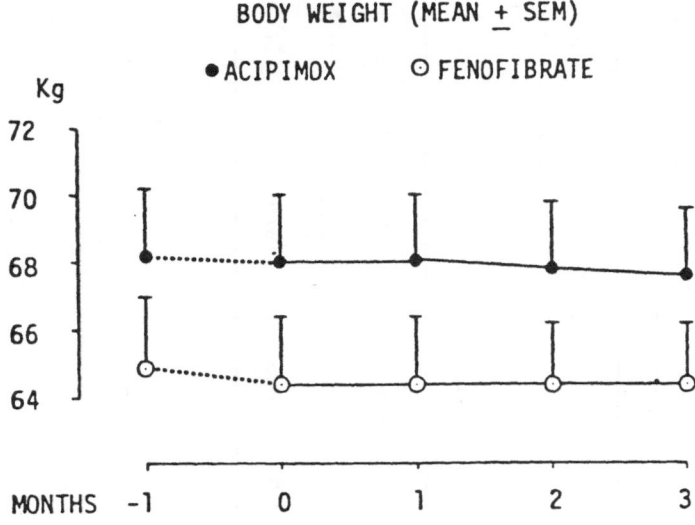

Figure 1 Body weight behaviour before and during A and F treatment.

During the F administration (Table 2) TC was reduced by 16% in IIA (p < 0.01) and 19% in IIB (p < 0.01) patients; in IIB also, the same 44% reduction was found in TG and VLDL-C (p < 0.01) values. LDL-C decreased significantly by 22% (p < 0.01) only in IIA; in IIB it decreased by 13% (N.S.), while HDL-C values were found unchanged after three months of drug administration in IIA, and increased by 10% (N.S.) in IIB.

Finally, (VLDL-C + LDL-C)/(HDL-C) ratios diminished from 6.12 to 4.80 in IIA and from 7.50 to 5.42 in IIB; these results were both highly significant (p < 0.01).

No side effects nor glycemia, uricemia and laboratory changes occurred during the three months of A or F treatment.

Table 1 Plasma lipids and lipoproteins variations in IIA (10) and IIB (8) patients one month before (-1), at the beginning (0) and three months (3) after ACIPIMOX administration. Values are given in mg/dl as mean ± standard error.

	TC		TG	VLDL-C	LDL-C		HDL-C		$\frac{\text{VLDL-C+LDL-C}}{\text{HDL-C}}$	
	IIA	IIB	IIB	IIB	IIA	IIB	IIA	IIB	IIA	IIB
-1	316 ± 15	332 ± 43	376 ± 89	69 ± 6	244 ± 19	236 ± 38	46.4 ± 4.3	35.6 ± 4.0	6.31 ± 0.71	9.34 ± 1.90
0	321* ± 16	329* ± 34	300* ± 31	68* ± 6	246* ± 15	222° ± 28	50.0° ± 5.4	35.1° ± 4.2	6.30** ± 0.75	9.11° ± 1.86
3	282* ± 15	273* ± 38	197* ± 31	49* ± 6	203* ± 12	183° ± 22	55.5° ± 5.7	37.6° ± 3.6	4.57** ± 0.19	6.31° ± 1.01

* p < 0.01; ** p < 0.05; ° N.S.

Table 2 Plasma lipids and lipoproteins variations in IIA (11) and IIB (7) patients one month before (-1), at the beginning (0) and three months (3) after FENOFIBRATE administration. Values are given in mg/dl as mean ± standard error.

	TC		TG	VLDL-C	LDL-C		HDL-C		VLDL-C+LDL-C / HDL-C	
	IIA	IIB	IIB	IIB	IIA	IIB	IIA	IIB	IIA	IIB
-1	312 ± 18	323 ± 13	315 ± 59	48 ± 6	242 ± 18	217 ± 21	46.1 ± 3.6	41.3 ± 7.0	6.07 ± 0.56	7.32 ± 1.21
0	308* ± 22	331* ± 25	275* ± 17	56* ± 5	238* ± 23	232° ± 32	45.5° ± 3.7	43.3° ± 6.6	6.12* ± 0.58	7.50* ± 1.53
3	257* ± 17	267* ± 29	143* ± 19	31* ± 4	185* ± 18	201° ± 30	46.4° ± 3.3	47.7° ± 6.9	4.80* ± 0.56	5.42* ± 1.03

* p < 0.01; ° N.S.

DISCUSSION

A has proved useful in a daily dose of 750 mg in IIA and in IIB HLP patients in lowering TC, TG and VLDL-C after three months of treatment; differences versus baseline values were significant (p < 0.01).

LDL-C decreased significantly in IIA (by 22%; 53 mg), not in IIB (by 13%; 31 mg). HDL-C increased in IIA by 11% (5.5 mg) after treatment, but the differences versus baseline values were not significant; in IIB patients HDL-C increase was very small (2.5 mg, + 7%).

These effects achieved with A almost correspond to the results obtained with Fenofibrate. F was given in a full dose of 300 mg/daily; as with A, the LDL-C decrease after three months of treatment was not significant; this finding could be due to IIB non-responders. A similar observation has been made for Clofibrate and analogous drugs[5,6,7,8].

The covariance analysis between the two different types of treatment did not show any significant difference. We have had four drop-outs during the wash-out period because of a bad compliance to the isocaloric diet and tablet intake; no side effects nor laboratory changes occurred during A or F treatment.

SUMMARY

Thirty six hyperlipoproteinemic patients randomized in equal group were administered Acipimox 750 mg t.i.d. (group A), 10 IIA, 8 IIB, or Fenofibrate 300 mg t.i.d. (group F), 11 IIA, 7 IIB. A one month isocaloric diet and placebo period preceded the three-month A or F period. TC decreased during A intake by 12% in IIA and 17% in IIB (p < 0.01); in IIB the TG and VLDL-C fell respectively by 34% and 28% (p < 0.01); LDL-C decreased by 17% in IIA (p < 0.01) and in IIB patients, although in the latter the difference was statistically not significant; HDL-C increased, but not significantly, by 11% in IIA and 7% in IIB. These effects achieved with A almost correspond to the results obtained with F.

The covariance analysis between the two different types of treatment did not show any significant difference. No side effects nor laboratory changes occurred during A or F treatment.

REFERENCES

1. Klose G., Mordasini R., Middelhoff G., Augustin J. and Gruten H. (1978). Medikamentose Behandlung Primarer Hyper-

lipoproteinamien. Klin. Wschr., 56, 99.

2. Berge K.G., Achor R.W.P., Christensen N.A, Mason H.L. and Barker N.W. (1961). Hypercholesterolemia and Nicotinic Acid. A long-term study. Am. J. Med., 31, 24.

3. Carlson L.A., Oro L. and Ostman J. (1968). Effect of Nicotinic Acid on Plasma Lipids in Patients with Hyper-lipoproteinemia During the First Week of Treatment. J. Atheroscler. Res., 8, 667.

4. Fuccella L.M., Goldaniga G., Lovisolo P.P., Maggi E., Musatti L., Mandelli V. and Sirtori C.R. (1980). Inhibition of Lipolysis by Nicotinic Acid and by Acipimox. Clin. Pharmacol. Ther., 28, 790.

5. Micheli H., Pometta D. and Gustafson A. (1979). Treatment of Hyperlipoproteinemia (HLP) Type IIA with a New Phenoxy-isobutiric Acid Derivative. Procetofen. Intern. J. Clin. Pharmacol. and Bioph., 17, 503.

6. Rossner S. and Oro L. (1981). Fenofibrate Therapy of Hyper-lipoproteinemia. A dose-response study and a comparison with clofibrate. Atherosclerosis, 38, 273.

7. Avogaro P., Bittolo Bon G., Belussi F., Pontoglio E. and Cazzolato G. (1983). Variations in Lipids and Proteins of Lipoproteins by Fenofibrate in Some Hyperliproteinemic States. Atherosclerosis, 47, 95.

8. Capurso A., Mogavero A.M., Taverniti R., Resta F., Pace L. and Bonomo L. (1984). Effect of Procetofen on Serum Lipids and Apoproteins. Intern. J. Clin. Pharmacol. and Toxicol., 22, 194.

61
Effect of Acipimox on serum lipids and apoproteins in type II hyperlipoproteinemia

A. Capurso, F. Resta, D. Ciancia, A.M. Mogavero,
M. Lavezzari, R. Taverniti, M. Di Tommaso, G. Siciliani
and S. Palmisano

INTRODUCTION

Acipimox is a nicotinic acid derivative which has a potent triglyceride (TG) lowering effect induced by sustained inhibition of adipose tissue lipolysis (Fuccella et al., 1980; Sirtori et al. 1981;
Stirling et al., 1985). The reduced free fatty acid flux to the liv̲
er, and the consequent reduction of the precursor pool of very low̲
density lipoprotein (VLDL)-triglycerides causes a diminution of
VLDL synthesis and a consequent lowering of plasma triglycerides.
Pantethine, defined as a natural hypolipidemic compound, is a vita-
min derivative and precursor of Co-A which has been show to modulate serum lipids, mostly triglycerides, in type IV hyperlipoproteinemia (Avogaro et al., 1983; Da Col et al., 1984; Gaddi et al.,
1984; Maggi et al., 1982).
The present study was undertaken to evaluate the effect of acipimox
and pantethine on lipids, lipoproteins and apoproteins, in patients
with type II-A and II-B hyperlipoproteinemias.

MATERIALS AND METHODS

Patients : Twenty outpatients (10 males and 10 females) attending
the Lipid Research Clinic of the University of Bari, all with primary type II-A and II-B hyperlipoproteinemia according to W.H.O.
criteria (Beaumont et al., 1970), partecipated in this study. The
mean age was 52 years (range 31-67) and the mean weight was 55 kg
(range 44-94).
All patients had been on a prudent isocaloric diet (35% fat, P/S
ratio 1.0; cholesterol intake less than 300 mg/day) for their lipid
disorder for not less than two months. Some of these patients had
previously received other drug therapies which, however, were discontinued at least two months before the start of the present trial.
All patients had stable weight and the prudent diet was followed
throughout the study.

Study design : The study was a controlled crossover open trial of
acipimox vs pantethine. After a two-month period of drug withdrawal
and dietary stabilization, the patients were given, in randomized
sequence, acipimox (250 mg tid) or pantethine (300 mg tid) for two
months, followed by a one-month wash-out interval then the drug

crossover for a further two months.

All patients were carefully monitored for subjective and objective side effects. Two patients out of 20 dropped out because of skin flushing. ECG, blood pressure, and palpatory assessment of liver size were recorded at intervals during the pre-trial treatment and throughout treatment. Lipids, apoproteins and standard laboratory tests (urinalysis, SGOT, SGPT, glucose, uric acid, bilirubin, alkaline phosphatase, prothrombin time and complete blood count) were made monthly intervals.

Methods : Blood samples were drawn after a 14-h overnight fast and divided into two aliquots, one collected in tubes containing EDTA (1 mg/ml) in order to separate plasma for preparative ultracentrifugation, the other collected without anticoagulants, to obtain serum for lipid and apoprotein assays.

Cholesterol and triglycerides were assayed by enzymatic methods (Boehringer, Mannheim, F.R.G.) in whole serum and in lipoprotein fractions isolated by sequential ultracentrifugation (Havel et al., 1955). HDL-cholesterol and HDL apo A-I were determined in whole serum precipitation of apo B-containing lipoproteins by the phosphotungstate-MgCl method (Burnstein et al., 1970).

Apoproteins (apo) were evaluated by radial immunodiffusion. Apo B was measured in Partigen B-lipoprotein plates (Behring, Marburg-Lahn, F.R.G.) using as reference standard a pool of 100 sera of normolipidemic individuals prepared by ourselves and calibrated with three different reference standards: a) a reference standard serum kindly provided by Dr. D. Grafnetter (WHO Collaborating Lipid Reference Centre, Prague, Czechoslovakia); b) a reference standard serum kindly provided by Dr. P. Alapovic (Oklahoma Medical Research Foundation, Oklahoma City, USA); c) isolated LDL (fraction d 1.030-1.063 g/ml NaCl-KBr) (apo B = total LDL proteins minus tetramethyl urea-soluble proteins of the same LDL sample). Apo A-I and apo C-III were assayed with antisera produced in our laboratory as described elsewhere (Capurso et al., 1984). Apo A-I was determined on native serum and on phosphotungstate-precipitated serum. Apo C-III was evaluated on native serum and on tetramethyl-extracted serum (v/v). The reference standards for apo A-I and apo C-III were those described elsewhere (Capurso et al., 1984).

Statistical methods : Student's t-test for paired data was used for this within-treatment preliminary analysis.

RESULTS

Reported here are the data regarding solely the determinations of lipid and apoprotein levels in whole serum.

Sequence Acipimox (A) ⟶ Pantethine (P) (Table 1 and Figure 1).

Given as a first drug acipimox lowered serum cholesterol by 11% (P < 0.001), serum triglycerides by 8.3% (P < 0.02), serum apo B by 6.6% (P < 0.01) and serum apo C-III by 7.3% (P < 0.02); serum apo A-I increased 1.8% (P < 0.05). The subsequent treatment with pantethine, after a one-month wash-out period, produced no significant changes in serum lipids and apoproteins.

Table 1. Lipid and apoprotein levels in whole serum
in 18 type II hyperlipoproteinemia patients

Sequence ACIPIMOX (A) ──────► PANTETHINE (P); (mg/dl, mean ± S.D.)

Serum	End w.o.	End (A)	p	End w.o.	End (P)	p
CH	346+47	305+45	<0.001	330+43	336+62	n.s.
TG	200+72	183+102	<0.02	204+100	200+92	n.s.
apo A-I	123+20	125+20	<0.05	125+17	123+18	n.s.
apo B	149+26	125+20	<0.01	146+22	152+27	n.s.
apo C-III	13.2+2.1	12.2+2.2	<0.02	12.9+2.3	13.2+2.3	n.s.

w.o. = wash-out; CH = cholesterol; TG = triglycerides;
apo = apoprotein

Sequence Pantethine ──────►Acipimox (Table 2, Figure 1)

Pantethine significantly reduced only serum triglycerides (-8.8%;
P <0.02); the other parameters were not affected. Acipimox given
after the wash-out period significantly reduced cholesterol (-5.2%;
P <0.01) and triglycerides (-18%; P <0.001). Apo B and Apo C-III
were not significantly changed. Apo A-I increased significantly,
by 6.8% (P <0.01).

Table 2. Lipid and apoprotein levels in whole serum
in 18 type II hyperlipoproteinemia patients

Sequence PANTETHINE (P) ──────► ACIPIMOX (A); (mg/dl, mean ± S.D.)

Serum	End w.o.	End (P)	p	End w.o.	End (A)	p
CH	342+53	334+74	n.s.	343+78	325+55	<0.01
TG	174+98	159+84	<0.02	175+85	143+66	<0.001
apo A-I	112+12	113+11	n.s.	114+10	122+11	<0.01
apo B	151+12	150+27	n.s.	152+28	148+23	n.s.
apo C-III	13.0+1.9	13.3+2.3	n.s.	13.5+2.0	12.7+1.9	n.s.

w.o. = wash-out; CH = cholesterol; TG = triglycerides;
apo = apoprotein

No changes were observed in routine laboratory tests. Except for
skin flushing in two patients during the first days of treatment
with acipimox, no side effects were reported.

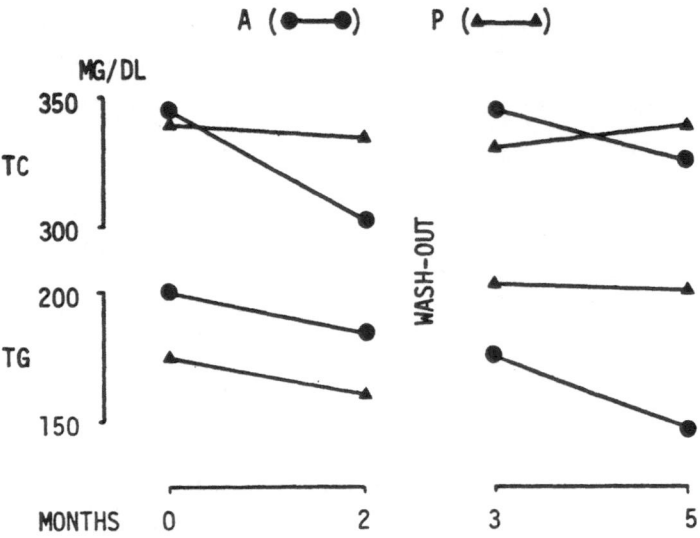

FIGURE 1   Serum cholesterol and triglycerides according to the sequence of treatment.

DISCUSSION

In this crossover trial in type II hyperlipoproteinemia patients, acipimox was more effective than pantethine in modifying serum lipids and apoproteins.
Acipimox induced a significant reduction of serum cholesterol and triglycerides and a significant rise in serum apo A-I. Serum apo B and apo C-III were significantly reduced only when acipimox was given as first treatment.
Pantethine significantly reduced only serum triglycerides.
Both drugs were well tolerated.

REFERENCES

Avogaro, P., Bittolo Bon, G., Fusello, M. (1983). Effect of pantethine on lipids, lipoproteins and apolipoproteins in man. Curr. Ther. Res. 33, 488.

Beaumont, J.L., Carlson, L.A., Cooper, J.R., et al. (1970). Classification of hyperlipidemias and hyperlipoproteinemias. Wld Hlth Org. Bull. 43, 891.

Burnstein, M., Scholnick, H.R., Morfin, R. (1970). Rapid method for the isolation of lipoproteins from human serum by precipitation with polyanions. J. Lipid Res. 11, 585.

Capurso, A., Mogavero, A.M., Taverniti, R. et al. (1984). Effect of procetofene on serum lipids and apoproteins. Int. J. Clin. Pharmacol. Ther. Toxicol. 22, 194.

Da Col, P.G., Cattin, L., Fonda, M. et al. (1984). Pantethine in the treatment of hypercholesterolemia: a randomized double-blind trial versus tiadenol. Curr. Ther. Res. 36, 314.

Fuccella, L.M., Goldaniga, G., Lovisolo, P.P. et al. (1980). Inhibition of lipolysis by nicotinic acid and by acipimox. Clin. Pharmacol. Ther. 28, 790.

Gaddi, A., Descovich, G.C., Noseda, G. et al. (1984). Controlled evaluation of pantethine, a natural hypolipidemic compound, in patients with different forms of hyperlipoproteinemia. Atherosclerosis 50, 73.

Havel, T.J., Eder, H.A., Bragdon, J.H. (1955). The distribution and chemical composition of ultracentrifugally separated lipoproteins in human serum. J. Clin. Invest. 34, 1345.

Maggi, G.C., Donati, C., Criscuoli, G. (1982). Pantethine: a physiological lipomodulating agent, in the treatment of hyperlipidemias. Curr. Ther. Res. 32, 380.

Sirtori, C.R., Gianfranceschi, G., Sirtori, M. et al. (1981). Reduced triglyceridemia and increased high density lipoprotein cholesterol levels after treatment with acipimox, a new inhibitor of lipolysis. Atherosclerosis 38, 267.

Stirling, C., McAleer, M., Reckless, J.P.D. et al. (1985). Effects of acipimox, a nicotinic acid derivative, on lipolysis in human adipose tissue and on cholesterol synthesis in human jejunal mucosa. Chem. Sci. 68, 83.

62
Long-term multicentre trial with acipimox in diabetic patients with hyperlipoproteinemia
M. Muggeo, M. Lavezzari, C. Montoro and G. Sacchetti

Acipimox is a new lipid-lowering agent with long-lasting antili-polytic activity chemically related to nicotinic acid (1,2).
The aim of the present trial was to study the effect of acipimox on plasma lipid levels and its tolerability during long-term treatment in diabetic patients with hyperlipoproteinemia. The trial included investigation of any influence of the drug on glucose tolerance.

MATERIALS AND METHODS

Twenty-nine Italian centres participated in this study. A group of 344 non-insulin dependent (NID) diabetic patients, in stable metabolic control, with type II and IV hyperlipoproteinemia were admitted to the trial. All patients had to present basal triglycerides levels $\geqslant 200$ mg/dl and/or cholesterol $\geqslant 250$ mg/dl.
After a 1-month run-in washout period on an isocaloric diet which was maintained throughout the study, the patients were given 250 mg acipimox 2-3 times daily for 6-12 months. At the end of the washout period (basal) and after 1, 2, 4, 6, 8, 10 and 12 months of treatment, total serum cholesterol (TC), serum triglycerides (TG), HDL-cholesterol, fasting blood glucose (FBG), glycosylated hemoblobin (HbA1), blood pressure (systolic and diastolic) and body weight were determined according to standard procedures. At the beginning and at 4-month intervals the following examinations were made: red blood count (RBC), white blood count (WBC), hemoglobin (Hb), serum creatinine, blood urea nitrogen, uric acid, transaminases (SGOT and SGPT) and alkaline phosphatase. Patient's compliance was assessed by periodic determinations of acipimox in urine.

RESULTS

Fifty-six patients withdrew from the trial before the end of treatment for adverse events or other reasons.
The remaining 288 patients were treated for at least 6 months. The results reported here are from analyses on 206 patients (101 F, 105 M) treated for 12 months. Fifty-eight percent of 206 patients had type IV hyperlipoproteinemia; 70% of cases were overweight or obese; 85% of cases were over 44 years.

In 90% of patients acipimox was used at the daily dosage of 500 mg
(250 mg b.i.d.). Concomitant antidiabetic treatments were diet
(28%) or diet and hypoglycemic drugs (sulfonylureas, biguanides or
both); with a few exceptions the antidiabetic treatment, was not
modified during the study.
Analysis of variance and Dunnett's test for multiple comparisons
were used as statistical procedures.

Table 1. Triglycerides (TG), Total Cholesterol (TC), HDL-Cholesterol (HDL-C), and body weight (mean, SEM) in 206 patients
given acipimox 250 mg b.i.d. for 12 months

Months	TG	TC	HDL-C	Body Weight
0	370.3, 15.9	283.9, 5.0	37.2, 0.8	76.1, 0.9
1	279.0, 12.5**	265.0, 4.9**	39.9, 0.9*	75.7, 0.8
2	254.7, 9.0**	254.4, 4.3**	41.8, 0.9**	75.4, 0.8
4	241.8, 9.8**	247.7, 3.8**	41.9, 0.9**	75.0, 0.8
6	224.2, 10.3**	239.8, 3.5**	43.5, 1.0**	75.0, 0.8
8	227.6, 8.9**	238.8, 3.7**	42.9, 0.9**	75.4, 0.8
10	217.8, 8.5**	238.6, 3.9**	43.0, 0.8**	75.3, 0.8
12	218.2, 10.9**	232.5, 3.6**	44.7, 0.9**	75.5, 0.8

Comparisons with baseline values: * $P < 0.05$; ** $P < 0.01$

Cholesterol and Triglycerides. An appreciable decrease of TG (24%)
and TC (7%) and an increase of HDL-C (11%) were already observed after 1 month of treatment (Table 1, Figure 1). At 6 and 12 months
the reductions were 40% and 15% for TG and TC respectively while
HDL-C increased by 20%. The differences in comparison to baseline
values were statistically significant at each control.

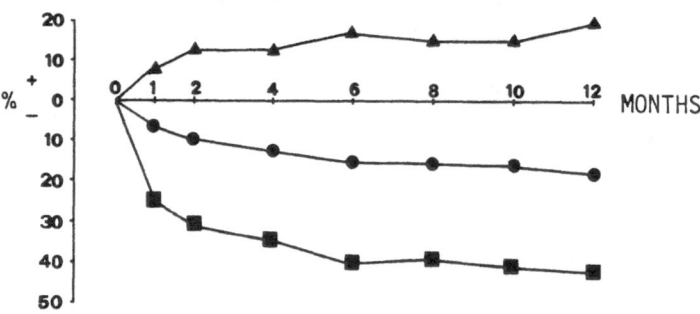

FIGURE 1   Mean percent changes in Total Cholesterol●
            Triglycerides■   and HDL-Cholesterol▲   in 206 cases
            given acipimox 250 mg b.i.d. for 12 months

FBG, HbA1. A slight, significant drop in FBG was observed at each control. HbA1 showed a progressive reduction, significant already from the 1st month (Figure 2)

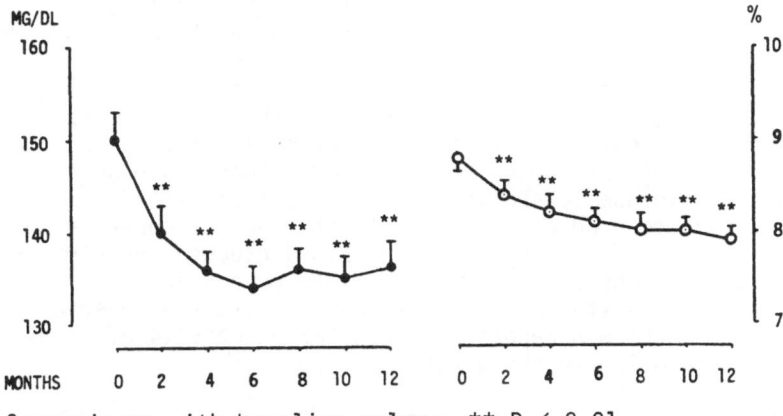

Comparisons with baseline values: ** P < 0.01

FIGURE 2.   Mean (SEM) of fasting blood glucose ● and glycosylated hemoglobin ○   in 206 cases given acipimox 250 mg b.i.d. for 12 months.

Hematology and biochemistry tests.   Sporadic and clinically insignificant changes of RBC, SGOT, Alkaline Phosphatase and BUN were observed. WBC, SGPT, uric and serum creatinine did not show any significant change. Hemoglobin levels presented statistically but not clinically significant increases.

Adverse reactions.   Transient episodes of flushing were observed during the first days of treatment in about 10% of cases. Drug administration was discontinued in 26 patients (Table 2), mainly because of mild G.I. disturbances (pyrosis, gastralgia) and skin reactions.

Table 2.   Discontinuation of treatment due to adverse events

Adverse events	No. Patients
Dyspepsia	8
Erythematous rash	5
Urticaria	3
Flushing	2
Itching	2
Vomiting	2
Headache	1
Dizziness	1
Gastritis	1
Abdominal pain	1
T o t a l	26 (7.5%)

DISCUSSION

The results of this study show that acipimox at the dosage of 250 mg b.i.d. significantly reduces cholesterol and triglycerides in NID diabetic patients with type II and IV hyperlipoproteinemia. The lipid lowering effect, maintained throughout the study, was combined with a significant increase of HDL-C.

Drug tolerance was satisfactory and adverse events, mainly mild G.I. disturbances and flushing, caused withdrawal of treatment in only 7% of patients. Monitoring of routine laboratory test confirmed the drugs biological safety. Compliance was good.

As regards glucose metabolism acipimox, unlike nicotinic acid (3,4), did not seem to produce negative effects. On the contrary a slight but significant decrease of fasting blood glucose and glycosylated hemoglobin was observed. This result, to be confirmed in double-blind controlled studies, is in agreement with the observations of Regat et al. (5) who reported a favourable activity of acipimox on glucose metabolism in obese patients.

Acipimox Cooperative Italian Group

Angileri G., Marsala; Antonini F.M., Firenze; Bartolomei G.,Pistoia; Benedetti G., Modena; Bentley R., Legnago; Cucurachi L., Lecce; D'Agostino A.W., Napoli; D'Onofrio F., Napoli; Erle G., Vicenza; Fumelli P., Ancona; Gentili G., Nemi; La Spada S., Palermo; Lomeo G., Palermo; Marinazzo A., Brindisi; Menci U.S., Grosseto; Morsiani M., Ferrara; Muggeo M., Verona; Mughini L., Catania; Mura C., Nuoro; Noacco C., Udine; Notarbartolo A., Palermo; Parodi F.A., Genova; Pedrazzi F., Verona; Saba P., Pescia; Savagnone E., Palermo; Squadrito G., Messina; Vannini P., Bologna; Vigna L., Castrovillari; Virgili F., Mestre.

References

1. Fuccella, L et al (1980). Inhibition of lipolysis by nicotinic acid and by acipimox. Clin.Pharmacol.Ther., 28, 790.

2. Stirling, C et al (1985). Effects of acipimox, a nicotinic acid derivative, on lipolysis in human adipose tissue and cholesterol synthesis in human jejunal mucosa. Clin.Sci., 68, 83.

3. Parsons, W B et al (1961). Studies of nicotinic acid use in hypercholesterolemia: changes in hepatic function, carbohydrate tolerance and uric acid metabolism. Arch.Int.Med., 107, 653.

4. Pollack, H (1962). Nicotinic acid and diabetics. Diabetes, 11, 144.

5. Regal, H et al (1984). Effect of a single oral dose of acipimox on glucose metabolism after intravenous glucose load in obese patients. Drugs Exptl.Clin.Res., 10, 621.

ACETYLCARNITINE AND AGEING BRAIN SYNDROMES

63
Experimental pharmacological aspects in brain aging

M.T. Ramacci, F.R. Patacchioli, O. Ghirardi,
L. Ferraris and L. Angelucci

INTRODUCTION

Aging of the whole organism can be viewed, at least partially, as the consequence of brain aging due to the loss of integration of the central aminergic, peptidergic and neuroendocrine systems and subsystems regulating peripheral functions of the body. Moreover, aging in social and medical terms must be pondered mostly in its behavioural aspects.

In consideration of this primary role of brain aging and of possible pharmacological interventions, a new branch of pharmacology, i.e. "biopharmacology" is expected to act as a preventive pharmacology in contrast to or at the side of traditional pharmacology.

"Biopharmacology" is envisaged to deal with those endogenous substances endowed with a fundamental role in the major biological processes, aimed at maintaining the homeostasis of complex systems, whose presence or action are gradually reduced or become completely absent with aging.

The activity of said substances is to be investigated on a well-integrated model or better still on " a living organism which can be studied as for a biological or behavioural aspect, typical of senescence; or investigated as for an age-dependent either spontaneous or induced pathological process; and where the phenomenon observed can be similar in one or more aspects to a phenomenon of senescence in the humans" (12). Acetyl-1-carnitine is one of such substances: it has a role in energy metabolism (7), in the turnover of the phospholipid component of the neuronal membrane (9) and in the cholinergic system (4, 6, 7, 11). Moreover, in long-term treatment studies, acetyl-1-carnitine improved bodily and behavioural general conditions of old rats (8).

Therefore, we propose the use of the aging rat as a valid experimental model and acetyl-1-carnitine as a prototypic biodrug.

Table 1. The effect of Acetyl-L-Carnitine on morphological, histochemical, histoenzymatic and neurochemical changes in some hippocampal and cerebral cortex areas, typical of senescence in the rat.

Age of rats (months)	3	22 control	22 treated
HIPPOCAMPUS			
°Nissl Pyramidal cells	71.95 ± 0.81^{d}	49.00 ± 0.72	54.39 ± 1.03^{d}
Granule cells	84.99 ± 0.92^{d}	51.49 ± 0.78	54.60 ± 0.80^{b}
§Lipofuscin	0	68.09 ± 2.64	53.54 ± 1.42^{d}
No. of CA1 neurons	327 ± 5^{d}	175 ± 6	257 ± 5^{d}
SDH Pyramidal cells	83.10 ± 0.59^{d}	63.90 ± 1.75	72.39 ± 1.47^{c}
Granule cells	86.56 ± 0.62^{d}	48.20 ± 2.94	60.13 ± 2.48^{c}
LDH Pyramidal cells	71.64 ± 0.81^{d}	65.28 ± 2.94	64.99 ± 1.04
Granule cells	65.58 ± 1.35^{d}	52.97 ± 0.92	55.77 ± 0.69^{a}
NADHD Pyramidal cells	94.87 ± 1.71^{d}	49.24 ± 1.60	74.32 ± 1.25^{d}
Granule cells	87.67 ± 1.64^{d}	40.02 ± 2.47	72.26 ± 1.94^{d}
GPDH Pyramidal cells	56.44 ± 1.12^{d}	4.02 ± 1.02	24.84 ± 1.59^{d}
Granule cells	47.98 ± 0.86^{d}	3.66 ± 0.90	27.60 ± 1.22^{d}
*DA	0.28 ± 0.06	0.19 ± 0.02	0.24 ± 0.03
*HVA	0.18 ± 0.04^{a}	0.09 ± 0.02	0.13 ± 0.06
*DOPAC	0.22 ± 0.05	0.14 ± 0.02	0.18 ± 0.03
CEREBRAL CORTEX			
°Nissl Pyramidal cells	75.70 ± 1.69^{d}	44.94 ± 1.06	53.33 ± 1.34^{d}
Granule cells	56.47 ± 1.38^{d}	34.65 ± 1.52	47.87 ± 1.30^{d}
§Lipofuscin	0	51.61 ± 2.41	41.34 ± 1.72^{c}
SDH Cells of 2nd layer	63.78 ± 1.11^{d}	52.54 ± 0.74	$56.44 - 0.78^{c}$
LDH Cells of 2nd layer	65.29 ± 0.80	58.90 ± 2.93	60.03 ± 1.08
NADHD Cells of 2nd layer	84.66 ± 1.19^{d}	46.07 ± 1.44	57.94 ± 0.85^{d}
GPDH Cells of 2nd layer	47.64 ± 2.09^{d}	24.81 ± 1.03	29.96 ± 1.01^{c}

$a = P \leqslant 0.05$; $b = P \leqslant 0.02$; $c = P \leqslant 0.01$; $d = P \leqslant 0.001$ compared with old controls.
° = arbitrary units of staining intensity
§ = arbitrary units of fluorescence
* = nmoles/g wet weight

MATERIALS AND METHODS

Young (3 months) and old (18-28 months), untreated and treated with acetyl-l-carnitine (75 mg/kg in drinking water for 3-6 months) were used to study the interactions between age and experimental treatment on some parameters currently assumed as indicative of brain aging. Namely, we adopted the following:
- morphological: lipofuscin and tigroid substance content, neuronal loss;
- biochemical: enzymes linked to oxido-reductase and energetic processes (SDH, LDH, NADHD, GPDH, in both pyramidal and granule cells, with histoenzymatic assays);
- neurochemical: neuroendocrinal activity at level of hypothalamo-pituitary adrenal axis (HPAA) (plasma corticosterone, 3H-corticosterone binding), dopamine (DA), homovanilic acid (HVA), 3,4-dihydroxyphenilacetic acid (DOPAC) contents;
- behavioural: learning and discriminative behaviour:
1) active avoidance in a shuttle box; 20 trials/10 min/day for 9 days: no. of avoidances;
2) T Maze in absence of external cues (opaque water in the vessel): occurrence of 5 correct choices over 6 for 2 consecutive sessions, in a total of 5 sessions;
3) spatial orientation in a circular vessel (filled with opaque water): 4 trials per daily session, 120 sec end point, 30 sec intertrial time, 9 consecutive sessions. Time spent in the vessel in the last session;
4) complex learning behaviour: discriminative behaviour in a skinner box, alternate 30 two-min light on, SD water rewarded, and light off, SΔ unrewarded. No. of lever pressings.

All morphological, biochemical and neurochemical measurements were observed in important functional areas (hippocampus, cerebral cortex) with respect to pyramidal and extrapyramidal activities.

RESULTS

Table 1 shows the effect of long-term treatment with acetyl-l-carnitine on some parameters of neuronal senescence in the hippocampus and cerebral cortex.

A clear-cut improvement was evident in the Nissl-reactive tigroid substance, in the cytoplasmic lipofuscin deposition, in the activity of enzymes of energy metabolism, indicating the presence of a more intense metabolic activity of ribonucleoprotein and phospholipids as well as an increased energy production.

477

Table 2. The effect of aging and Acetyl-L-Carnitine treatment on some behavioural parameters in the rat.

	3 months	23 months control	23 months treated
(+) Active Avoidance	$32.5+4.2^{d}$(12)	2.2 ± 0.6(12)	13.4 ± 3.9^{c}(12)
(°) T Water Maze	1.9 ± 0.1(15)	3.4 ± 0.4(14)	2.3 ± 0.3^{a}(11)
(') Spatial Orientation	$33.\pm9.1^{a}$(12)	54.2 ± 9.6(12)	23.8 ± 4.5^{a}(6)
(§) Discriminative Behaviour	SD 509 ± 42(10)^{c*} SΔ 190 ± 14	302 ± 39(18) 205 ± 37	416 ± 50(11) $202\pm15^{a*}$

(+) total avoidances over 9 sessions, 20 trials per session

(°) no. of sessions required to score at least 5 correct choices out of 6

(') time in sec spent in the vessel at the last session

(§) no. of lever pressings: SD=rewarded; SΔ=unrewarded periods

In parentheses, no. of animals. Student's "t" test: a=P≤0.5; c=P≤0.1; d=P≤0.01 versus controls; * paired "t" test: SΔ versus SD.

The above effects are strictly correlated with a retarded loss of neurons in the CA1 areas, with a minor decrease in dopaminergic activity in the hippocampus.

Table 2 shows that acetyl-l-carnitine treatment improved learning (increased performances in the shuttle box) of active avoidance and the ability to solve maze problems in the absence of external cues (faster performances). Spatial orientation capacity was preserved also (less time spent in the maze), and the discriminative behaviour in a relative complex task pointed out by a higher reward and a lesser rewarded activity in comparison with their aged-matched controls.

Direct evidence of disinhibition of the HPAA in the aged rat was the reduced suppression of the response to a psychic stress by feed-back from a previous cold stress, in comparison with young rats; the decrease in binding capacity for 3H-corticosterone in basal conditions; and the absence of a reduction in binding capacity following stress. Thus, because of the loss of functional plasticity of the hippocampal glucocorticoid receptor, the activity of the HPAA is amplified and becomes a marker of the aging process in the brain (3).

In aged rats, the activity of HPAA was beneficially affected by the treatment with acetyl-l-carnitine: basal and psychic stress levels of plasma corticosterone were close to those exhibited by adult rats; most important, feedback regulation of the axis was partially preserved. It is to be noted that lesser degree of disinhibition of the axis in the treated rats was accompanied with a glucocorticoid binding capacity in the hippocampus of the same degree as that in the adult rats (3).

The behavioural deficit observed in the old rat, especially in simple (maze) and complex (light discrimination for reinforcement) learning and in spatial orientation, could be connected to the changes in number of hippocampal pyramidal neurones and in their endocrine competence. In the old rat, behavioural functions of the hippocampus and the inhibitory control by this structure on HPAA are strongly deteriorated. The adrenocortical activity progressively increases with aging in the rat, both with regard to basal level (1), stress level and duration of nicthemeral increase (5). Concomitantly, binding capacity for 3H-corticosterone in the hippocampus is reduced, due to absolute loss of glucocorticoid receptors (1). By the way of these receptors, the hippocampus controls the activation of HPAA; during stress, their glucocorticoid binding capacity is transitoroly down-regulated, with a consequent attenuation of the endocrine response (2, 10).

The difference observed with old rats, treated and untreated with acetyl-l-carnitine, leads to justify the better quality of life shown by the animals, not so much because of the improvement of one parameter or the other, but mainly because of a slow-down of the normal degrading process linked to aging.

By that, we do not mean to indicate a connection between experimental aspects in the rat and the results obtainable in man; however, it is important to notice the consistency of the respective results. All parameters are likely to have common mechanisms ascribable to alterating processes of the membrane, chemical physical structures, fluidity, and consequently to factors of cellular regulations (neuro-hormones, steroid-hormones, metabolic co-factors).

It is possible to identify the experimental model of the aged rat as a valid means to single out the modifications of parameters in the aging processes and to assess the efficacity of experimental treatments with compounds to be used as a preventive therapy.

REFERENCES

1. Angelucci, L, Valeri, P, Grossi, E, Veldhuis, HD, Bolus, B and De Kloet, R (1980). Involvement of hippocampal corticosterone receptors in behavioral phenomena. In: Brambilla, F, Racagni, G and De Wield, G (eds.) "Progress in psychoneuroendocrinology". p. 177-185. (Amsterdam: Elsevier/North Holland)

2. Angelucci, L and Patacchioli, FR (1984). Brain glucocorticoid receptor, serotonin and pituitary-adrenocortical activity in stress. In: Usdin, E and Kvetnansky, R (eds.) "Catecholamines and other neurotransmitters and stress". p.731-740. (Amsterdam: Elsevier/North Holland)

3. Angelucci, L, Patacchiolo, FR, Taglialatela, G, Maccari, S, Ramacci, MT, and Ghirardi, O (1986). Brain glucorticoid receptor and adrenocortical activity are sensitive markers of senescence-retarding treatment in the rat. In: Biggio, G, Spano, PF, Toffano, G and Gessa, GL (eds.) "Modulation of Central and Peripheral Transmitter Function". p. 337-343. (Padova: Liviana Press)

4. Blum, K, Seifter, E and Seifter, J (1971). The pharmacology of d- and l-carnitine and d- and l-acetylcarnitine comparison with choline and acetylcholine. J Pharmacol Exp Ther, 178, 331

5. DeKosky, ST, Scheff, SW and Cotman, CW (1984). Elevated corticosterone levels. Neuroendocrinology, 38, 33-38

6. Falchetto, S, Kato, G and Provini, L (1971). The action of carnitines on cortical neurons. Can J Physiol Pharmacol, 49, 1

7. Fritz, IB (1963). Carnitine and its role in fatty acid metabolism. Adv Lip Res, 1, 285

8.   Ghirardi, O, Milano, S, Peschechera, A, Ramacci, MT and Angelucci, L (1985). Learning and brain monoamines in aging rats: effect of chronic treatment with acetyl-l-carnitine. Br J Pharmacol, 86, 683P. Proceedings Suppl.

9.   Morris, AJ and Carey, EM (1983). Postnatal changes in the concentration of carnitine and acetylcarnitine in rat brain. Dev Brain Res, 8, 381-384

10. Patacchioli, FR, Capasso M, Chiappini, P, Chierichetti, C, Scaccianoce, S, Tozzi, W and Angelucci, L (1983). Variations of hippocampal cytosol glucocorticoid binding capacity as an after effect of physiological increases in brain and blood corticosterone concentrations. In: Endröczi, E, De Wied, D, Angelucci, L and Scapagnini, U (eds.) "Integrative neurohumoral mechanisms". p.165-172. (Amsterdam, Elsevier Biomedical)

11. Tempesta, E, Janiri, L, Pirrongelli, C and Ancona, L (1982). The effect of microiontophoretically applied d, l-, l- and d-acetylcarnitine on single central neurons. Neuropharmacology, 21, 1207-1210

12. Animal Models for Research on Aging (1981) Expert Committee of the National Academy of Science, USA.

64
Acute effects of L-acetylcarnetine (LAC) on quantitative EEG (QEEG) and visual evoked potentials (VEPS) in patients affected by senile, presenile and alcoholic dementia. Comparison with L-carnetine

D. Gambi, M. Onofrj, M. Basciani, C. Censoni and
A. Faricelli

INTRODUCTION

On the basis of experimental and clinical studies, e-
lectrical activities of the brain have displayed close
coupling with nervous cell methabolism and cerebral blood
flow.

These relationships have produced new informations
about some disfunctions which characterize brain diseases
in aging, expecially senile dementias and cerebral infarc
tions.

To study brain electric activities, Q EEGs were recorded with a variety of sophisticated techniques, provid
ing the identification of EEG patterns typical of pathological conditions.

Furthermore studies on cerebral cortex properties
have been performed by means Evoked Potentials (EPs) tech
niques, to elucidate the regional responsiveness to visual, acoustic and somathosensory stimuli.

The aim of oru work was to investigate QEEG and VEP
findings in patients with presenile adn senile dementias
and with alcoholic dementia.

Different patterns of brain electric activities were
studied after administration of L-Acetyl-Carnitine, and
were compared with those obtained in basal conditions.

QEEG and VEP changes were signaled by different studies on experimental models (1, 2, 3), and on human diseases (4, 5, 6).

These changes may occur 90 min. after drug administra
tion (1, 3, 6), eventhough protracted modifications of
VEPs were reported several days after in rats (1) and in
men (5).

The LAC effects on brain activities are ascribed to direct or mediated activities of the drug on cholinergic (1, 3) or serotoninergic (7) brain receptors.

These effects can be utilized following three main therapeutic perspectives:
 a) evaluation of LAC effects on the electric brain activities in patients with EEG abnormalities;
 b) evaluation of LAC cholinergic effects using non-invasive methodologies;
 c) evaluation of physiologic performance improvements occurring in patients after LAC administration.

The brain electric activities were studied using EEG power spectral analysis with Fast Fourier Transform (FFT) and VEPs by gratings of several spatial frequencies.

These studies were performed before and after LAC administration and the frequency following response (FFR) was calculated to evaluate cholinergic activity reductions of the brain cortex occurring in patients with dementia (8, 9, 10).

The modifications of the EEG during FFR were measured after LAC and after Carnitine administration, to confirm the specificity of effects.

MATERIALS AND METHODS

8 patients with Senile (5) and Pre-senile (3) Alzheimer's Disease (Group A: 290.00-30 and 290.10-13 DSM 111) and 10 patients with Alcoholic Dementia (Group B: 291.23 DSM 111) were studied. CT scan (diffuse cortical atrophy and ventricle enlargements) and neuropsychological tests produced the main laboratory findings to confirm the diagnosis of dementia.

All the patients were submitted to the study protocol as follows:
A) Basal conditions: EEG recordings (8 channels; 10-20 International EEG System) were performed before LAC administration with FFR at 5,10 and 20 Hz. The test duration was 30 min. for baseline EEG and 30 min. for EEG during FFR.
B) Pharmachological test: 10 mg/kg LAC were injected in 30 min. intravenously, following EEG recordings in basal conditions, on the first day of the test. EEG recordings (30 min. baseline and 30 min. on FFR) were performed immediately after LAC injection and again 60 min. later.
A second intravenously LAC injection was performed 3 days after the aforementioned procedures. VEPs were in these

cases recorded before LAC injection, in basal conditions, and 60 min. after for 2 hours. VEPs were recorded by means Ag/AgCl disc electrodes placed in occipital region (15), Monocular pattern reversal stimuli (vertical gratings) were used of 1 cpd (cycle per degree),50% contrast and 4 cpd, 50% contrast.

6 days after the first pharmacological test, 10 mg/kg Carnitine were intravenously injected in 30 min. EEG and VEPs recordings were performed following the procedures of LAC tests.

EEG and VEP recordings were transfered to Hp 3968A tape recorder, and were analyzed by Berg Fourier 12440TE apparatus to obtain power spectral quantifications. The following EEG bands were selected: 0.5-3.5 Hz, 3.5-7.5 Hz, 7.5-12.5 hz, 12.5-16.5 Hz, 16.5-18.5 Hz, 18.5-22.5 Hz, 22.5-30 Hz; and 0.5-3.5 Hz, 3.5-7.5 Hz, 7.5-12.5 Hz,3-7 Hz, 8-12 Hz, 13-17 Hz, 18-22 Hz in EEG under FFR at 5-10-20 Hz.

The mean amplitude of FFT-EEG power spectra were calculated of 30 sec. for 120 EEG recording segments before LAC and for 60 segments after LAC (20 segments from 0 to 40 min., 20 segments from 40 to 80 min., 20 segments from 80 to 120 min.). The same calculations were performed before and after Carnitine.

The 1st, 2nd, 3rd and 4th harmonic amplitudes were summed up for the 5 Hz stimulation FFR. The 1st and 2nd harmonic amplitudes were summed up for 10 Hz stimulation and only the amplitude of the 1st harmonic was calculated for 20 Hz stimulation.

The mean values of 40 recording segments in basal conditions and those of 12 segments in periods of 0-40, 40-80, and 80-120 min. after the drug administration were calculated.

Statistical tests (Anova and Paired Wilcoxon tests) were calculated for EEG power spectra and VEP Amplitudes. EEG correlation indexes were obtained for basal conditions vs. 1 hour LAC pharmacological test, basal conditions vs. 2 hour LAC pharmacological test, 1 hour LAC pharmacological test vs. 2 hour LAC pharmacological test. Furthermore results of LAC pharmacological tests were compared with Carnitine tests.

Pattern VEPs were obtained using a Medelec ST 10 stimuli generator. VEPs were recorded by means of a Sensor Medelec Apparatus (1-15 Hz bandpass filters; 128-256 reversal stimuli) and plotted with Hp 7470A. VEPs were submitted to the frequency cross correlation test of the

Stolberg program. Furthermore amplitude and latency of
P100 VEP were measured before and after the pharmacological test.

RESULTS

A) Frequency analysis of EEG recordings - FFT - QEEG.
      In the early periods of the LAC test (0-40 min.) pa-
tients of both Groups A and B showed amplitude increments
of EEG alpha bands. These increments decreased progressively in the following periods of the test: 40-80 min. and
80-120 min. Amplitude increments were also observed for
theta and beta EEG bands, in early periods of the test,
similarly to alpha increments. ANOVA and Paired Wilcoxon
tests reported statistically significant differences with
basal condition recordings in the period from 10 to 70
min. following the LAC administration.
Fig. 1 shows the variations of EEG power spectra for the
        theta, beta and alpha bands and of FFR amplitudes
        following LAC administration in comparison with ba
        seline values.
        The scale for each analysed band or FFR indicates
        per cent variations of the amplitudes in compari-
        son with basal condition recordings.
        The arrows point to values of 0.05 or less of the
        p during the ANOVA comparisons.
        The circles mark p significances of 0.01 or less.
        The horizontal scale reports the time elapsed from
        the LAC i.v. injection. As reported in the figure
        high levels of statistical significance were ob-
        tained for amplitude increments of EEG tetha, beta
        bands and for 5 and 20 Hz FFR.
        THe significant amplitude increments were obtained
        in both Groups of patients, for the same periods
        following the drug injection.
        Carnitine administration did not induce any stati-
        stically relevant modification of QEEG and FFR.
B) Visual Evoked Poterntials (VEPs)
      The LAC administration induced an amplitude increment
of VEPs (P100 wave) obtained by 4 cpd pattern stimuli
both in Group A and in Group B. The increment of VEPs ap
peared 20 min. after LAC injection and disappeared 70
min. after LAC injection.
      On the contrary VEPs, obtained with 1 cpd pattern sti
muli, showed amplitude decrements at 20 min. after LAC
administration.

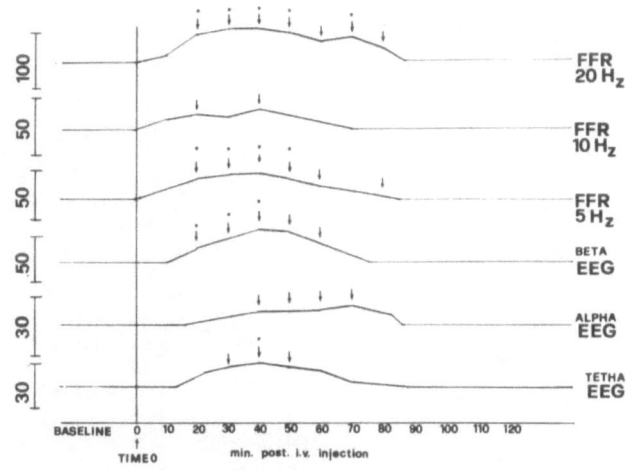

Fig. 1. See text for explainations.

The administration of Carnitine did not induce any changes of VEP amplitudes.
Fig. 2 shows the mean values of VEP amplitudes in basal conditions, and at 40, 80, 120 min. from the LAC i.v. injection, and at 60 and 120 min. from the Carnitine administration, in the two different groups of patients.

CONCLUSIONS

1) LAC administration may induce changes of the brain electric activities. This effect is observed using low doses of LAC, intravenously injected in man.
The timing of the brain electric modifications shown with QEEG and VEP amplitude changes indicates LAC effects in the first 40 min. after the i.v. administration. Early effects appear in the first 10 min. and the latest effects are reported sist 60-90 min. after the injection.
2) The modifications of VEPs induced by LAC are dependent on spatial frequencies of the grating pattern stimuli. The P100 amplitude increases after LAC when 4 cpd stimuli are used, is scarcely modified or decreases when 1 cpd stimuli are used. This finfing resembles VEP modifi-

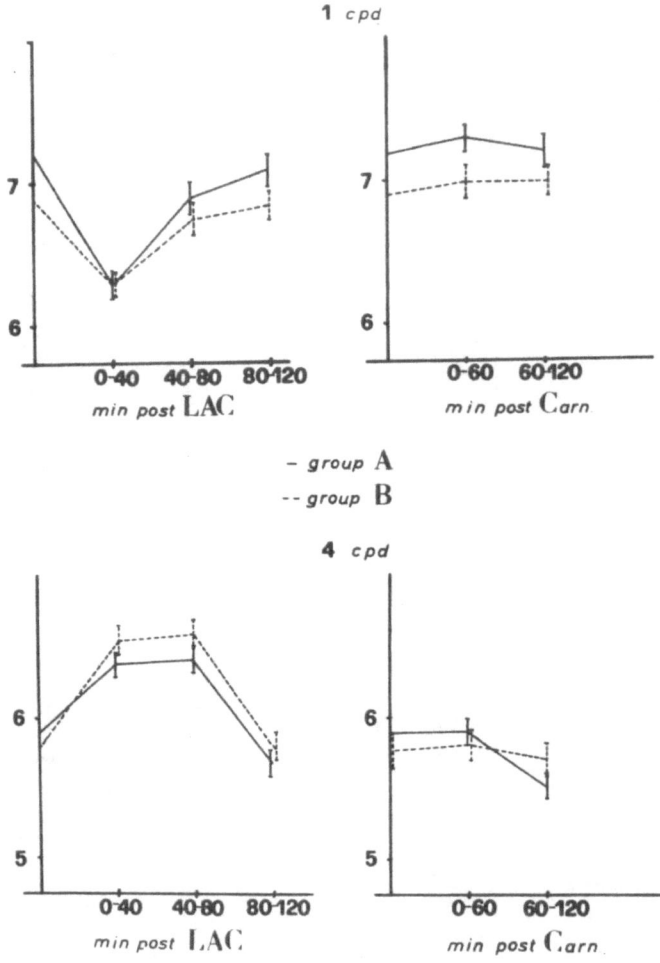

Fig. 2. Effects of LAC (Levo-Acetyl-Carnitine) and Carn
(Carnitine) on VEPs amplitude obtained with Coarse
(1 cpd) and fine (4 cpd stimuli) in the two groups of
patients. (A: senile and presenile dementia, B: alcoholic dementia). Notice the increment of VEPs amplitude to fine stimuli at 40-80 min. after LAC injection, and, coversly the decrement of amplitude to
coarse stimuli. The effect is the same for the two
groups of patients. The numbers on the vertical scale
report amplitude values in micro V. Horizontal scale
reports the time elapsed from the i.v. injection.

cations induced by physostigmine (8, 9) in animals. These data may suggest a physiologic effect of LAC which is related with the function of retinal or cortical structures, rather than with pre-existing histopathologic damages of CNS.

Recent reports indicate that acetylcholine blokade or defects selectively increases the amplitude of VEPs to low spatial frequency stimuli (10).

All in all the specific variations of QEEG and VEPs induced by LAC might suggest a proper use of this and of similar drugs in curologic degenerative diseases.

REFERENCES

1) Onofrj M., Bodis-Wollner I., Pola P., Calvani M.
   Drugs Expl. Clin. Res. 9 : 161 - 169, 1983
2) Falchetto S., Kato G., Provini L.
   Can. J. Physiol. Pharmacol. 49 : 1 - 6, 1971
3) Fariello R.S., Zeeman E., Golden G.T., Reyes P.T., Ramacci M.T.
   Neuropharmacology 23 : 585 - 587, 1984
4) Bertolino A., Papagno G.
   Clin. Europea 22 : 384 - 395, 1983
5) Pierelli F., Lazzari R., Calvani M., Burla F., Rizzo P.A., Morocutti C.
   Riv. Ital. EEG Neurofisiol. Clin. 1 : 45 - 46, 1981
6) Rossini P.M., Di Stefano E., Febbo A., Gambi D., Calvani M.
   Europ. Neurol. 24 : 262 - 271, 1985
7) Tempesta E., Ianiri L., Pirrongelli C.
   Neuropharmacology 24 : 43 - 50, 1985
8) Kirby A.W., Wiley R.W., Harding T.H. in: RQ Cracco, I. Bodis-Wollner ed.s Evoked Potentials. Frontiers of Clinical neuroscience Vol. 3. A.R. Liss, New York pp. 296 - 306, 1986
9) Harding T.H., Wiley R.W., Kirby A.W.
   Science 221 : 1076 - 1078; 1983
10) Bajalan A.A., Wright C.E., Van Der Vliet V.J.
   J. Neurol. Neurosurg.Psychiat. 49 : 175 - 182, 1986

65
The pharmacology of cognitive disturbances: problems and perspectives

S. Giaquinto

Before entering into the topic of this article, one should bear in mind that the treatment of the normal elderly is not supported by any current neurobiological issue. A normal brain function is unlikely to be sensitive to cure and on the other hand there is no evidence that a preventive pharmacological management in absence of clinical reasons may overcome a possible mental deterioration. On the other side, the medical prescription of useless compounds might lull the physician in a state of false safety, thus obscuring a deeper and more reasonable intervention (1).

The elderly is generally a staunch consumer of drugs and a motivated follower of endless therapies. One may note the success of compounds in water solution, that allow meticulous ceremonial of drop counting. The increasing percentages of the elderly all over the occidental world may easily account for the industrial interest in this field. This trend is by no means negative,because the private policy will support basic as well as applied research,giving in such a way a contribution to institutions and knowledges. A liberal observer might argue that private firms do not support research for philanthropy's sake,but we think that more funds are welcome,in a field where Government funds are limited compared to the urgent necessity of coping with the Alzheimer's disease and other causes of mental deterioration in the late age (2).

On this topic, we should say that a therapeutical protocol is still lacking. On the other hand, even the utmost criticism has to recognize the recent achievements in the field of aging and dementia. The policy of renunciation just at the beginning of new trends seems to me an anti-scientific and unfruitful attitude. At the end of the eighties we cannot foresee when and how the control of third D in the triplet Depression, Delirium and Dementia will represented an achievement of Science, but certainly have a better knowledge than in the recent past. We are now aware of possibilities and energetic campaigns against dementia are in progress.

Active drugs on brain circulation are of wide use. They are classified as follows (3):

1) drugs with a mainly eumetabolic action
2) drugs with a vasoactive and eumetabolic action
3) drugs with a main alphalitic action
4) drugs with a main betafacilitating action
5) drugs with a mainly myolitic action

Many of them are not placebo and can be usefully applied either to mild subjective symptoms as headache, dizziness, drowsiness on circulatory basis or to more serious consequences of cerebrovascular diseases. However, they are not really "cognitive drugs". This heading should be reserved to those drugs inducing positive changes at the level of the higher mental functions, changes which are considered useful for medical treatment. Recent reviews present the reasons for both pessimism and optimism (4,5).

At the time being, three lines of research are in progress for the aging brain. The first one is focused on the neurotransmitters. Since a fall of choline-acetyltransferas is known to occur in the Alzheimer's disease, an obvious approach is the endeavour to stimulate acetil - choline synthesis. Precursors have been given to patients, such as choline, deanol and lecithin, but scientific evidence for positive results is still lacking Moreover, the physostigmine has been applied in order to counteract the breakdown of the neurotransmitter as well as the arecholine, a post-synaptic cholinergic agonist. Although musca-rinic receptor is known to survive in the brain wasting of the Alzheimer's disease, the final outcome has been disappointing (6), in spite of some positive results. On the basis of the favorable outcome in the case of Parkinson's disease, some relief was expected in the case of dementia and other cognitive disturbances, where a dopaminergic loss is known to occur. Again, the use of L-Dopa has been disappointing and the addition of the agonist, such as bromocriptine and lisuride, has not improved the therapeutical trials. Some positive effects, expecially at emotional level, were seen in patients treated with alaprociate, a selective drug on the re-uptake of serotonin in the synaptic cleft (6).

The second research trend is focused on the so-called "nootropic" drugs, that have effects on the neurons. Their use in dementia is suggested by the telencephalic site of action, the protective effect on ATP and remarkable results in animals. The first nootropic drug to appear on the market was the piracetam,a gabaergic compound. A new nootropic drug, the oxiracetam appeared to be active in restoring the EEG profile at fronto-temporal level in patients previously treated with diazepam (7). Studies are in progress in demented with the assistance of the Positron Emitted Tomography.

The third research line is that one based on the neuromodulation in the domain of the phospholipids. According to this view,a strong action at synaptic level is unprofitable in demented patients for the amount of the side effects and the modulation of receptors is considered a more practical approach. The gangliosides are compounds that may work in this line. Acetyl-L-carnitine is a natural compound having a role in the cellular acetylation systems homeostasis, which has shown positive results mainly in cognitive and memory functions of senile patients in a double-blind study (8). Severe Alzheimer patients showed a favorable trend on the computerized EEG following a 3-month therapy at the dosage of 1,5 gr/die, with a reduction of the delta + theta/alpha ratio,compared to placebo (9). Positive effects induced by acetyl-L-carnitine were seen in rats with a histological and histochemical counterpart (10).

Obsolete treatments are briefly reported here,as psychostimulants, which were widely used in past (pentylenetetrazole,methylphenidate) but are now outdated because of both lack of beneficial effects and,on the contrary, vegetative symptoms. The well-known Gerovital is also an obsolete treatment, i.e. procaine in a suitable preparation for i.m. administration; because local inactivation the amount of drug reaching the central nervous system is probably scanty. The hyperbaric oxygen was hypothesized to improve cerebral oxygenation,but the results were disappointing. Moreover, worsening of ischemic cerebrovascular accidents may happen.

Many researchers chide the field of experimental therapy of cogni - tive defects for its inattention to a fundamental problem:namely, when a common protocol will be brought about ? It has been argued that the partial results obtained so far are due to a threefold problem: a) groups of patients are not homogeneous and often un- selected; b) instruments are inadequate in many cases; c) approach is naive, because in dementia it is not possible to single out one neurotransmitter system as the primary locus of impairment (8).

According to this view, the ideal methodology would be a tailored treatment for each patient after a careful check, including biochemical studies of the spinal fluid. In agreement with the statement of a combined treatment, it has also been suggested (11) to improve the glycolitic and tricarboxylic acid turnover capacity, which seems to be the most important metabolic system in the acetylcholine synthesis.

There are two more issues of primary interest. The first one is the steep course of the Alzheimer's disease, a highly progressive brain wasting. The medical treatment has therefore to go against such a trend. The second trouble comes from psychological considerations: if an effectful drug restored at once the impaired neurochemical milieau, the memory stores of the patients would be devoid of previous information, language texture, thinking, abstract reasoning. The patient would probably have incomplete benefit. Thus each pharmacological treatment should bear in parallel a neuropsycho - logical training.

In the past, conflicting results were found to depend on either the various experimental settings or the confused composition of the groups, where normal elderly were intermingled with deteriorated subjects.

A strict protocol is therefore necessary for the future research. For obvious reasons it will be impossible to cover the complete field of information, but it is convenient to start the discussion from a defined point. Until recently, pharmacological treatment of the aging brain and related cognitive diseases has therefore been insufficient. The clinical model was over-semplified. Nowadays, studies may amplify a narrow visual field, by differentiating more precise patterns in the protocol. The study is not so easy as it may appear, owing to the many variables. The following one is just an attempt to present the questions rather than the answers.

Subject: patient, out-patient, normal; age, sex, social class, income, hometown, living-together, education, job.
Illness: normal aging, AD/SD, MID, other diseases, beginning, evolution, cognitive damage, risk factors.
Environment: stimulation, indifference, hostility, recent changes of house, recent losses, climate, diet, intoxications.

Internal medicine: subjective symptoms, heart and vessels, lungs, liver, kidney.
Neurology: clinical signs, CT scan, CBF, PET, NMR, EEG,event-related potentials, spinal fluid, biopsy, neuropsychological testing, video-tape.
Psichiatry: testing for anxiety and depression , Rorschach.
Parallel therapies: neuroleptics, antidepressants, nootropics, vaso-active and antiparkinson drugs.
Protocol: observing rate, place, time, statistics, observers.
Drug: dosage, administration, duration, double-blind, monitoring, enhancement by training.

More questions are ahead.   What is the best neuropsychological testing ? What are the most reliable electrophysiological correlates ? What are the proper markers in the cerebral spinal fluid ? what is the minimal requirement for a therapy to be considered as effective ? The lack of accuracy may change results False positive as well as false negative can be reached in neuropharmacological trials.

Summing up, we can say that a long avenue is in front of the actual neurochemistry and neuropharmacology. Although spectacular results have not accomplished yet, some active molecules do exist. Probably, the day is not far off for an improvement of our diagnosis and consequently of our therapeutical means. No possibility should be neglected for alleviating the burden of the Alzheimer's disease and other forms of mental decay, moving this time from care to cure.

Chemistry was born in the XVI century, but four more centuries were necessary in order to get the first antiepileptic molecule.   Nowadays more than two thirds of epileptic patients are controlled by medical therapy, whereas our great Colleagues of the last century were unable to gather professional gratification in this field. Probably, some of them had to believe that epilepsy was really an untreatable disease.

REFERENCES

1) Mac Donald E.T., Mac Donald J.B. Drug treatment of the elderly.
John Wiley & Sons, New York, 1982 .

2) Hollister L.E. Pharmacotherapy of mental disorders of old age. In "Aging 2000: our health care and destiny". C. M. Gaitz, T. Samorajski Eds. Springer Verlag, Berlin,1985,303-315

3) Passeri M., Cucinotta D. Principles and methods of evaluating mental disorders in the aged and the modification following drug administration. In "The aging brain". Barbagallo-Sangiorgi G., Exton-Smith A.N. Eds. Plenum Press, New York, 1980,275-293.

4) Galizia V. Pharmacotherapy of memory loss in the geriatric patient. Drug Intell. Clin. Pharmacol. 18:784-791,1984.

5) Goodnick P.J., Gershon S. Chemotherapy of cognitive disorders. In "Aging" vol. 22 . Samuel D. et al. Eds. Raven Press, New York, 1983, 349-361.

6) Gottfries C.G. Rationale for the use of therapeutic agents in affective disorders (AD) and senile dementia of the Alzheimer type (SDAT). In "Aging 2000:our health, care,destiny". C.M. Gaitz, T. Samorajski Eds. Springer Verlag, Berlin, 1985, 327-338.

7) Giaquinto S., G. Nolfe, S. Vitali. EEG changes induced by oxiracetam on diazepam-medicated volunteers. Clin. Neuropharmacol. 7:786-787, 1984.

8) Agnoli A. Discussion on the therapeutical effect of acetyl-L-carnitine in psycho-orhanic syndrome and senile dementia. IVth World Congress of Biological Psychiatry, Philadelphia, 1985.

9) Giaquinto S. unpublished observations.

10) Angelucci L., Ramacci M.T. Acetyl-L-carnitine: neuropharmacological potentialities in senescent rats. IVth World Congress of Biological Psychiatry, Philadelphia, 1985.

11) Meyer-Ruge W. New prospects in neuropharmacology of senile dementia. In "Aging". vol. 21. J. Cervos-Navarro, H.I. Sarkander, Eds. Raven Press, New York, 1983, 391-399.

66
L-Acetylcarnetine prevents the parkinsonian syndrome induced by MPTP in monkeys

M. Onofrj, M.F. Ghilardi and I. Bodis-Wollner

1-Methyl-4-phenyl-1,2,3,6 tetrahydropyridine (MPTP) destroys dopaminergic nigrostriatal neurons and induces a ParKinsonian-like state in humans and in monkeys (1, 2). This finding has stimulated speculations that specific environmental or endogenous toxins may underlie most causes of Parkinson's Disease (3, 4).

MPTP binds with high affinity to receptor-like sites which appear to be identical to the enzyme monoaminoxidase (MAO)B found in glial cells (5). MAOB transforms MPTP into the toxic form having an unsaturated pyridine ring, N-methyl-4phenyl pyridine (MPP +), which is accumulated via the pump-like cathecolamine uptake system into dopamine neurons (6). MPP+ is converted into its saturated form and this process induces the production of toxicfree radicals which are held responsible for driving the senescense and death of monoaminergic neurons.

Based on this probable mechanism of action, several drugs were evaluated to assess teir effectiveness in preventing the MPTP toxicity. Cathecolamine uptake inhibitors, like mazindol and bupropyone were shown to be ineffective (7, 8). MAO inhibitors, like pargyline,Deprenyl and RO-166491 (a benzamide derivative) prevented MPTP effects in mice and in monkeys (9). Ascorbate, -tocoferol and -carotene (which are active in redox reactions)were shown to be only moderately effective in mice (10).

In this paper we describe the protective effect on MPTP toxicity of the administration of an endogenous compound, L-acetyl-carnitine (LAC). In previous studies (11, 12), we had shown the effect of MPTP on visual evoked potentials (VEPs) and on P-300-like evoked potentials of the cynomolgus monkey. In the present paper we show a protective effect of LAC on behavioral, evoked potentials biochemical and neuropatological manifestations of MPTP toxicity. The protective effect of LAC was studied for as long as one year since recent reports suggest that MPTP can induce a Parkinsonian state even following exposure to low toxic levels or in subjects who are asymptomatic shortly after contamination (3).

MATERIALS AND METHODS

10 cynomolgus monkeys (macaca fascicularis), mean weight 2.1 kg + 0.1; 5 males , 5 females underwent our study. In 4 monkeys, 0.35 mg/kg of MPTP were administered i.v. once per day for 3 consecutive days following a protocol used in our department (11) and reported in previous studies (13, 14). These animals were classified as "MPTP monkeys". In 4 monkeys 20 mg/kg LAC were administered i.m. every day for 30 days. On the 8th, 9th and 10th days of LAC administration, MPTP was injected i.v. following the aforementioned protocol. These animals were classified as "MPTP + LAC monkeys". In one monkey, "Lac prior MPTP", a single dose of LAC was administered i.m. prior to the first MPTP injection and the normal MPTP protocol was followed. In one monkey, "LAC post MPTP", MPTP was administered for 3 days and LAC was injected i.m. for 20 days beginning on the 3rd day after the last MPTP administation. In all the monkeys, daily observations reported food intake, necessity of nosogastric tube feeding, brady kinesia, posture, standing ability, masked face, rigidity vocalization, tremor and impairment of eye movements.

5-10 times in a 4 month period, prior to the drug administration, VEPs, ERGs, somatosensory evoked potentials (SEPs), brainstem evoked potentials (BAEPs) and endogenous P300-like evoked potentials were recorded in 8 monkeys. In 2 "MPTP + LAC" monkeys, recording electrodes were not implanted. EP recordings were repeated every 3 days for 27-350 days following the last MPTP administration.

EPs were recorded by stainless steel, self-tapping electrodes placed onto pre-drilled holes in the same positions. Needle electrodes placed at the earlobes served as the reference and the grounding electrode was alternated for Fz and Oz. Needle electrodes or silver silver chloride electrodes placed in the inferior orbital bones recorded ERGs (11, 12). Interelectrode resistance was below 5 K. Three bolts were placed in the head and secured with dental acrylic to maintain head position during the recordings. The monkeys were comfortably restrained in a primate chair. Monocular VEPs and ERGs were simultaneously obtained by means of vertical grating stimuli with a square wave luminance profile presented in the counterphase mode. The stimulus was produced by means of a Digitimer Stimulator on a screen subtending 45 degrees of visual angle, with mean luminance of 56 cd/m^2 and contrast of 90%. Temporal frequency of the stimulus was 1 Hz, and 0.5, 1, 2 and 3.5 cpd spatial frequency stimuli were used. The signals were amplified 20,000 times and filter settings were .3-100 Hz. The transient responses (1 Hz) were summated by a Nicolet 1170 averager and plotted by an X-Y plotter.

BAEPs were obtained by means of monaural clicks at 70 dB intensity and 10 Hz frequency signals recorded for Cz electrodes were amplified 20,000 times and filter settings were 100-3000 Hz. SEPs were obtained by square wave electric pulses of .2 msec duration applied at the right sciatico-popliteal nerve. Signals were recorded for a Cz-Fz derivation, amplification was 20,000 times, filter settings were 3-3000 Hz. P300-like potentials were obtained by a method previously developed in our laboratory (13) following an auditory "oddball" paradigm. Frequent stimuli were pure tones at 500 Hz and rare stimuli were pure tones at 4000 Hz. A reinforcing electric pulse followed the rare tone after 600-800 msec. Frequent to odd ratio was 1/10. The clearest potentials were recorded from "Cz" The intensity of tones was 50 dB. The amplifiers were set for 10,000 amplifications and filter settings were 1-300 Hz.

The "MPTP monkeys" were sacrificed 90-180 days after the last injection. The "LAC prior MPTP monkey" was sacridiced 30 days after the last injection. The "LAC post MPTP monkey" was sacrificed 60 days after the last MPTP injection. The "MPTP + LAC monkeys" were sacrificed 60-350 days after the last injection. On the day of sacrifice the animals were killed by sodium pentobarbital, the brains and eyes were excised and homognized in 0.32 M sucrore. Standard Methods were used for analyses of homovanillic acid (HVA) and dopamine by HPLC.

RESULTS

"MPTP monkeys" developed symptoms shortly after the administration of the drug. The time of appearance and

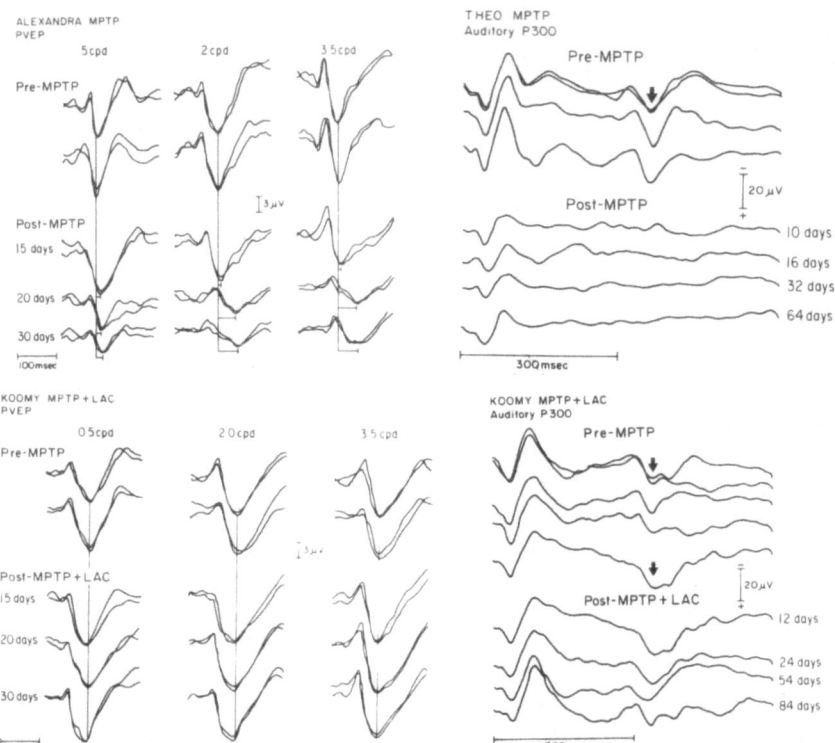

Fig. 1. On the left are reported VEPs to different spatial frequencies (0.5, 2, 3.5 cpd) recorded in two
sessions prior to MPTP injection and in 3 different
periods following MPTP injection (15, 20, 30 days) in
a monkey treated only with MPTP (upper quadrant) and
in a monkey protected with LAC (lower quadrant). Noti
ce that MPTP delayed mainly VEPs to fine spatial frequency in the unprotected "MPTP" monkey. Notice also
the VEP amplitude reduction induced by MPTP. This
finding is similar to VEP alterations reported in Par
kinson's Disease patients (14). The MPTP + LAC monkey
did not develop any alteration of VEPs. The two right
quadrants report auditory potentials to rare stimuli
of oddball paradigm, and the P300 like potentials (ar
rows). Top quadrant reports traces of the "MPTP" monkey, botton quadrant reports traces of the "MPTP +
LAC" monkey. Notice that in the "MPTP" monkey the pri
mary auditory EP undergoes an amplitude decrement and
P300 disappears. Notice that the "MPTP + LAC" monkey
does not develop any alteration of EPs.

500

Table 1. Mean Values of PERG, VEP and P300 measurements in control monkeys, monkeys treated only with MPTP, monkeys protected with LAC from the MPTP toxicity.

	PERG (Amp. u V)	VEP (Amp. u V)	(Lat msec.)	P300 (Amp. u V)
Ctl.	3.8 + 0.4	15.6 + 1.8	104.1 + 2.7	24.5 + 4.2
"MPTP"	1.2 + 0.2	6.8 + 1.7	150.3 +11.3	- - - -
"MPTP + LAC"	3.7 + 0.3	16.9 + 1.3	103.9 + 2.8	25.6 + 3.1

Table caption. PERG (pattern electroretinogram) and VEP (Visual Evoked Potentials measurements) are reported only for responses recorded with 2 cycle per degree stimuli. P300 indicates the amplitude of the P300-like endogenous component recorded in monkeys with an auditory "oddball" paradigm (13). Ctl indicates results obtained in control conditions. + indicates the standard deviations of the mean.
Notice absence of P300 component in "MPTP" monkeys.

- - - - - - -

Table 2. Endogenous dopamine and homovanillic acid in the head of the caudate in control, "MPTP" and "MPTP + LAC" monkeys.

Group	Dopamine (ng/g)	HVA (ng/g)
Ctl.	11.4 + 1.0	9.1 + 0.7
MPTP	0.2 + 0.2	less than 0.2
MPTP + LAC	10.9 + 0.6	9.0 + 0.6

No statistical differences were observed between the control and "MPTP + LAC" Groups. Data are the mean + S.D. for n = 4.

intensity of symptoms was overlapping to the disease cour
se reported by other researchers (1 - 10) and in our previous studies (11, 12). "MPTP + LAC" monkeys showed to be
immune from MPTP toxicity: we did not observe any behavio
ral modification in these monkeys for the entire perio of
our study. In the " LAC prior MPTP" monkey, symptoms appeared 2-7 days later than in "MPTP" monkeys, but in 12
days, the Parkinsonian Syndrome was totally developed. In
the "LAC post MPTP" monkey, decrement of food intake and
bradykinesia appeared as early as in MPTP monkeys, but a
reduction of symptoms was reported already on the 12th
day following the last MPTP injection.

Of the different neurophysiological parameters measur
ed in our study, as reported in previous publications
(11, 12) only ERG amplitudes, VEP latencies and amplitudes and P300 potential amplitudes underwent consistent
modification in "MPTP" monkeys. VEP latencies increased
concurrently with the course of behavioral symptms (11).
PERG and VEP amplitudes decreased after MPTP administration and VEP latencies increased. The alterations were
greatest when 2 and 3.5 cpd stimuli were used as compared
to 0.5 stimuli VEPs and PERGs. This finding is similar to
recently described VEP alterations in human Parkinson's
Disease (14). In "MPTP + LAC" monkeys and in the "MPTP
post   LAC" monkey, PERGs, VEPs and P300 potentials o-
scillated inside the range of normal variations. In the
"LAC prior MPTP" monkey, evoked potentials underwent the
same changes as in "MPTP" monkeys.

Table 1 reports measurements of PERGs and VEPs obtain
ed with 2 cpd stimuli and of the amplitude of the P300 in
all the monkeys of our study. P300 potential was unreco-
gnizable after "MPTP" in our monkeys. Fig. 1 shows a comparison of VEPs to 1-4cpd stimuli and of P300 potentials
in one "MPTP" monkey and in one "MPTP + LAC" monkey. Notice the characteristic modifications of VEPs and the disappearance of the P300 potential in the "MPTP" monkey
and the absence of alterations in the "MPTP + LAC" monkey.

Biochemical and neuropathological studies performed in
the sacrificed animals showed a decrement of dopamine and
homovanilic acid in the caudate, striatum and neuronal .
loss of as much as 90% in "MPTP" monkey and in the "LAC
prior MPTP" monkey.

The same measurements were inside normal limits in
"MPTP + LAC" monkeys. In the "LAC post MPTP" monkey, post
mortem measurements showed a 40% decrement of dopamine in

the striatum and 30% neuronal loss in the nigra.

Table 2 reports measurements of Dopamine and HVA in Control monkeys of previous studies, "MPTP monkey" and "MPTP + LAC monkeys".

DISCUSSION

Our study shows that LAC intramuscular administration prevents behavioral and neurophysiological alterations in duced by MPTP in monkeys. The protective effect of LAC is confirmed by post mortem studies which show no altera- tions of dopamine content or neuronal loss in the brain. Since MPTP exerts its toxicity via oxidative and up- take mechanisms of the CNS (7, 10), it is likely that LAC exerted its protective effects inside the CNS. Since our study involved both monkeys with chronic electrodes and without surgical manipulations, we were confident that LAC did not enter the CNS through alterations of the blood-brain barrier. A precise biochemical pathway, throu gh which LAC protected the brain from MPTP toxicitu, has yet to be established.It is known that LAC can increase the firing rate of cholinergic and serotoninergic neurons (15, 16) has structural resemblances to cholinergic neuro transmitters (17) and can alter behavioral and neurophy- siological activities related to cholinergic mechanisms (15, 18).

Besides this mechanism of action related to synaptic transmission, it was reported that LAC can modify mito- chondrial respiratory activities (19) and could figure as an energy supplying substrate, parallel to glucose oxida- tion. Our finding in MPTP + LAC monkeys shows an unsu- spected therapeutic effecr of LAC on a disease dependent on neurotransmitter alteration and cell senescence and death mechanisms. If, as it was recently hypothesized (1, 2, 3), MPTP induced desease and Parkinson's Disease sha- re a similar etiology, the common pathway of which is the oxidation of monoamines, LAC could represent the new frontier of drugs designed to treat neurological degenera tive diseases.

REFERENCES

1) Langston J.W., Forno L.S., Rebert C.S., Irwin I. Brain Res. 1984; 292: 390-4
2) Burns R.S., Chieuli C.C., Markey S.P., Ebert M.H. Proc. Natl. Acad. Sci. 1983; 80: 4546-50
3) Barbeau A. Canad. J. Neurol. Sci. 1983; 11: 24-28
4) Collins M.A., Neafsey E.J. Neurosci. Letters 1985; 55: 179-84
5) Chiba K., Trevor A., Castagnoli N. Biochem. Biophys. Res. Commun. 1984; 120: 574-8
6) Javitch J.A., D'Amato R.J., Strittmatter S.M., Snyder S.H. Proc. Natl. Acad. Sci. 1985; 82: 2173-7
7) Langston J.W., Irwin I., Langston E.B. Science. 1984; 225: 1480-2
8) Snyder S.H., D'Amato R.J. Neurology 1986; 36: 250-8
9) Cohen G. et al. Eur. Jou. Pharmaco. 1984; 106: 209-10
10) Kopin I.J. et al. In: Markey S.P., Castagnoli N., Trevor A., Kopin I.J. eds "MPTP: a neurotoxin producing a parkinsonian Syndrome". Acad. Press. (California) 1986; p 8-24
11) Onofrj M. et al. In: Markey S.P., Castagnoli N., Trevor A., Kopin I.J. eds "MPTP: a neurotoxin producing a parkinsonian Syndrome. Acad. Press. (California) 1986; p 683-8
12) Glover A., Ghilardi M.F., Onofrj M., Bodis-Wollner I. In: Markey S.P., Castagnoli N., Trevor A., Kopin I.J. eds "MPTP: a neurotoxin producing a parkinsonian Syndrome" Acad. Press. (California) 1986; p 667-72
13) Glover A., Onofrj M., Ghilardi M.F., Bodis-Wollner I. Electroenceph. Clin. Neurophysicl. 1986; 65: 231-35
14) Onofrj M., Ghilardi M.F., Basciani M., Gambi D. J. Neurol. Neurosurg. Psychiat. 1986; 49: 1161-71
15) Onofrj M., Bodis-Wollner I., Pola P., Calvani M. Drugs Expl. Clin. Res. 1983; 9: 161-69
16) Tempesta E., Ianiri L., Pirrongelli C. Neuropharmacology 1985; 24: 43-50
17) Reed K.W., Murray J.W., Roche E.B. J. Pharm. Sci. 1980; 69: 1065-67
18) Fariello R.G., Zeeman E., Golden G.T., Reyes P.T., Ramacci M.T. Neuropharmacology 1984; 23: 585-87
19) Siliprandi N., Siliprandi D., Ciman N. Biochem. J. 1965; 96: 77-81

NON-INVASIVE INVESTIGATIONS OF THE CARDIOVASCULAR SYSTEM

67
Nuclear magnetic resonance in the detection of the atherosclerotic lesion

L. Lalloni, A. Bucci and P. Ricci

In recent years, several investigators have concentrated on detecting a diagnostic tool which would allow the structural analysis, classification and quantitative evaluation of the atherosclerotic lesion in vivo.

These findings will aid in defining the presence/absence and progression/regression of lesions.

Non invasiveness, validity, accuracy and precision are the basic requirements wich such tecniques must possess.

Although ultrasonography is the most commonly used tecnique since it meets the above mentioned charateristics, ultrasonography (doppler cw, b-mode, duplex-scan) is still far from being thoroughly satisfactory.

More recently, a major interest has been focused on the applications of Nuclear Magnetic Resonance (NMR), which holds considerable promise in the study of the atherosclerotic lesion.

GENERAL PRINCIPLES OF NUCLEAR MAGNETIC RESONANCE

NMR phenomenon was first described by Felix Bloch (Stanford University) and Edward M. Purcell (Harvard University) in 1943.

Atomic nuclei consist mainly of protons and neutrons possessing spin. When protons and neutrons are present in such nuclei in an even number, spins couple two by two and neutralize; otherwise spins produce a resultant different from zero, with a consequent internal rotation of the nucleus which behaves like a rotating particle, whose magnetic moment is randomly oriented. If nuclei possessing spin are

immersed in an external magnetic field,they undergo two different phenomena.
a) nuclei abandon their random assembly and tend to align themselves in a parallel fashion with respect to the external magnetic field,while only a very small number will orientate in an antiparallel fashion;
b) production of a gyration (precession),whose frequency depends on the applied field strength.

Nuclear magnetization,which is at equilibrium in the static magnetic field, is altered by the application of an alternating electromagnetic field (radio frequency impulse).
This stimulus brings about two basic phenomena:
a) phase uniformization in the precession,induced by the external magnetic field so that all the nuclei align themselves in the same spatial position;
b) gradual deviation of the axis of the internal magnetic field until it is positioned at 90' or 180' with respect to the external magnetic field (depending on duration and intensity of the radio frequency impulse).

Interruption of radio-frequency impulses makes the excited nuclei return to starting conditions (relaxation) and release energy within the range of radio-frequencies,in such a way as to be recognizable by the source itself.
Two different relaxation processes can occur for nuclei previously excited by the radio-frequency impulse:
a) T1,determined by the time the internal magnetic fields of nuclei previously deviated by the radio-frequency impulse take to re-align themselves on the axis of the external magnetic field.
Nuclear realignement is dependent on the gradual energy release to the surrounding microenvironment (spin-lattice relaxation);this time is shorter than T2;
b) T2,the time individual nuclei take to recover the same circumference rotation as the one previous to the radio-frequency impulse.The different circumference rotation of nuclei is determined by the spin-spin interaction (spin-spin relaxation).

Both T1 and T2 have a quantitative and qualitative effect on the signal underlying magnetic resonance.Another fundamental MR signal is produced by the registration,subsequent to the interruption of the MR impulse, of signals emitted by excited nuclei.Since the signal intensity depends on the number of excited nuclei ,it is known as "nuclear density" ,or "proton density when speaking of hydrogen.

In the '50s and '60s the main parameters for measuring NMR (proton density,T1 and T2) used mainly in the fields of physics and chemistry to characterize inorganic systems.

In the early '70s,systematic studies carried out on the proton of biological systems revealed the possibility of characterizing biological tissues of laboratory animals,in vitro at first and then in vivo,through the measurement of proton density and relaxation times of the hydrogen nucleus.

It was in 1973 that Lauterbur made the first attempt at representing the NMR signal through images.

In building up NMR images,the possibility of determining the spatial position of each signal has been obtained by the application of a magnetic field variable in space and time,overlapping a constant magnetic field;therefore,the resonance frequency will not be the same in each spatial point and will be characteristic in every point of the sample examined.

In NMR systems available today,the magnet can be either of the permanent or resistive type.

The permanent type requires amounts of iron andferromagnetic material and has low energy consumption.On the other hand,it is heavy,the magnetic field stromgly depends on temperature and great care must be taken to obtain uniform fields.It has a maximum operating field of 3,000 Gauss.

Resistive systems,consisting in classical windings,are more easily designed and have a maximum operating field of about 2.000 Gauss (above these values their use is uneconomic because of high current consumption).

Superconducting magnets,i.e. formed from material which at a given temperature has no resistance,are more costly than resistive magnets operating at low field strengths,but can reach fields of 15,000-20,000 Gauss,so that images can be formed also with spectra of less sensitive nuclei at low concentration in biological tissues,such as Phosphorus 31.

With such magnets high resolution spectra can be obtained also in vivo,focusing a constant and homogenous magnetic field in a small region.

NMR AND ATHEROSCLEROTIC LESIONS

Today NMR,which permits the analysis of at least 2 mm thick body slices,independently of their spatial orientation,has a minimum resolution power of 0.5 mm.

The high contrast between the weak blood resonance signal,at least under physiological conditions,and the stronger signal of the vesse walls account for the good NMR definition of these structures,particularly at the level of large vessels (aorta,iliac,femoral and carotid arteries),where atherosclerotic lesions have been identified as eccentric thickening of the wall or as formations projecting into the lumen.

The lipid constituent of the atherosclerotic lesion is revealed by a high resonance signal.Reduction or loss of the intraluminal signal tahe place under physiological conditions – since in their going forth and back the excited blood protons are replaced,upon receipt of the signal,by protons from the adjacent sections,which are not excited and therefore are not able to emit radio-frequency impulses.

The weak or nearly absent signal when blood flow is laminar and its speed normal (10-25 cm/sec) already gives evidence of a qualitative analysis ,being the lumen signal stronger when blood flow is either absent or reduced or turbulent.

Studies are now being made on the quantitative evaluation of blood flow,although mostly in animal models.

CONCLUSIONS

So far,preliminary studies on the vascular system,although promising,do not allow drawing definite conclusions on specificity and sensitivity of NMR for the detection of atherosclerotic disease,nor do they permit the exact evaluation of its validity as compared to other non invasive tecniques.

   Nonetheless,a few general observations can be made,which are reported in Table 1.

Table 1

_____

NON INVASIVENESS

COST

EXAMINATION TIME

OPERATOR'S VARIABILITY

_____

   Both tecniques are safe and non invasive.Ultrasonography is cheaper from the point of view of purchasing,installation and running costs,and the examination time is considerably shorter.

   The introduction of paramagnetic contrast media,currently under study,will undoubtedly help in better understanding the vascular system.

   The application of NMR spectroscopy "in vivo" for the study of tissue metabolism represents one of its most interesting perspectives.

REFERENCES

1-Bore P.J. :"Principles and applications of phosphorus magnetic resonance spectroscopy". MAGNETIC RESONANCE ANNUAL 1985,edited by Herbert Y.Kressel.Raven Press,New York 1985.

2-Budinger T.F :"Nuclear Magnetic Resonance in the study of atherosclerosis". NONINVASIVE TECHNIQUE FOR ASSESSMENT OF ATHEROSCLEROSIS IN PERIPHERAL,CAROTID AND CORONARY ARTERIES, edited by Thomas F.Budinger et al. Raven Press,New York 1985.

3-Kaufman L. , Crooks L.E. , Margulis A.R :" Nuclear Magnetic Resonance Imaging in Medicine".IGAKU-SHOIN Ltd.,Tokyo 1983.

4-Kaufman L.,Crooks L.E.,Sheldon P.E.,Rowan W,Miller T.:"Evaluation of NMR imaging for detection and quantification of obstructions in vessels".INVEST.RADIOL. 17:554,1982.

5-Kaufman L.,Crooks L.E.,Sheldon P.E. et al.:"The potential impact of nuclear magnetic resonance imaging on cardiovascular diagnosis." CIRCULATION 67:251,1983.

6- Herfkens R.J.,Higgins C.B.,Crooks L.E. :"Nuclear magnetic resonance imaging of the cardiovascular system:normal and pathologic findings".RADIOLOGY 147:749,1983.

7-Herfkens R.J.,Higgins C.B.,Crooks L.E.:"Nuclear magnetic resonance:imaging of atherosclerotic disease".RADIOLOGY 148:161,1983.

8-James E.M.,Earnest F.,Forbes G.S. et al.:"High-resolution dynamic ultrasound imaging of the carotid bifurcation:a prospective evaluation".RADIOLOGY 144:853,1982.

9-Battocletti J.H.,Halback R.E.,Salles-Cunha S.X.,Sances A.Jr.:"NMR blood flowmeter:theory and history". MED.PHYS.8:435,1980.

10-Bradley W.,Tosteson H.:"Basic Physics of NMR".in NUCLEAR MAGNETIC IMAGING IN MEDICINE.Igaku-Shoin, Tokyo 1981.

68
Perspective and limits of emission tomography in cerebrovascular disorders

G.L. Lenzi, P. Pantano, C. Pozzilli, V. Di Piero
and F. Giubilei

A technique is helpful to clinician when it helps to explain the clinical presentation and when it helps to predict the future decourse.

Neuroimaging techniques are, in this respect, a classical example. The more widely known of them, the TCT scan, is not helpful to explain depression or schizophrenia or anxiousness, but it is however dramatically relevant in the identification and follow-up of many organic brain syndromes, from tumors to hydrocephalus to cerebrovascular disorders. Other neuroimaging techniques are more intended toward the representation of functional aspects of the brain, and thus are theoretically of a potential wider usefulness for clinicians, filling a space not explored by TCT scan.

These techniques are the Positron Emission Tomography (PET) and the Single Photon Emission Computerized Tomography (SPECT), branches of the Emission Computerized Tomography general approach.

Main aim of the present short review is the analysis of the results obtained to date with PET and SPECT, on the light of the revenue offered to clinicians and in particular of the real advantages for the management of the cerebrovascular patients. And, from the analysis of the results, to focus the perspectives and the limits of these techniques.

No room will be spent for technical details on the two techniques, referring the interested reader to the chapter "Evaluation of CVD by emission tomography" by C. FIESCHI and G.L. LENZI in the Handbook of Neurology (1987).

OUTLINE OF PHYSIOPATHOLOGY OF CEREBRAL ISCHEMIA

The major acquisition, so far, of the PET techniques in the field of CVD has been a deeper knowledge of the mechanisms under-lying the pathophysiology of acute human cerebral ischemia.

In particular, the simultaneous measurements of cerebral blood flow (CBF), cerebral oxygen metabolism (CMRO2), cerebral oxygen extraction (OER) and cerebral blood volume (CBV), obtained in many PET centers, have led to a better understanding of this extremely relevant clinical entity. In fact, the treatment of cerebral ischemia is being addressed more and more toward the very early hours, and it requires the knowledge of the time-course of the transition between a potentially recoverable ischemia and the completed infarction.

Also the preventive treatment of the patients "at risk" needs a more complete assessment and consideration of their haemodinamic conditions, in order to recognize the correct sub-populations that could really benefit from a particular therapy which may otherwise appear as uneffective if applied to an un-selected population.

In pathophysiological terms, cerebral ischemia is a condition in which cerebral energy metabolism becomes impaired by an inade-quate blood supply.

In physiological conditions, the local CBF is metabolism-dependent, while in ischemia the metabolism becomes flow-rate dependent. Normally a considerable excess of energy substrates is delivered to the brain: the oxygen is 2-3 times and the glucose is 7 times the normal requirement of the nervous tissue per minute. Active neurons burn more substrates and the close relation-ship between metabolism and flow leads to an increase in rCBF in the active regions. This regional coupling is expressed by the fractional extraction of oxygen (OER).

This variable indicates that by increasing extraction, a twofold increase in metabolic activity (or vice-versa a comparable decrease in blood supply) can be accomodated. It follows that CBF and CMRO2 are linearly related, but that the angular coefficient of their linear relationship may change a great deal. Only when the hypoperfusion cannot be compensated for and therefore affects local metabolism, is there a true ischemia. In this sense, the situation of "compensated hypoperfusion" is a condition at risk of haemodynamic imbalance. The recognition and the understanding of this situation represent one of the major achievements of the emission tomography techniques.

However, a fundamental role appears to be played also by the changes in the peripheral resistance of the cerebral vascular tree. The measurements of the cerebral blood volume (CBV) have shown how the main mechanism of autoregulation acts through increase or decrease of CBV in order to maintain constant CBF. A rise in systemic blood pressure results in a vasoconscriction and in an increase in peripheral resistance. Thus the decrease in CBV is the counterpart of the stability of CBF. Vice-versa, as the systemic blood pressure falls, CBV increases and CBF again remains constant.

Gibbs et al.(5) have underlined the sensitivity of the index CBV/CBF (that expresses the transit time of blood flow through the cerebral vascular tree) to point out conditions of pre-clinical ischemia, an impairment of perfusion reserve.

CLINICAL RESULTS OF PET AND SPECT IN CVD

In patients with RIA, studies with PET and SPECT have been mainly performed out of the symptomatic phase. Only one case has been reported (11) during the symptomatic period. In general, when the patient presents with a normal TCT scan and without large vessel disease, the PET and SPECT landscapes are normal. However, these cases are few.

Many cases with clinical RIA showed in fact a TCT scan hypodensity and/or had a significant pathology of the large neck vessels and they have been studied with respect to the procedure of revascularization (EC-IC by-pass).

In the series of patients studied by Gibbs et al.(5) and by Powers et al.(12), the evaluation of cerebral blood volume (CBV) has provided further information on the consequences of ICA occlusion. In fact, many patients showed an increase in rCBV, pointing to an impaired autoregulation and a maximal vaso-dilation of resistance vessels distal to the occluded ICA. rCBV may be increased in the affected territory without any detectable change in CBF and OER, as well as a decrease of rCBF in the symptomatic hemisphere may occur together with an increase of OER. This latter situation, termed misery perfusion, indicates a loss of the normal coupling between flow and metabolism, and rCMRO2 is maintained by an increase in rOER, with progressively higher extraction needed as flow decreased. The general meaning is that PET may help to identify those stroke-prone patients who are at increased risk of stroke on a low-flow basis by de-monstrating focal regions of diminished cerebral perfusion.

The PET data have helped to estabilish the threshold for normal functioning of the brain. The minimum rCBF and rCMRO2 levels observed in viable brain tissue were 15 and 1.3 mls/100g/min respectively (12). However, rCBF values showed high variability, while rCMRO2 data reflects more consistently the tissue functions.

In addition to these data, which point towards the identifica-tion of a haemodynamic unbalance, a parallel reduction in flow and metabolism, with normal OER, has been reported in the cortical territory distal to an ICA or MCA occlusion (6,3,15). This condition of metabolic depression could be due either to neuronal loss, or to functional deactivation or to both, affecting these cortical

515

areas.

For stroke, the studies performed with PET and SPECT are not very much larger in respect to those performed on TIAs, in particular if considering only the very early phase.

Our review of the available literature has collected 10 patients studied during the first 24 hours, 9 studied during the 2nd day, 14 during the 3rd day and 11 during the 4th and 5th day. Apart from the scanty amount of data, the results have brought about a better understanding of events taking place in acute cerebral ischemia. The role of CBF, apart from initiating the cascade of events has been reduced to a very secondary and fluctuating variable.

PET studies have indicated that in the very early phase of cerebral ischemia, cerebral tissue in and around the area of depressed flow exibits an increased oxygen extraction, that is a state of "critical perfusion". This indicates that at the onset of a major reduction of CBF, trespassing the threshold of 15 ml/100g/min for a period of time lasting probably well over a few minutes, mitochondrial function remains intact, resulting in a maximal extraction of oxygen from the residual trickle of arterial blood. And, as previously stated, the metabolism becomes flow-dependent and flow-limited. In the early hours, practically all the patients show this marked focal elevation of oxygen extraction. Within the following hours, rOER tends to fall, indicating that the balance between oxygen supply and demand is tilting in favour of the former. That is, the tissue becomes hyperaemic relative to its underlying metabolic demands, whatever the absolute level of blood flow. The frequent fall in rOER below the normal value may simply imply reperfusion of the infarcted tissue or indicate a further progressive decline in the tissue metabolism, perhaps because of delayed cell death following a critical degree or duration of ischemia. Thus, the OER per se is not a reliable predictor of tissue viability. It is the combination of rOER and rCMRO2 evaluations which is highly predictive: a low rOER together with a low rCMRO2 indicates irreversible infarction.

A regional pattern of differential tissue vulnerability becomes apparent in the first hours: cortical regions supplied by the occluded arterial branch show a very high OER, whereas deep regions, (basal grey and subcortical white matter) show an early decrease in OER. This finding has been considered as indicative of an early change from ischemia to infarction in the deep tissue, probably related to the anatomy of the microvasculature. The only irreversible changes occurring in deep cerebral structures may limit the potential clinical benefit derived from maintenance of cortical function. Therapy has to be administered in a very short time interval: the therapeutical window. However, together with the experimental data, PET studies have shown that this window is definitely larger than the few minutes reported in classical text-books. Further studies, performed with stroke units, working in close proximity to a fast PET camera, may be crucial in order to fully clarify this point.

During this period, rCMRGlu is not as depressed as the oxygen metabolism. Within the infarct, regional oxygen consumption and glucose metabolism are significantly correlated, with a ratio of two moles of oxygen per mole of glucose (1/3 that of normal tissue). This finding has led Wise et al. (17) to suggest that the metabolising tissue of a recent cerebral infarct utilizes anaerobic glycolysis. This (relatively) increased glucose consumption could be due to the migration of phagocytic cells in the lesion (13).

In chronic infarction, PET measurements show that blood flow and oxidative metabolism are reduced in and around the lesion, while the coupling between the two reverts to the balance found in normal cerebral tissue. Studies of chronic multi-infarct dementia patients have shown focal reductions in cerebral oxygen and glucose utilization, which have a normal coupling to tissue blood flow. However, the findings indicating a coupled decrease of CBF and metabolism in otherwise unimpaired cerebral regions may also be due to the occurrence of disconnection effects (diaschisis).

Frackowiak et al. (4) have described no significant elevation of the OER in mild or severe dementia of the vascular type, thus supporting the hypothesis of Hachinski et al. (7) that chronic global cerebral ischemia is not a major pathogenetic mechanism in dementia. Further evidence that flow meets regional tissue metabolism demands comes from the PET study of the effect of a vasodilator drug in M.I.D. patients (5). Measurements performed after six months of treatment have failed to show any changes in blood flow and/or oxygen extraction.

For SPECT, the first studies, performed with IMP, showed a reduction of the tracer's uptake, that in general largely outpassed the structural alterations detected by TCT scan. This discrepancy has been confirmed by SPECT studies performed with other radiopharmaceuticals (HIPDM, HM-PAO), and it makes a relevant contrast with results obtained with PET.

The discrepancy between hypodense regions at TCT scan and hypoperfused regions with SPECT has been interpreted by Holmann et al. (9) to indicate that the IMP study "is depicting both areas of infarction and viable cerebral tissue that has decreased blood flow but sufficient metabolism to sustain the tissue". In other words, SPECT studies may be able to detect the extension of the "ischemic penumbra".

It must be remembered that a large contrast still exists between the supporters of the "penumbra" and the supporters of the "partial infarction" (14). That is, does the infarction terminate abruptly, with clear-cut borders between dead neurons and healthy neurons? Pathological SPECT and PET data are still contraversial, as are the clinical reports.

Argentino et al. (1) have studied with SPECT 20 patients presenting with acute stroke, with a follow-up after 1-2 weeks and after 1 month. In general, there is a reduction of the CBF defect with time in respect to the early SPECT study. The extent of the early SPECT defect correlates better with the neurological conditions at the one-month follow-up than it does with the early TCT scan.

Let us remember that transneural depression of function resulting from a distant brain lesion was first described by Von Monakow, in 1914, and named "diaschisis" (16). The phenomenon consists in a transient dysfunction of some cortical regions in the cerebral hemisphere contralateral to the actual brain infarct. The dysfunction may be initially profound and widespread, then slowly recovering. Kempisky in 1957 (10) provided electrophysiological experimental evidence of decreased neuronal activity in the homotopic points of the cerebral hemisphere contralateral to the cortical ablation.

In stroke, the first reports were presented by Hoedt-Rasmussen and Skinhoj (8), who found a bilateral decrease in CBF after stroke. The phenomenon of a decreased rCBF distant from the actual lesion was reported by other scientists working with the 2-D CBF techniques, without, however, much recognition from the neurological world, probably because of lack od anatomical and/or clinical correlations. It is due to the introduction of PET and to the report from Baron et al. (7) of a decreased metabolic activity in the cerebellar hemisphere contralateral to the cerebral ischemic stroke that the "remote-effects" or "diaschisis" re-enter the scene with a certain importance.

The description of crossed cerebellar diaschisis (CCD) was widely recognized also because it gave an explanation to the old findings of crossed cerebellar atrophy in long-standing unilateral brain damage. The basic explanation for the decreased metabolic activity in an otherwise intact brain structure is the decrease in the synaptic input leading to a decreased functioning of the target neuron. In this respect, SPECT studies of rCBF may probably have a meaning closer to that of the PET data on rCMRO2 or rCMRGlu, once the structure under scrutiny appears normal to TCT, or now, to MRI.

Diaschisis must be differentiated from diffuse metabolic

depression in patients with large cerebral lesions; a depression that correlates, in general, with the level of consciousness, tends to recover with time. A parallel comparison with the general recovery of patients with completed stroke seems noteworthy: in fact, besides the fact that the neurological deficit remains unmodified, the general status of the patient improves with a similar time course.

CONCLUSION

From all the data summarized above, what are the perspective and limits of PET and SPECT in the field of cerebrovascular disorders?

The neuroimaging modalities have two faces. The "qualitative" face (SPECT) is appealing but does not answer the quantitative questions raised by scientific medicine in the field of patho-physiology. The "quantitative" face (PET), on the other hand, should not be inbellished by the niceties of the color images which can hide the problems still present that present their correct interpretation. In particular the application of tracer's models to pathological tissue.

In spite of these limitations, the pathophysiological in-formation obtained by Emission Computerized Tomography is highly relevant. This is especially true in critical situations where the tissue morphology is intact, in spite of radical changes in haemodynamic reserve and/or energy metabolism. The area where the largest gains are expected is in the selecting of patients for specific therapeutical protocols and in monitoring in "real time" the therapeutical efficacy. Both goals very relevant for clinicians.

The major problems in this direction are two-fold: one is the limited access of acute cerebrovascular patients to PET facilities. These facilities are, in fact, seldom "clinically" oriented to acute neurological problems, problems in which one might expect to find the newest information. Hopefully SPECT technologies will be more easily applied to those circumstances, as our group does routinarily. The second aspect is not so much a limitation of the technologies on hand but rather the modesty of therapeutical proposals available in the acute phase of cerebral ischemia so far. This is a clinical-pharmacological "black-spot" that optimistically will be deleted by new pathophysiological and experimental knowledge.

Improved technologies, more specific development of radio-pharmaceuticals and of kinetic models with which to study metabolic aspects of functional relevance, but, more than all, a closer collaboration with clinical centers and an active partecipation of clinicians to these studies are the basis for some cautious optimism that with this shot review, has to be inspired.

REFERENCES

1   Argentino C, Bozzao L, Canal N, Candelise L, Di Piero V, Fazio F, Fieschi C, Franceschi M, Giubilei F, Lenzi GL, Pantano P, Perani D, Rango M, Rasura M and Rossetti, C (1986). Acute brain ischemia in humans: a follow-up study with CT scan, angiography and SPECT. (submitted for publication)

2   Baron JC, Bousser MG, Comar D and Castaigne, P (1980). Crossed cerebellar diaschisis in human supratentorial brain infarction. Trans Am Neurol Ass, 105, 459-461

3   Baron JC, Bousser MG, Rey A, Guillard A, Comar D and Castaigne, P (1981). Reversal of focal "misery-perfusion syndrome" by extra-intracranial arterial bypass in haemodynamic cerebral ischemia. Stroke, 12, 454-459

4   Frackowiak RSJ, Pozzilli C, Legg NJ, Du Boulay GH, Marshall J, Lenzi GL and Jones, T (1981). Regional cerebral oxygen supply and utilization in dementia: a clinical and physiological study with oxygen-15 and positron tomography. Brain, 104, 753-778

5   Gibbs, JM (1984). Cerebral blood flow and metabolism in dementia, with reference to the effects of pharmacological intervention. In: Trimble, M (ed) "Proceedings of British Association of Psychopharmacology Meeting". (Oxford: Pergamon Press)

6   Grubb RL, Ratcheson RA, Raichle ME, Kliefoth AB and Gado, MH (1979). Regional cerebral blood flow and oxygen utilization in superficial temporal middle cerebral artery anastomosis patients: an exploratory definition of clinical problems. J Neurosurg, 50, 733-741

7   Hachinski VC, Lassen NA, Marshall J (1974). Multi-infarct dementia. A cause of mental deterioration in the elderly. Lancet, 2, 207-209

8   Hoedt-Rasmussen,K and Skinhoj, E (1964). Transneural depression of the cerebral hemispheric metabolism in man. Acta Neurol Scand, 40, 41-46

9   Holmann BL, Hill TC, Polak JF, Lee RGL, Royal HD and O'Leary, DH (1984). Cerebral perfusion imaging with iodine 123 labeled amines. Arch Neurol, 41, 1060-1063

10   Kempisky, WH (1957). Experimental study of distant effects of acute local injury: a study of diaschisis. Acta Neurol Psychiatr, 79, 376-389

11   Perani D, Di Piero V, Lucignani G, Pantano P, Gilardi MC, Rossetti C, Pozzilli C, Gerundini P, Lenzi GL and Fazio, F (1986). Cortical blood flow in small subcortical cerebro-vascular lesions: a clinical-SPECT correlation study (submitted for publication)

12   Powers WJ, Grubb RL, Darriet D and Raichle, ME (1985). Cerebral blood flow and cerebral metabolic rate of oxygen requirements for cerebral function and viability in humans. J Cerebr Blood Flow Metab,5, 600–608

13   Pozzilli C, Lenzi GL, Argentino C, Carolei A, Rasura M, Signore A, Bozzao L and Pozzilli, P (1985). Imaging of leukocytic infiltration in human cerebral infarcts. Stroke, 16, 251–255

14   Pozzilli C, Itoh M, Matzuawa T, Fukuda H, Takeda S, Sato S and Ido, M (1986). PET in minor stroke. Cerb blood flow metabol (in press)

15   Sgouropoulos P, Baron JC, Samson Y, Bousser MG, Comar D and Castaigne, P (1985). Stenoses serrees et occlusions persistantes de l'artere cerebrale moyenne: consequences hemo-dynamiques et metaboliques: etudes par tomographie a positron. Rev Neurol, 141, 698–705

16   Von Monakow, C (1914). Die Lokalisation im Groohirn und der Abban der Funktion durch Korticale Herde.(Wiesbaden: Bergmann JF)

17   Wise RJS, Bernardi S, Frackowiak RSJ, Legg NJ and Jones, T (1983). Serial observations on the pathophysiology of acute stroke. Brain, 106, 197–222

69
The real utility of nuclear magnetic resonance in cardiovascular diseases

C. Gaudio

In the last few decades cardiovascular imaging techniques have been employed mostly for diagnosis. Later, through such techniques, cardiac pathophysiology was studied for a more functional assessment of patients with established disease. More recently this trend has developed and researchers focused on new and sophisticated techniques for the study of myocardial metabolism in vivo.(1,2)

Nuclear Magnetic Resonance (NMR) is a technique capable of providing both sets of information needed by the cardiologist:

A) STRUCTURAL INFORMATION

The technique allows visualization of the cardiovascular system providing high resolution tomographies in every spatial direction, including three-dimensional reconstructions. Magnetic Resonance Imaging (MRI), based on resonance of hydrogen nuclei, can produce in a relatively short time (1-3 minutes) from 1 to 9 tomographies about 1 centimeter thick, clearly showing heart chambers and large vessels (Fig.1), wall and septum thickness. In particular MRI allows accurate measurements of apical and lateral walls of left ventricle (LV), that are areas not well visualized by other imaging techniques, with a high definition of endocardium (Fig.2). (3,4)

Considering that two dimensional echocardiography (2D Echo) provides a great number of structural information in real time and at relatively low costs, the use of MRI should be limited to the following groups of diseases and diagnostic examinations:

1. Hypertrophic cardiomyopathies and in particular those forms localized in the apical and lateral areas, not satisfactorily imaged by echocardiography (Fig.3, 4); (5,6)

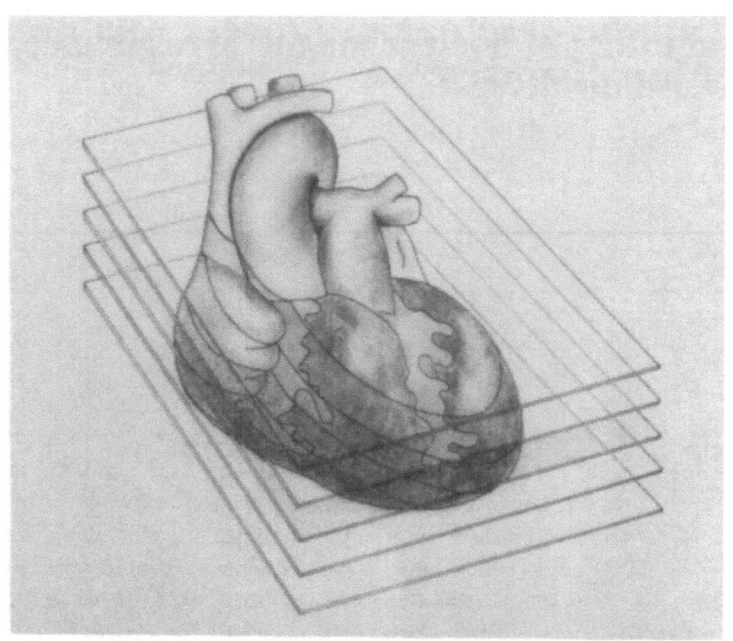

FIGURE 1 Three-dimensional reconstruction by multislice technique.

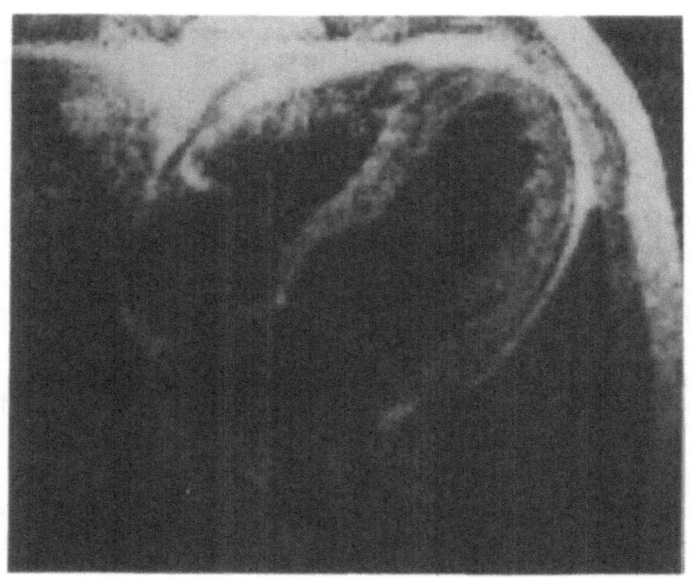

FIGURE 2 The "Four Chambers" NMR.

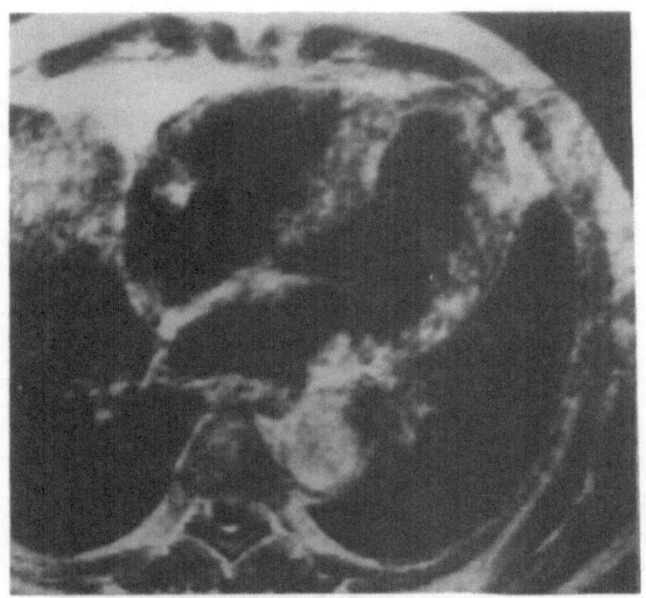

FIGURE 3 Hypertrophic cardiomyopathy involving interventricular septum and the lateral wall of LV.

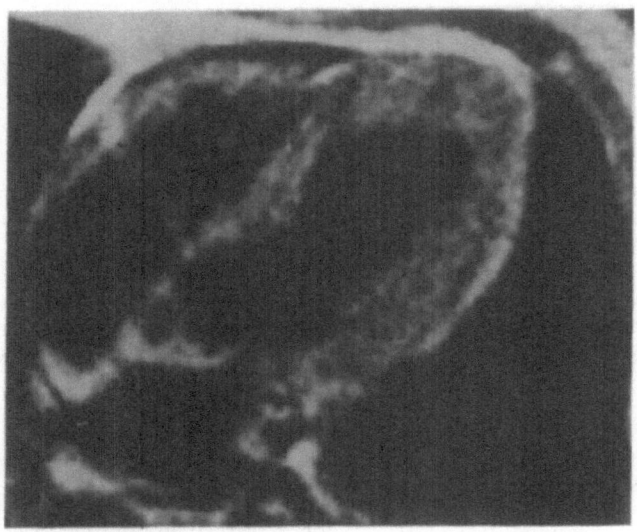

FIGURE 4 Hypertrophic cardiomyopathy localized in the apical wall of LV.

2. Congestive cardiomyopathies (Fig.5);

3. Visualization of proximal and middle tracts of coronaries;

4. Angiographies without contrast, with good visualization of atherosclerotic plaques;(7,8)

5. Research on infarct extension, with myocardial tissue characterization of infarctual and peri-infarctual areas; (9)

6. Morphological research on those patients who cannot be examined by echocardiography owing to technical difficulties.

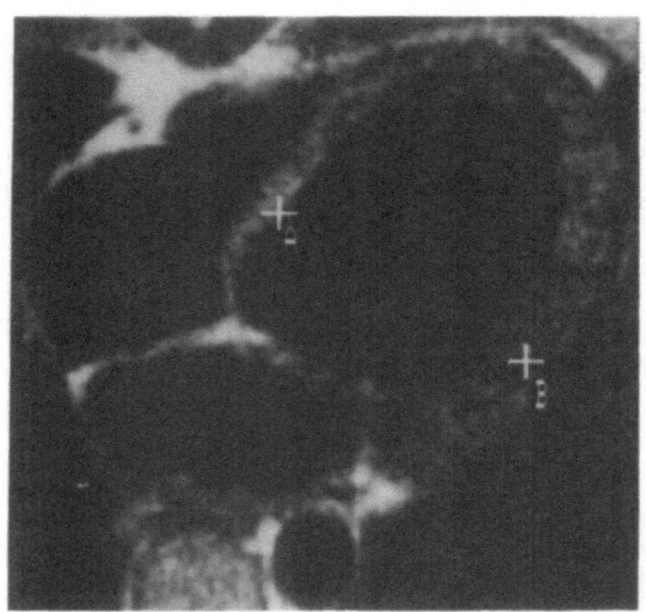

FIGURE 5 Congestive cardiomyopathy.

B) METABOLIC INFORMATION

Magnetic Resonance Spectroscopy (MRS), based on physical properties of some natural isotopes, such as 31P, 13C and 23Na, allows monitoring in vivo of the metabolic functions of myocardium.

Firstly because energy reserve of myocardial fibrocell consists of phosphates (ATP, ADP, PC). Secondly because cell capacity to preserve adequate levels of high energy phosphates is itself a metabolic integrity marker. Research by 31P-MRS has been carried out both in vivo and on excised and perfused hearts. Variations of high energy phosphates content can provide important information in the field of myocardial ischemia:

    a. Regional variations of phosphates concentration in ischemia and reperfusion, also during drug administration;(10)
    b. The efficacy of myocardial protection techniques on excised hearts after cardioplegic arrest and reperfusion;
    c. High energy phosphates concentration and intracellular pH variation of infarctual and peri-infarctual areas, before and after drug administration;
    d. Myocardial tissue characterization, by measuring relaxation time T1 and T2.(11)

31P-MRS has also allowed to determine in vivo the anomalous metabolism of high energy phosphates in an infant with hypertrophic cardiomyopathy.(12)

By 13C-MRS and 23Na-MRS we can also go into the study of:

    - Metabolic flows and level variations of some C metabolites, after acetate infusion marked with 13C;
    - Blood pool of excised and perfused hearts (23Na-MRS);
    - Na levels of fibrocells damaged by ischemia.

CONCLUSION

The use of NMR techniques in cardiology is still in its early stage. However, the results obtained so far show that this noninvasive technique can play a great role in providing structural information and in studying cardiac metabolism in vivo, in a well defined spectrum of pathological states.

REFERENCES

1.   Brown JJ, Peterson TM, Slutsky RA (1985). Regional myocardial blood flow, edema formation, and magnetic relaxation times during acute myocardial ischemia in the canine. Invest Radiol, 20, 5,465-471

2.   Wilson JR, Fink L, Maris J, Ferraro N, Power-Vanwart J, Eleff S, Chance B (1985). Evaluation of energy metabolism in skeletal muscle of patients with heart failure with gated phosphorus-31 nuclear magnetic resonance. Circulation, 71, 1, 57-62

3.   Fisher MR, Von Schulthess GK, Higgins CB (1985). Multiphasic cardiac Magnetic Resonance Imaging: normal regional left ventricular wall thickening. Am Journ Rad, 145, 27-30

4.   Friedman BJ, Waters J, Kwan OL, De Maria AN (1985). Comparison of magnetic resonance imaging and echocardiography in determination of cardiac dimension in normal subjects. JACC, 5, 6, 1369-1376

5.   Maron JB, Dwyer AJ, Knop R, Bonow RO, Doppman JL (1985). Efficacy of nuclear magnetic resonance in the diagnosis and the identification of distribution of left ventricular hypertrophy in hypertrophic cardiomyiopathy. JACC, 5, 2, 434

6.   Higgins CB, Byrd III BF, Stark D, McNamara M, Lanzer P, Lipton MJ, Schiller NB, Botvnick E, Chatterjee K (1985). Magnetic Resonance Imaging in hypertrophic cardiomyopathy. Am J Cardiol, 55, 1121-1126

7.   Flak B, Li DKB, Ho BYB, Knickerbocker WJ, Fache S, Mayo J, Chung W (1985). Magnetic Resonance Imaging of aneurysm of the abdominal aorta. Am Journ Radiol, 144, 991-996

8.   Rehr RB, Filipchuk NG, Malloy CR, Peshock RM (1985). Magnetic Resonance Imaging in aortic valve, ascending aortic and isthmic aortic disease. Am J Cardiol, 55, 1243-1244

9.   Johnston DL, Thompson RC, Liu P, Dinsmore RE, Wismer GL, Saini S, Kaul S, Rosen BR, Brady TJ, Okada RD (1986). Magnetic Resonance Imaging during acute myocardial infarction. Am J Cardiol 57, 1059-1065

10.   Brown JJ, Strich G, Higgins CB, Gerber KH, Slutskj RA (1985). Nuclear Magnetic Resonance analysis of acute myocardial infarction in dogs: the effects of transient coronary ischemia of varying duration and reperfusion on spin lattice relaxation times. AHJ, 109, 3 (1), 486-490

11.   Farmer D, Higgins CB, Yee E, Lipton MJ, Wahr D, Ports T (1985). Tissue characterization by magnetic resonance imaging in hypertrophic cardiomyopathy. AJC, 55, 230-232

12.   Whitman GJR, Chance B, Bode H, Maris J, Haselgrove J, Kelley R, Clark B, Harken AH (1985). Diagnosis and therapeutic evaluation of a pediatric case of cardiomyopathy using phosphorus-31 nuclear magnetic resonance spectroscopy. JACC, 5 (3), 745-749.

70
B-Mode echography: a new approach to the epidemiology of atherosclerotic disease?

A. Bucci, L. Lalloni, C. Chiaromonte, C. Stefanutti,
A. Scarno, P. Ricci, L. Azzarri and G. Ricci

Since the 1950s a large body of evidence concerning epidemiological studies aimed at identifying the subjects at high risk of developing atherosclerotic disease and its complications has accumulated.

Among these studies, the most famous is the Framingham Heart Study, which firmly established the relationship between some risk factors and the development of clinical events which can be attributed to atherosclerotic disease. The main limitation of this approach is represented by the difficulty to understand if a clinical end-point (e.g. myocardial infarction, coronary death) is always related to the extension of an unvisualized coronary obstruction.

In fact the possibility that risk factors may act independently of the arterial stenosis and/or obstruction of the vascular bed is a still open question.

In the late 1970s, the introduction of non-invasive diagnostic methods deeply changed the traditional approach to the study of atherosclerosis and its ischaemic sequelae. For a long time the intra-arterial events which occur during the exposure to the established cardiovascular risk factors have been virtually ignored, the overwhelming difficulty being represented by the fact that arterial angiography cannot be proposed to screen and follow large numbers of subjects.

Furthermore, the atherogenic process develops after decades, so that clinical complications involving several vascular beds may occur.

The imaging of the arterial vessel wall with high-resolution real-time B-mode echography can be performed with great accuracy, particularly in the carotid, ilio-femoral and popliteal vascular beds, moreover, the early detection of non-stenosing atherosclerotic lesions can be detected at an early stage.

The atherosclerotic lesion can be studied along longitudinal and cross-sectional scanning planes with respect to the major axis of the vessel.

A dimensional evaluation of the plaque can be attempted.

Data (pictures) can be easily recorded on paper and/or video-cassettes.

Examination of the vascular tree can be easily repeated over time, the lesion evolution can be followed and an attempt to describe the natural history, the progression and/or regression of the atherosclerotic lesion can be made.

The time and size modification of the previously detected echogenic formation during intervention trials with diets and/or drugs can be monitored.

Furthermore, the high-resolution real-time B-mode ultrasonography is substantially safe, non-invasive, quick, relatively inexpensive and can be performed regardless of the individual's body mass index and age.

In 1980, D.H.Blankenhorn suggested that serial angiographies carried out in order to evaluate the size of the atherosclerotic plaque before complications (CHD, CVD, PVD) occur, might potentially decrease the number of subjects to be enrolled in a study aimed at evaluating how modifications of the classical risk factors can change the course of atherosclerosis.

In fact, the classical epidemiological approach requires large samples which are followed for a long time (at least 5-10 years).

The aim is to establish a cause-effect relationship between the characteristics of the subjects enrolled at the beginning of the study and the subsequent development of clinical events.

This is essentially due to the long evolution of the atherosclerotic lesion before haemodynamic effects occur.

The use of high-resolution real-time B-mode echography might potentially change the above-mentioned approach by reducing the number of subjects to be followed.

The dynamic evolution of the plaque could be related to the time-trend of each cardiovascular risk factor. The crucial factors involved in a study devoted to the size evaluation of the atherosclerotic lesion are:

- sample size
- observation period
- measure variability
- size changes of the lesion (progression, regression, no change).

  Bearing in mind these variables we tried to calculate the number of subjects to be followed over time (Table 1).

The following parameters have been taken into account:

- an observation period lasting 1 or 2 years
- a 5% variability of the measure
- a change in plaque size in the range of 1, 2, 4, 6, 8, 10, 15% per year
- correlation between subsequent measures of 0.6 ($r = 0.6$)
- stenosis degree ranging from 5 to 40% (10, 15, 20, 25, 30, 35, 40%).

  These values were chosen on the basis of evidence suggesting that low degree stenoses can change in a relatively short time.

  The accepted statistical significance - one-tailed t-test - was set at $p < 0.05$ (type I error), the statistical power at 0.95% (type II error = 0.05).

Table 1: Number of subjects to be followed for 1 or 2 years to detect changes in lesion size (see text).

%	Yrs	Delta						
		1	2	4	6	8	10	15
5	1	10828,7	2707,2	676,8	300,8	169,2	108,3	48,1
	2	2707,2	676,8	169,2	75,2	42,3	27,1	12,0
10	1	2707,2	676,8	169,2	75,2	42,3	27,1	12,0
	2	676,8	169,2	42,3	18,8	10,6	6,8	3,0
15	1	1203,2	300,8	75,2	33,4	18,8	12,0	5,3
	2	300,8	75,2	18,8	8,3	4,7	3,0	1,3
20	1	676,8	169,2	42,3	18,8	10,6	6,8	3,0
	2	169,2	42,3	10,6	4,7	2,6	1,7	*
25	1	433,1	108,3	27,1	12,0	6,7	4,3	1,9
	2	108,3	27,1	6,8	3,0	1,7	1,1	*
30	1	300,8	75,2	18,8	8,4	4,7	3,0	1,3
	2	75,2	18,8	11,3	2,1	1,2	*	*
35	1	221,0	55,3	13,8	6,1	3,5	2,2	*
	2	55,3	13,8	3,5	1,5	*	*	*
40	1	169,1	42,3	10,6	4,7	2,6	1,7	*
	2	42,3	10,6	2,6	1,2	*	*	*

%: stenosis percent
*: less than 1 subject

Table 2 shows the multiplying-factors to be applied to the number of subjects, taking into account a variability of 10-15-20% and different correlation between measures of (r = 0.7,0.8,0.9).

Table 2 (see text)

r	Variability (%)			
	5	10	15	20
0,6	1	4	9	16
0,7	1,3	5,3	12	21,3
0,8	2	8	18	32
0,9	4	16	32	64

It is clear from Tables 1 and 2 that the number of subjects to be followed is generally lower than that ordinarily needed in classical epidemiological studies for any of the hypotheses assumed.

Bearing in mind the above considerations, in 1984 we carried out a cross-sectional study of the atherosclerotic lesion in the carotid vascular bed of a randomly selected sample, representative of a free-living population in Central Italy (Priverno, Latina).

473 male and female subjects aged 45-64 years were screened with B-mode echography.

This work was supported by a grant from the Italian National Research Council - Special Project: Preventive Medicine and Rehabilitation - SP4; Research Line: Progression and regression of the atherosclerotic lesion.

Tables 3 and 4 show the age-related prevalence, by age groups of the atherosclerotic lesion in the carotid vascular bed.

Table 3: Male subjects: age-related prevalence of atherosclerotic lesions in carotid vascular beds

Age (years)	Lesions (n)	Absence of lesions (n)	Prevalence (%)
45-54	23	96	19.32
55-64	26	62	29.54
45-64	49	158	23.78

In 1987 these subjects will be submitted to a new examination to assess the incidence of the atherosclerotic lesion in the same vascular beds and, if possible, the progression and/or regression of the previously detected lesions.

Table 4: Female subjects: age-related prevalence of atherosclerotic lesions in carotid vascular beds.

Age (years)	Lesions (n)	Absence of lesions (n)	Prevalence (%)
45-54	26	108	19.40
55-64	32	77	29.35
45-64	58	185	23.86

ACKNOWLEDGEMENT

This work was partially supported by a grant from the Italian National Research Council (C.N.R. - Progetto Finalizzato "Medicina Preventiva e Riabilitativa", Sottoprogetto SP4 "Malattie degenerative", Obiettivo 44).

References

1. Blankenhorn, DH, Brooks, SH, Seltzer, RH, and Barndt, R (1978). The rate of atherosclerosis change during treatment of hyperlipoproteinemia. Circulation, 57, 355

2. Blankenhorn, DH and Curry, PI (1982). The accuracy of arteriography and ultrasound imaging for atherosclerosis measurement: a review. Arch. Pathol. Lab. Med., 106, 483

3. Cohen, J (1977). Statistical Power Analysis for the Behavioural Sciences. (New York: Academic Press)

4. Harlan, WR and Landis, JR (1981). What the epidemiologist and clinical interventionist expect and need for studies of atherosclerotic disease. In: Budinger, TE, Besson, AS, Ringqvist, I, Mock, MB, Watson, JT and Pawell, RS, (eds) Non Invasive Diagnostic Techniques for Assessment of Atherosclerosis in Peripheral, Carotid and Coronary Arteries. (New York: Raven Press)

5. Karmel, WB, Gordon, T and Sorlie, P (1971). The Framingham study: an epidemiological investigation of cardiovascular disease. Section 27: coronary heart disease, atherosclerotic brain infarction, intermittent claudication - a multivariate analysis of some factors related to their incidence: Framingham study, 16 year follow up. (Washington D.C.: Government Printing Office)

6. Peterson, RE, Livingstone, KE and Escobar, H (1960). Development and distribution of gross atherosclerotic lesions at cervical carotid bifurcation. Neurology, 10, 955

7. Schwarts, CJ and Mitchell, JRA (1962). Observation on localization of arterial plaques. Circ. Res., 11, 63
8. Solberg, LA and Strong, JP (1983). Risk factors and atherosclerotic lesions. Arteriosclerosis, 3, 187
9. Solberg, LA, Strong, JP, Holme, I, Helgeland, A, Hsermann, I, Leren, P and Mogensen, SvB (1985). Stenosis in the coronary arteries. Relation to atherosclerotic lesions, coronary heart disease and risk factors. The Oslo Study. Lab. Invest., 6, 648

71
Cardiac doppler in the assessment of aortic valvular diseases
T. Bombardini, C.F. Manetti and F. Zacà

Doppler method allows an exact evaluation of flow velocity curves inside arterial and venous vessels.The maximal flow velocity along the direction of the exploring beam is measured by continous wave doppler. The velocity in the section explored by sample volume is measured by pulsed wave doppler.If we consider doppler formula:

(1) Doppler shift=2F0*(V Cosϑ)/C

in order to exactly measure blood flow velocity it is necessary to get an exact alignment between the exploring beam and the flow direction.

Blood flow velocity can be measured also in ascending and descending aorta and in heart chambers. Using the following formula:

(2) P2-P1=(V2^2-V1^2) (Modified Bernoulli)

and measuring transaortic flow velocity by cardiac doppler we can exactly calculate the pressure drop(mmhg) in correspondence of an aortic stenosis(1-2).

The exploring probe is generally positioned on the thoracic wall using the apical window:this approach allows a good alignment between the exploring beam and the flow direction in aortic stenosis.The suprasternal window is generally used only in young patients because the verticality of ascending aorta makes this kind of approach useful.The right parasternal window is used in patients with orizontal or ecthasic ascending aorta.

Using the flow velocity curve we calculate instantaneous peak pressure drop by means of the above mentioned formula(2);a further criterium of evaluation of an aortic stenosis is considering the time to peak on the velocity curve in ascending aorta:the longer it is,greater is entity of the stenosis.

In cath.laboratories the peak-to-peak pressure drop is used for the evaluation of an aortic stenosis:this measured pressure drop is not an instantaneous gradient because sistolic peak pressure isn't reached in the

same moment in left ventricle as in the ascending aorta(3).
Instantaneous peak pressure drops measured by cardiac doppler are generally greater than peak-to-peak pressure drops measured by heart catheterization(4).
Many authors have proved a good correlation between cath.peak-to-peak pressure drop and mean pressure drop as measured by the doppler method(5-6).Doppler mean pressure drop is calculated using the following formula:
    (3)   Mean PD(mmhg)=4(V1^2+V2^2+V3^2+...Vn^2)/n
in this formula is utilized the mean value of isntantaneous squared peak flow velocity during the entire sistolic ejection time(Fig.1).

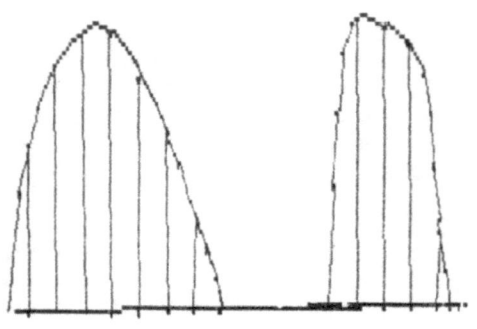

$$\text{Mean P.D.(mm.Hg)} = 4\ \frac{(V1^2 + V2^2 + V3^2 + \ldots Vn^2)}{N}$$

Fig.1-DOPPLER MEAN PRESSURE DROP.

We studied by cardiac doppler method thirty patients who already underwent to heart catheterization;we compared cath.peak-to-peak pressure drops to peak doppler and to mean doppler pressure drops by statistical analysis with simple linear regression tests and we found the following regression equations:
    Cath.peak-to-peakPD(mmhg)=0.8*peak dopplerPD-10.5
    Cath.peak-to-peakPD(mmhg)=0.97*mean dopplerPD+6.6
    Doppler meanPD   (mmhg)=0.8 *peak dopplerPD-14.9
In our study too we found a good correlation (R=0.87)between cath.peak-to-peak pressure drops and mean doppler pressure drops(Fig.2):that's why in daily clinical practice we use mean doppler gradients for the

evaluation of the gravity of an aortic stenosis.
In the evaluation of the transaortic pressure drop we
must consider the variations of cardiac output;in fact
also little variations of cardiac output cause sensible
modifications of transaortic gradients,especially in
closed stenoses(AVA <0.6CM2);therefore the most useful
date in aortic stenosis is the AVA(7-8-9-10).
In cardiac doppler method Gorlin formula:
    (4)   AVA=CO/44.5*SEP*V P2-P1
can be utilized measuring the cardiac output in LVOT
and calculating the SEP on aortic velocity curves.

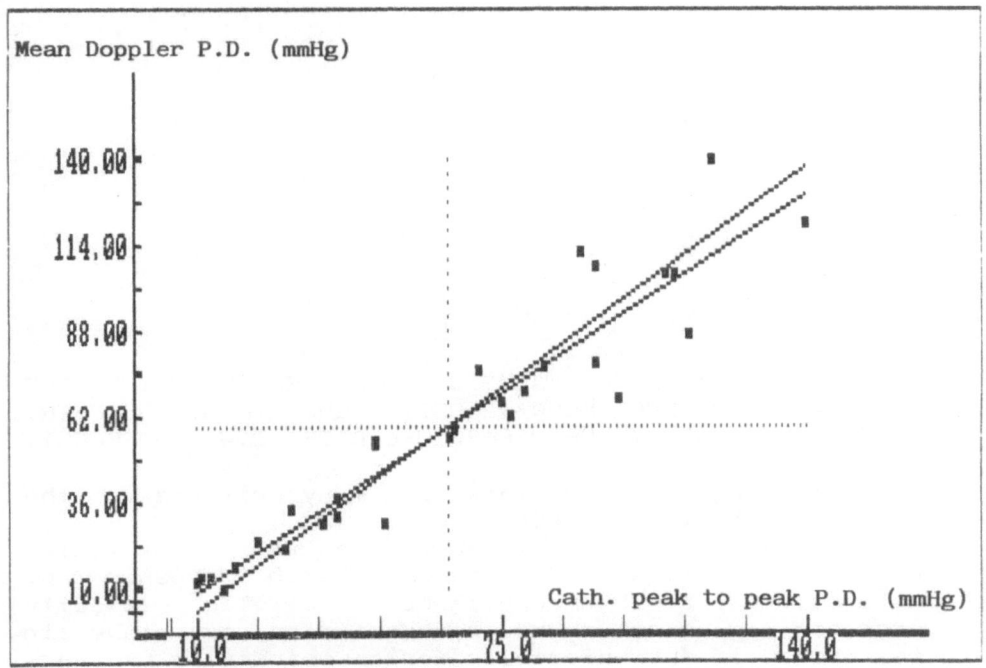

Fig.2-CORRELATION BETWEEN CATH. PEAK TO PEAK PRESSURE
DROPS AND DOPPLER MEAN PRESSURE DROPS IN 30 PATIENS
WITH AORTIC STENOSIS.

Others authors suggest the use of the following
formula:
    (5)   AVA=A*INT.V(t)/INT.V1(t)
AVA=aortic valve area   A =LVOT area
introducing a correction factor because in presence of
laminar flow with a flat profile we can consider

instantaneous maximal velocity=instantaneous mean
velocity:on the contrary in the presence of an aortic
jet it is necessary to have instantaneous mean
velocities(11-12-13)(Fig.3).

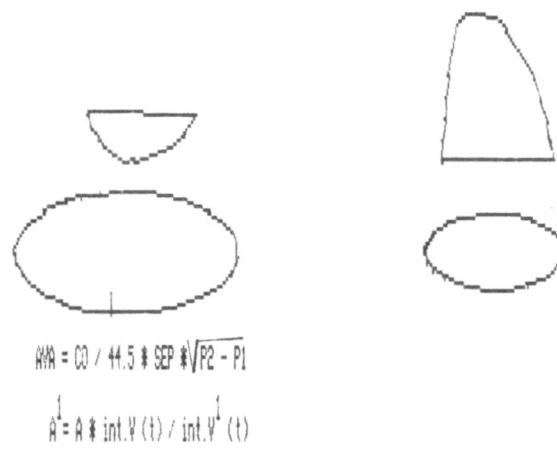

$$AVA = CO / 44.5 * SEP * \sqrt{P2 - P1}$$

$$A^1 = A * int.V(t) / int.V^1(t)$$

Fig.3-CALCULATION OF AORTIC VALVE AREA MEASURING THE
LVOT AREA,THE LVOT FLOW VELOCITY CURVE(P.W. DOPPLER)
AND THE TRANSAORTIC MEAN PRESSURE DROP (C.W. DOPPLER).

In aortic regurgitation there are many criteria for the
evaluation of the disease:
I-We analize the diastolic aorta ventricular
regurgitant flow velocity curve:in absence of
alterations of LV compliance diastolic velocity
decrease is greater when regurgitation is higher;in
this case in fact diastolic aorto-ventricular pressure
drop decreases faster.
II-By P.W. doppler we explore LVOT and LV from aortic
anulus to ventricular apex:thelonger the distance
reached by the regurgitant jet from aortic anulus
the higher is the valvular insufficiency.
III-We evaluate the transmitralic diastolic flow
velocity curve and protodiastolic and telediastolic
peak velocities:in presence of higher aortic
regurgitation with increased LVEDP atrial contribution
to ventricular filling becomes more important than
usual and telediastolic flow velocity increases.
IV-We perform by P.W. doppler a scanning of ascending
and descending aorta testing the presence,the entity
and the distance from the valvular anulus of the

diastolic reverse flow.
V-We test the presence of diastolic reverse flow in
subclavian arteries and in common carotid arteries.
By using the above mentioned methods it is possible to
classify aortic regurgitation in four classes
corresponding to the angiocardiographic data in our
patients.
Different methods are suggested for a quantifying
evaluation of aortic regurgitations(14-15-16):we utlize
the ratio of diastolic time velocity integral to
sistolic time velocity integral ratio as measured by
P.W.doppler in aortic isthmus to calculate ARF(Fig.4).

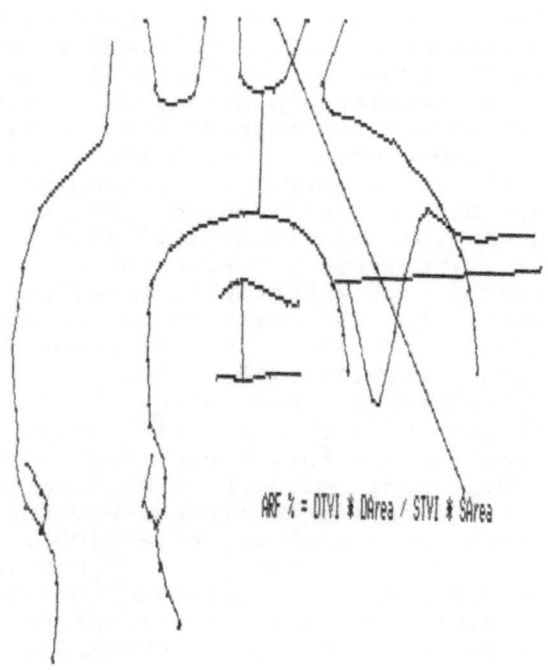

ARF % = DTVI * DArea / STVI * SArea

Fig.4-CALCULATION OF AORTIC REGURGITANT FRACTION BY
MEASURING SYSTOLIC TIME VELOCITY INTEGRAL AND DIASTOLIC
TIME VELOCITY INTEGRAL.

REFERENCES:
1)Hatle L.,Angelsen B.:Doppler Ultrasound in
Cardiology.Phisical Principles and Clinical

Applications.Second Edition.Lea & Febiger.
Philadelphia.1985.
2)Hatle L.,Angelsen B.,Tromsdal A.:Non-invasive
assesment of aortic stenosis by Doppler
ultrasound.British Heart Journal 43:284,1980.
3)Currie P.J.,Seward B.J.,Reeder G.S.,Vliestra
R.E.,Bresnahan D.R.,Bresnahan J.F.,Smith H.C.,Hagler
D.J.,and Tajik A.J.:Continuous-wave Doppler
echocardiographic assesment of severity of calcific
aortic stenosis:a simultaneous Doppler-catheter
correlative study in 100 adult patients.Circulation
71:1162,1985.
4)Krafchek J.,Robertson J.H.,Radford M.,Adams D.,Kisslo
J:A reconsideration of Doppler assessed gradients in
suspected aortic stenosis.Am Heart J 110:765,1985.
5)Agatson A.S.,Chengot M.,Rao A.,Hildner F.,Samet
P:Doppler diagnosis of valvular aortic stenosis in
patients over 60 years of age.Am J Cardiol 56:106,1985.
6)Smith M.D.,Dawson P.L.,Elion J.L.,Wisenbaugh T.,Kwan
O.L.,Handshoe S.,DeMaria A.N.:Systematic correlation of
continous-wave Doppler and hemodynamic measurements in
patients with aortic stenosis.Am Heart J 111:245,1986.
7)Skiarpe T.,Hegrenaes L.,Hatle L.:Noninvasive
estimation of valve area in patients with aortic
stenosis by Doppler ultrasound and two-dimensional
echocardiography.Circulation 72:810,1985.
8)Seitz W.S.,McIlroy M.B.,Kline H.,Operschall
J.,and Kashani I.A:Echographic application of the
Gorlin formula for assessment of aortic stenosis:
Correlation with cardiac catheterization in pediatric
patients. Am Heart J 111:1118, 1986.
9)Warth D.C.,Stewart W.J.,Block P.C.,and Weyman
A.E:A new method to calculate aortic valve area without
left heart catheterization. Circulation 70:978,1984.
10)Ramirez M.L.,Wong M.,Shah P.M: Subcostal Window:A
New Portal for Recording Continuous-Wave Doppler Aortic
Flow Velocities. Am J Cardiol 56:199,1985.
11)Kawanishi D.T.,McKay C.R.,Chandraratna
P.A.N.,Nanna M.,Reid C.L.,Elkayam U.,Siegel M.,and
Rahimtoola S.H: Cardiovascular response to dynamic
exercise in patients with chronic symptomatic mild-to-
moderate and severe aortic regurgitation. Circulation
73:62,1986.
12)Wallmeyer K.,Wann L.S.,Sagar K.B.,Kalbfleisch
J.,and Klopfenstein S:The influence of preload and
heart rate on Doppler echocardiographic indexes of left
ventricular performance: comparison with invasive
indexes in an experimental preparation. Circulation
74:181,1986.
13)Wisenbaugh T.,Booth D.,DeMaria A.,Nissen S.,and
Waters J:Relationship of concractile state to ejection
performance in patients with chronic aortic valve
disease. Circulation 73:47,1986.

14)Goldberg   S.J.,and   Allen   H.D.:Quantitative Assessment by Doppler Echocardiography of Pulmonary or Aortic Regurgitation. Am J Cardiol 56:131:1985.
15)Touche   T.,Prasquier   R.,Nitenberg   A.,Zuttere D.,and Gourgon R.:Assessment and follow-up of patients with   aortic regurgitation by an updated Doppler echocardiographic   measurement of   the   regurgitant fraction in the aortic arch. Circulation 72:819,1985.
16)Kitabatake   A.,Ito   H.,Inoue   M.,Tanouchi J.,Ishihara   K.,Morita   T.,Fujii   K.,Yoshida Y.,Masuyama   T.,Yoshima H.,Hori M.,and Kamada   T.:A new   approach to noninvasive evaluation of aortic regurgitant   fraction   by   two-dimensional   Doppler echocardiography. Circulation 72:523,1985.

72
Myocardial ischemia in pediatric age: clinical pictures and non-invasive assessment

D. Prandstraller, F.M. Picchio, P.M. Benenati,
M. Ferlito, C. Rapezzi, F. Tartagni and B. Magnani

SUMMARY

From 1978 to 1986 we reviewed clinical, noninvasive and angiographic data of 734 pts with congenital heart disease (CHD), looking for evidence of myocardial ischemia (MI). Thirteen pts (= 1.8%) were identified: 3 pts with abnormal congenital coronary origin (ACCO), 7 pts with transient neonatal myocardial ischemia (TNMI) and 3 pts with pulmonary atresia with intact ventricular septum (PAIVS).

The usefulness of the various noninvasive techniques in the evaluation of MI, and in particular of basal electrocardiogram, BD-echocardiogram and Tl 201 angioscintigraphy is discussed.

INTRODUCTION

Notwithstanding its lack of precise pathopysiological characterization, MI is fairly common in pediatric age and rather important in affecting the natural history of many different situations [1,3,4,8,9,10,11] (Table I).

In the last few years the improved survival of critically ill newborns and the better surgical changes in complex CHD have required a highly accurate definition of MI. Noninvasive techniques have proven to be most useful because of their accuracy and repeatibility [1,12]. Aim of the present study is the definition of frequency and clinical significance of MI in pediatric age.

Table I. Myocardial ischemia in pediatric age

<u>MI associated with coronary arteries anomalies</u>

- abnormal congenital coronary origin
- coronary fistulae

<u>Mi associated with structural malformations of the heart</u>

- pulmonary atresia with intact ventricular septum
- truncus arteriosus communis
- aortic stenosis
- cyanotic congenital heart disease
- jatrogenic (surgical) coronary lesions
- others

<u>MI without structural malformations of the heart</u>

- transient neonatal myocardial ischemia
- perinatal asphyxia and hypoxemia
- persistence of fetal circulation
- primary coronary thrombosis
- venous thromboembolism
- erythroblastosis
- disseminated intravascular coagulation

- Kawasaki's syndrome
- familial hypercholesterolemia
- progeria

MATERIALS AND METHODS

From 1978 to 1985 we reviewed 734 consecutive pediatric pts, referred to the Cardiology Institute of the University of Bologna for CHD. All of them underwent complete clinical evaluation, Chest X ray, electrocardiogram and BD-echocardiogram. Tl 201 angioscintigraphy was also performed when indicated.

We have defined MI according to the following restrictive criteria:
- myocardial infarction (M. inf.) patterns and/or acute MI on basal electrocardiogram;
- reversible perfusion defects on Tl 201 angioscintigraphy;
- segmental contraction abnormalities related to a definite coronary anomaly.

544

RESULTS

Thirteen pts, aging 1 day to 14 years, met the criteria for MI and were divided into three groups.

GROUP 1: 3 pts with ACCO. They presented with quite different clinical problems and their data are summarized in table II. All pts revealed segmental, reversible, hypocaptation on Tl 201 angioscintigraphy, spatially related to M. inf. areas on basal electrocardiogram. BD-echocardiogram showed a huge antero-lateral and apical left ventricular aneurysm in one pt, a severe left atrial and ventricular dilatation in another and a trivial subaortic diaphragm without abnormality of contraction in the third pt. All pts underwent successful revascularization procedures (subclavian-coronary artery bypass) with 0% mortality. On post-operative control all pts showed an improvement of Tl 201 uptake. In particular 2 out of 3 pts, normali zed Tl 201 patterns, while a small apical defect persisted in the third pt (case 2).

GROUP 2: 7 pts with TNMI. All pts showed acute MI on basal electrocardiogram: acute inferior M. inf. in 1 pt; acute anterior M. inf. in 1 pt; acute subendocardial MI (V_3R-V_4) in 4 pts and acute subepicardial MI in 1 pt. Clinical and laboratory data are summarized in Table III In all cases echocardiogram ruled out the presence of cardiac malformations. Medical treatment with digitalis diuretics and O_2 led to a successful clinical improvement in 6/7 pts (86%) with gradual normalization of the electrocardiogram. Only 1 pt died because of refractory heart failure.

GROUP 3: we identified 3 pts with PAIVS and evidence of sinusoids causing perfusion anomalies of left ventricle. They represented 43% of all pts with PAIVS observed. Deeply cyanosed at birth they all had a complete BD-echocardiogram and angiographic evaluation. Hypokinetic areas of one or two segments of left ventricle were present at angiography together with myocardial sinusoids with left ventricle to right coronary artery fistulae. The electrocardiogram showed ischemic patterns in all pts with PAIVS regardless of the presence of sinusoids. No Tl 201 study was performed in neonatal age. 2 pts died following palliative procedures. 1 pts is alive 15 months later and is waiting for corrective surgery.

Table III: Clinical data of pts with TNMI

7 pts: 6 ♀   1 ♂
Age at onset of symptoms:
Basal PaO$_2$ (mmHg):   33-49   (47$\pm$11)
   "   PaCO$_2$ "   :   31-49   (38.8+9.5)
   "   pH   :7.08-7.30 (7.24$\pm$0.10)
pts with tricuspid insufficiency: 4/7 (57%)
   "   "   heart failure: 5/7 (71%)
   "   "   respiratory distress: 4/7 (57%)
Time of normalization of ECG (days): 6,38 (18.7$\pm$18)

Outcome: 6 pts alive without signs of heart disease (86%)
         1 pt died at 6 days of refractory heart failure

DISCUSSION AND CONCLUSIONS
     The presence of MI is a rare but not exceptional
problem. In the pts of groups 1 e 2, ischemia is
the main determinant of the entire clinical picture.
Generally speaking, MI in pediatric age can have
three different types of clinical presentation.
Beside angina and heart failure, which are typical
ischemic pictures also in adults, cyanosis can
be a direct consequence of ischemia in TNMI because:
A) Many of these newborns present with predominant
   respiratory distress [10];
B) High mean right atrial pressure, which is constant
   in TNMI, determines tricuspid insufficiency
   and right to left shunt through foramen ovale.
Differential diagnosis (d.d.) is particularly challenging
in ACCO and TNMI.
ACCO has to be distinguished from early onset dilatati-
ve cardiomyopathy (DCMP) and from congenital mitral
insufficiency. BD-ecocardiogram is of little value
whereas Tl 201-scan plays a more important role.
We tested the diagnostic accuracy and specificity
of Tl 201 in the d.d. between ACCO and DCMP (10
pediatric pts). Two out of 10 pts with DCMP (=20%)
showed perfusion defects but in no case was the
defect reversible, while the 3 pts with ACCO had
reversible perfusion defects (100% specificity).
In ACCO left ventricular failure is due to volume
overload (aorto-pulmonary shunt though intracoronary
anastomoses) and chronic ischemia (territory of
distribution of left coronary artery). Revascularization procedures are followed by a brilliant functional

TABLE II: Clinical data of pts with ACCO

Pt	Age	Diagnosis	Clinical picture	ECG	BD-Echo	Tl 201 scintigraphy
Case S.G.♂ 1	3 m	LCA from PA	Heart failure	Acute M.inf. (extensive anterior)	LV aneurysm (antero-la-teral apical)	↓uptake (antero-lateral apical)
Case E.G.♂ 2	6 m	LCA from PA	Heart failure mitral insuffi-ciency	M.inf. (late-ral) LV hy-pertrophy	LA+LV dilata-tion	↓uptake (antero-lateral apical)
Case P.F.♂ 3	14 a	Circumflex from PA subaortic diaphragm	Exertional an-gina	LV hypertro-phy and strain	Subaortic dia-phragm normal contraction	↓uptake (poste-ro lateral)

LCA = left coronary artery; PA = pulmonary artery; LV = left ventricular; ↓ = decreased

recovery provided that no extensive M. inf. has occurred [5,6,7].
In TNMI the diagnostic goal is the d.d. with cyanotic congenital heart defects. Echocardiogram has the highest sensibility [12], while Tl 201 scintigraphy results in diffuse omogeneous perfusion defect 2 . TNMI often presents as a complex clinical picture with respiratory problems and must always be taken into account in the newborn with cyanosis and/or heart failure [10].
In PAIVS MI is essentially due to sinusoids [3,9]. Right ventricular pressure exceeds systemic pressure, thus conditioning intramyocardial sinusoids persistence and anastomoses with the coronary district [4,8]. In this way the abnormal perfusion pattern affects left ventricle and can influence the natural history of the disease. Ecocardiogram and angiography are essential in neonatal age, while Tl 201 scintigraphy has the greatest importance in long term evaluation of pts, especially before corrective surgery.

REFERENCES
1. Bernstein D, Finkbeiner WE, Soifer S and Teitel D(1986) Perinatal myocardial infarction: a case report and review of the literature. Pediatr Cardiol, 6, 313
2. Finley JP, Howman Giles RB, Gilday PL and Rowe RD(1979) Transient myocardial ischaemia in the newborn infant demonstrated by thallium imaging. J Pediatr, 94, 263
3. Freedom RM and Harringhton DP (1974). Contributions of intramyocardial sinusoids in pulmonary atresia and intact ventricular septum to a right-sided circular shunt Br Heart J, 36, 1061
4. Gobel FL, Anderson CF, Baltaxe HA, Amplatz K and Wang Y (1970). Shunt between the coronary and pulmonary arteries with normal origin of the coronary arteries. Am J Cardiol, 25, 655
5. Laborde F, Marchand M, Leca F, Jarreau NM, Dequirot A and Hazan E (1981). Surgical treatment of anomalous origin of the left coronary artery in infancy and chilwood: early and late results in 20 consecutive cases.J Thorac Cardiovasc Surg 82, 423
6. Levitsky S, Van Der Horst RL, Hastreiter AR and Fisher EA (1980). Anomalous left coronary artery in the infant. Recovery of ventricular function following early direct aortic implantation. J Thorac Cardiovasc Surg, 70, 598
7. Pursky WW, Fagan LR, Mudd JFG and William VL (1976)

Subclavian-coronary artery anastomosis in infancy for
the Bland-White-Garland Syndrome. A three year and five
year follow-up. J Thorac Cardiovasc Surg, 72, 15
8. Rose AG (1978). Multiple coronary arterioventricular
fistulae. Circulation, 57, 178
9. Rowe GG (1970). Inequalities of myocardial perfusion
in coronary disease ("coronary steal"). Circulation, 42,
193
10. Rowe AD, Izukawa T, Olley PM, Freedom RM and Swyer
PR (1981). Abnormalities of the cardiovascular transition of the newborn: current views on vascular and myocardial responses. In: Godman MJ (ed)."Paediatric Cardiology" vol. 4 p.236 (Churcill Livingstone Press)
11. Thiene G, Angelini A, Carini A, Cefis F, Frescura C
and Baroldi G (1986). Juvenile Atherosclerosis in
Northen Italy: a post morten study. In: Doyle EF, Engle
MA, Gersony WM, Rashkind W and Talner NS (eds.) "Pediatric Cardiology" p. 1187 (New York: Springer-Verlag
Press.)
12. Williams RG and Tucker CR (1977). "Echocardiographic
diagnosis of congenital heart disease". (Boston: Little
Brown and Co. Press.)

73
Extracranial carotid atherosclerosis evolution and stroke occurrence: Role of the echotomographic analysis

U. Senin, L. Parnetti, G. Lupattelli, A. Susta,
M. Mercuri and G. Ciuffetti

INTRODUCTION

Thrombo-embolism caused by atheromasic plaques in the carotid artery has been recognized as one of the many causes of ischemic stroke (De Bono and Warlow, 1981).

The carotid atheromasic plaque is most frequently localized in the extracranial tract, especially at the bifurcation (Hass et al., 1968). This is why endoarterectomy is often proposed for stroke prevention in patients affected by plaques located in this area (Barnet 1984). Since the efficacy of this type of surgery in stroke prevention is not really understood, the identification of lesions most prone to progression is of extreme importance. This is possible today because of the availability of ultrasound imaging systems for vascular diagnosis, which are particularly suitable for the study of this vascular tract (Comerota et al., 1981).

We report here the results of a 2 year longitudinal study using real-time B-mode ultrasound echotomography on patients affected by atheromasic plaques in the extracranial carotid tract.

MATERIALS AND METHODS

This study was carried out on 118 extracranial carotid tract lesions observed in 70 patients (59 male, 11 female, average age 61 ± 7 years) referred to our Centre for Non-Invasive Vascular Diagnosis for TIA, CHD, PAD, cervical bruits. 19 patients were affected by only one of these conditions, 51 patients by two or more.

61 patients were suffering from one or more of the major atherosclerosis risk factors (hypercholesterolemia, diabetes mellitus, hypertension, cigarette smoking).

Exclusion criteria were atheromatous lesions causing a degree of vascular stenosis greater than 60% and cholesterol levels >300 mg/dl because those patients were admitted to pharmaceutical and/or surgical trials. We have also excluded lesions with a stenosis degree of less than 15%, because, in our experience, their echo-structure could not always be well defined. Treatment of the patients admitted to our follow-up was left to the discretion of the referring physician. Particular attention was paid to 10 (9 male, 1 female) patients who during the follow-up suffered a clinical cerebrovascular episode and/or carotid occlusion. The attendant risk factors for atherosclerosis and the nature of the plaques present were carefully analysed in these cases. During the 2 year follow-up ultrasound studies were performed every six months and in any case, immediately after the clinical event.

Instrumental Equipment:

The echotomographic analysis of the lesions was carried out using a Biosound with an electromechanical probe of 4 cm/8 MHz, the axial resolution being 0.3 mm and the lateral resolution 0.5 mm.

During the two year follow-up ultrasound studies were carried out at least every six months, and in any case, immediately after the clinical event.

The patient's position and the scanning planes used were standard for the ultrasound imaging of the carotid bifurcation (Wolverson et al., 1983).

Lesion Characteristics Monitored: echogenicity, surface aspects and stenosis degree.

Echogenicity: Plaques were subdivided into 4 echogenic patterns - "soft", "intermediate", "mixed" and "hard". The "soft" were low-reflecting lesions, the "intermediate" reflected moderately, the "mixed" showed a non-homogenous echogenicity with or without a shadow cone, the "hard" were extremely high-reflecting accompanied by a black shadow.

Surface aspects: Regular or irregular.

Stenosis Degree: This was calculated using the following formula:

$$\frac{D_t - D_r}{D_t} \times 100$$

where D_t = the total diameter of the vessel lumen and
D_r = the residual diameter, both being calculated at the maximal extrinsic point of the lesion.

The lesions were then subdivided into three classes of stenosis: 15 - 30%, 31 - 50% and 51 - 60%.

Validation Study on Real-time (B-Mode) Ultrasound

This method of defining the stenosis degree was validated by a comparison with both angiographic findings (Senin et al., 1986) and histomorphometric tests on endoarterectomy samples (Tanganelli et al., 1986; Weber et al., 1986). Intra- and inter-observed reliability for both the stenosis degree and the echogenic characteristics of the lesions, through 'blind' readings of the video echographic images was calculated using the variation coefficient.

Evolution Index

Lesions were considered modified if the echogenic pattern changed and/or if the percentage variation of the stenosis was at least ± 8%. (Intra- and inter-observer variation coefficient for the stenosis degree ± 5%).

RESULTS

8 of the 70 patients studied (7 male, 1 female, average age 61 ± 5) suffered a clinical cerebrovascular episode: 5 TIAs, 2 strokes, 1 multi-infarct dementia (MID) in the course of the follow-up. Table 1 reports the extracranial carotid atherosclerosis profile observed immediately after the clinical event and/or occlusion.

TAB.1 EXTRACRANIAL CAROTID ATHEROSCLEROSIS PROFILE OBSERVED AT THE CLINICAL EVENT.

N.	Pts.	Clinical Events	Echopattern			% stenosis degree
1	B.D.	TIA	unilat	inter	regular	21 - 30
2	M.P.E.	TIA	unilat	inter	irregular*	31 - 40
3	S.An	TIA	unilat	inter	regular	21 - 30
4	S.Al.	TIA	bilat	hard	irregular*	31 - 40
			"	inter	regular	31 - 40
5	A.A.	TIA	unilat	inter	regular	51 - 60
6	C.R.	Stroke	unilat	inter	regular	31 - 40
7	F.F.	Stroke	unilat		occlusion*	
8	F.I.	MID	bilat		occlusion	
				inter	regular	31 - 40
				hard	regular	10 - 20
9	B.U.	/	bilat	inter	regular	41 - 50
					occlusion	
10	R.G.	/	unilat	inter	occlusion	

* ipselateral to the ischemic event

We therefore analysed the behaviour of plaques probably related to clinical events and/or occlusion, and Table 2 gives the results of our analysis. As one can see, 5 of the 6 lesions were mixed and 4 of these had irregular surfaces; 3 had a stenosis degree of more than 50%. In the first case reported in the table, the plaque modification from regular to irregular is worth noting. A general analysis was therefore performed on the 118 plaques under observation with the aim of identifying the importance of the echogenic pattern in lesion growth. Lesions most prone to modifications in their echogenic pattern are low-reflecting (soft, 70%), but their stenosis degree remained quite stable (in fact, 65% of the soft and 80% of the intermediate were unchanged). On the other hand, plaques least subject to echogenic pattern changes were high-reflecting lesions (mixed and hard). A strong tendency to increase the stenosis degree was observed in these plaques.(In 46% of the mixed and in 50% of the hard the stenosis degree increased during our 2 year follow-up). The influence of surface characteristics must not be underestimated. In fact, in 42% of the plaques with an irregular surface the stenosis degree increased, but this increase was documented in only 27% of the regular surfaced lesions. Finally, an initial stenosis degree >50% seems to lead to a greater plaque progression even if we studied few cases in this category (N.6).

TAB. 2 BEHAVIOUR OF PLAQUES PROBABLY RELATED TO CLINICAL EVENTS AND/ OR OCCLUSION

N.	Pts.	Clinical Events	Plaque Profile	
			Last check-up	At the clinical events and/or occlusion
2	M.P.E.	TIA	intermediate regular 21 - 30%	intermediate irregular 31 - 40%
4	S.A1	TIA	mixed irregular 31 - 40%	hard irregular 31 - 40%
7	F.F.	Stroke	mixed regular 31 - 40%	occlusion
8	F.I.	MID	mixed irregular 51 - 60%	occlusion
9	B.U.		mixed irregular 51 - 60%	occlusion
10	R.G.		irregular 51 - 60%	occlusion

We considered age and the major atherosclerotic risk factors as possible extrinsic influences on plaque progression and echogenic pattern modifications. In the former, patients with progressed lesions were significantly older (64 ± 7 years vs. 58 ± 7, $p<0.01$) and 59% of them were affected by two or more risk factors; in the second case the most important fact emerging is that diabetes mellitus is recurrent in patients with mixed and hard plaques, which are the complicated lesions.

CONCLUSIONS

The results we have presented permit two speculations. The first is that different evolutive trend may be defined on the basis of the echogenic characteristics of the plaque under observation. The regular surfaced intermediate plaque usually shows a slight progressive trend; this becomes marked for irregular surfaced and mixed plaques.

The second speculation lies in our attempt to delineate the risk profile for clinical events and/or occlusions for patients with extracranial carotid atherosclerosis. The elements of this profile are the presence of irregular surfaced and mixed plaques, bilateral atheromasic lesions, especially if multiple; two or more of the major atherosclerosis risk factors and, perhaps, being over 60 years of age.

REFERENCES

1. Barnet, HJM, Plum, F and Walton, JN (1984).Carotid endarterectomy-An expression of concern.Stroke, 15, 941.
2. Comerota, A, Cranley, J and Cook, S (1981).Real time B-Mode carotid imaging in diagnosis of cerebrovascular disease.Surgery, 86, 718.
3. De Bono, DP and Warlow, CP (1981).Potential sources of emboli in patients with presumed transient cerebral or retinal ischaemia. Lancet, 1, 343.
4. Hass, WK, Fields, WS, North, RR, Kricheff, II, Chase, NE and Bauer, RB (1968).Joint study of extracranial arterial occlusion. II.Arteriography, techniques, sites and complications.JAMA, 203, 961.
5. Senin, U, Mannarino, E, Susta, A, Ciuffetti, G, Parnetti, L, Floridi, P, Pelliccioli, P and Signorini, E (1986).Echotomographic extracranial carotid evaluation in amaurosis fugax, hemispheric TIA and stroke patients.In: Ventura, A, Crepaldi, G and Senin, U (eds)"Extracoronary atherosclerosis".p 94.(Basel: Karger).
6. Tanganelli, P, Bianciardi, G, Cao, PG, Centi, L, Moggi, L, Novelli, MT, Pelliccioli, G, Senin, U, Signorini, E, Susta, A, Tazza, D and Toti, P (1986).Carotid atherosclerotic lesions: comparati-

ve evaluation of echotomographic, histomorphometric and angio-
graphic data of endoarterectomy samples.In: Ventura, A, Crepaldi
G and Senin, U (eds)"Extracoronary atherosclerosis".p.189.(Basel
Karger).

7. Weber, G, Bianciardi, G, Centi, L, Novelli, MT, Reri, L, Salvi,
    M, Toti, p and Tanganelli, P (1986).Comparative studies of cere-
    bral atherosclerosis: observation on endoarterectomy in man.In:
    Fidge, NH and Nestel, PJ (eds)"Atherosclerosis VII".p.593.(Amst-
    erdam: Excerpta medica).
8. Wolverson, MK, Bashiti, HM and Peterson, GJ (1983).Ultrasonic
    tissue characterization of atheromatous plaques using a high re-
    solution real time scanner.Ultrasound in med. & biol., 9, 599.

Acknowledgments:the Authors would like to thank Mrs.G.A.BOYD - MAN-
              CINELLI B.A. (hons) for her help in the translation
              of this paper.

74
Pre- and post-operative echotomography and aortic endoarterectomy

A. Stella, B.I. Cifiello, M. Gessardi, M. Mirelli,
M. Trianni and R. Angelini

The application of noninvasive techniques is expecially attractive in diagnosis of vascular disease (1).

The duplex scanner combines high resolution, real time B-mode ultrasonic arterial imaging with sound spectrum analysis, thus enabling the technique to accurately detect disease ranging from minimal arterial wall irregularities to total arterial occlusion with a high degree of accuracy (2).

The real time imaging is corrently used in the study of cerebro-vascular disease (1). Because of safety and low cost features we use duplex scanner in surgical decision and also in postoperative follow up.

Recently ecotomography has been also used to study abdominal aorta and visceral and pelvic vessels (3-4).

Ultrasonografic imaging permits morphologic definition of arterial wall and the study of degeneration of atherosclerotic plaque (5-6).

Thromboendoarterectomy (TEA) is one of the most performed vascular procedure for treatment of carotid and aortic lesions.

Both in aorta and carotid artery there is an evolution in morphology of the vessel wall with a thickness increasing after operation.

CAROTID ENDOARTERECTOMY
Preoperative

The clinicopathological studies of carotid atheroma have implicated plaque structure as an etiologic factor in the production of cerebro-vascular symptoms (7-8).

Real-time imaging may prove useful in characterizing the nature of the plaque, most notably the presence of ulceration or intraplaque hemorrage (5-6).

To evaluate the ability of duplex scanner in the assesment of the vessel wall characteristics, a study that compared specimen pathology with the ultrasonic plaque structure. 122 carotid findings obtained from 111 patients submitted to carotid TEA were available for correlation with the B-mode imaging. Preoperatively, all the patients underwent B-mode ultrasound examination and arteriography.

The carotid was examined in the anterior, lateral and posterior views and then studied in the transverse plane. The character of the carotid artery plaque was defined as follow (Table 1):

Table 1: Echogenicity pattern and surface characteristics of the different atherosclerotic plaques.

	N. cases	Echogenicity pattern	Surface
Fibrous plaques	27	homogeneous soft	regular
Irregular plaques	32	heterogeneous mixed-hard	irregular
Ulcerated plaques	41	heterogeneous mixed-hard	irregular crater – proximal and distal lipping
hemorrage plaques	22	heterogeneous soft hard – mixed	irregular

- FIBROTIC PLAQUES (27 cases - 22%): these plaques are characterized by homogeneous ultrasound pattern with soft ecogenicity and without evidence of surface irregularities. In only 4 cases (14%) there were acoustic shadowing, diagnosed as calcifications.
- IRREGULAR PLAQUES (32 cases - 26,3%): the ultrasound pattern was heterogeneous with mixed or hard ecogenicity. The plaque surface was irregular, but the pathological study didn't show intimal ulceration.
- ULCERATED PLAQUES (41 cases - 33,7%): the echogenic pattern was mixed or hard. Ulcers were diagnosed by the presence of isolated crater or with a proximal and distal lipping with sharp demarcation of echogenic borders. The lesion was well recognized in the transverse plane.
- HEMORRAGE PLAQUES (22 cases - 18%): the diagnosis of plaque hemorrage was made for the presence of echolucent area within the plaque, which results in heterogeneous echogenicity. In the maiority of cases there were high-grade stenotic lesions and in 5 cases (22,7%) there were both haemorrhage plaques and surface ulceration.

Our data suggest that duplex scanner can be used to characterized plaque composition with good accuracy. The study is particularly indicated in bilateral stenosis and also in asymptomatic patients.

It may be of considerable value in identifying clinical significant carotid artery plaques and it may be essential in choice
of medical or surgical therapy.

Postoperative

Actually noninvasive studies are employed in long-term follow-
up of the patients submitted to carotid TEA.

We followed up 1 year a series of 54 consecutive patients submitted to 65 carotid TEA. 46 were male, (85.2%), and 8 female
(14.8%); their age ranged from 45 and 76 years (mean 62.6 y.). Only 5 (9.2%) were symptomatics, at follow-up but in all the cases
there were not specific symptoms (vertigo, dizziness, headache).

The 65 arteries were subdivided on the basis of B-mode examination performed 1 year after operation in:

- NORMAL (28 cases - 43%): the B-mode examination showed a thin,
weakly echoreflective strip overlying the normal, hightly echogenic adventitia. A shelflike step-off was observed below the endarterectomy site in the common carotid artery.

- MILD PLAQUE DISEASE (24 cases - 37%): the B-mode examination
showed an increase in the internal/medial layer to > 3 mm. In all
the cases there were a regular surface and a soft plaque without
evidence of calcification.

- RESTENOSIS OF THE INTERNAL CAROTID ARTERY (3 cases - 4.6%): there were a low echogenic plaque with regular surface at the origin
of the internal carotid artery in the site of the previous TEA.
One patient of this group underwent a re-operation because of a
progressively increasing of internal carotid stenosis. The intraoperative examination showed the features of myointimal hyperplasia, confirmed also by hystological study.

- RESTENOSIS (> 50%) OF THE COMMON CAROTID ARTERY (7 cases - 10.8%):
the recurrent disease below the endarterectomy site showed a
highly echogenic plaque, probably indicative of accentuation of
preexisting atheroma of the common carotid artery. Also in this
group there were not evidence of degeneration in plaque composition.

- ECTASIA OF THE INTERNAL CAROTID ARTERY (3 cases - 4.6%): in these cases there were a dilatation of the internal carotid artery,
due to the presence of a patch angioplasty in PTFE. In the carotid
artery there were a regular surface without evidence of recurrent
disease.

The sequence of events which follow from TEA are deposition

of platelet-fibrin-trombus, which undergoing to marked regression after 7 days, when endotelial regeneration begins.

The pathologic features of the early restenotic lesion and recurrent atherosclerosis are now well recognized (9-10): the lesion that occurs within 24 months represents neointimal hyperplasia, whereas redevelopment of an atherosclerotic lesion occurs later.

The intimal hyperplasia is characterized by an uniform surface, with increasing in the intimal/media layer > 3 mm. (2) while in recurrent carotid restenosis there is an uniform, homogeneous low echogenicity, as observed in fibrous plaque.

Recurrent stenosis in common carotid artery below the site of TEA are characterized by highly echogenic pattern, as observed in irregular plaques.

In our experience ultrasonographic scanning must be made in patients submitted to carotid TEA after 1, 6 months and every year.

AORTIC ENDARTERECTOMY

The aortic endarterectomy is indicated for atherosclerotic aorto-iliac disease expecially in young patients or in segmentary lesions (11-12).

Also in the aortic plaque, as in the carotid artery, the atherosclerotic degeneration can give distal microemboli (13-14). Diagnosis and treatment should be directed toward location and eradication of the aorto-iliac source of embolization (15).

Preoperative

The duplex scanner can be used preoperatively to study aortic wall characteristics and morphology of aortic plaque. Nowadays the duplex scanner is also used for noninvasive evaluation of mesenteric blood flow (4), of renal arteries (16) and of pelvic vessels (3), precluding the need for angiography.

Postoperative

There is an evolution with increased thickness of the wall after aortic endoarterectomy.

We studied a group of 44 patients submitted to aortic TEA and followed up from 6 months to 12 years after operation. 37 were male, 7 female. Their age ranged from 33 to 67 years (mean 48.6 y.). Only 3 patients (6.8%) were symptomatic with mild claudication at follow-up (> 300 m.). In all the cases claudication was due to a distally atherosclerotic progression with obstruction of the femoral artery.

The follow-up included a clinical evaluation, an angiographic study and an ecotomography of abdominal aorta with study in B-mode and M-mode.

A thickned wall within 3 mm. was considered normal (2); 21 patients (47.7%) showed a pathologic evolution in the thickning of the aortic wall.

Then we made correlation with sex, age, smoke habits and hyperlipemia and we didn't find significative results.

The evolution of the aortic thickening showed a significant correlation with the time from operation: there is a 8.3% (1/12) of thickening > 3 mm. after 2 years, that arise to 81.2% (13/16) after 5 years (Tab. 2).

Table 2: Correlation between distance from TEA and thickening> 3 mm.

Follow up	N° cases	Thickening > 3 mm.	
< 2 years	12	1	(8.3%)
between 2 and 5 years	16	7	(43.7%)
> 5 years	16	13	(81.2%)

The evolution was also marked influenced by anticoagulant drugs: there is a 35.7% (10/28) of augmented thickening of the aortic wall in patients which were submitted to anticoagulant drugs, against a 68.7% (11/16) of the patients without theraphy (Tab. 3).

Table 3: Correlation between anticoagulant therapy and thickening > 3 mm.

Anticoagulant drugs	N° cases	Thickening > 3 mm.	
Yes	28	10	(35.7%)
No	16	11	(68.7%)

It is particularly interesting to study the way of evolution of the endoarterectomized aorta. In all the cases there is an increased thickening of the hind aortic wall after 6 months from operation, that only in few cases are > 3 mm.

Subsequently the thickening of the aortic wall can stop or have a progressive increasing laterally and priorly with a reduction of the aortic diameter.

CONCLUSION

It is well recognized that B-mode ultrasound presents significant advantage in studying the extracranial carotid artery (2).

Its importance is in detecting residual lumen, but also in detailing the arterial surface and wall composition (6).

The ultrasonic image permits also to detect noninvasively the morphology of the atherosclerotic plaque (5).

The endarterectomy site is not a biologically static segment, but an area of great cellular activity. There is an interdipendence between recostitution of the endotelial lining and formation of a fibrocellular intimal thickening. The early recurrent myointimal hyperplastic lesion may be consequence of an accelerate responce to de-endothelization of the arterial wall (9).

Ultrastructural study of the early recurrent lesions showed features of smooth muscle cells, while the later recurrent disease showed atherosclerotic features (17).

The appearance of recurrent disease in the site below endarterectomy suggests a different features of the lesion. The preexisting atherosclerosis may have been accentuated by hemodinamic or by persistence of atherosclerosis risk factors (hypertension, cigarette abuse, diabetes, lipid disorder).

Factors that are cause of recurrent stenosis after endarterectomy are not well known. A number of clinical studies have studied the role of aspirin and antiplatelet drugs in proliferative reaction of arterial wall after endarterectomy (17).

Also clinical findings don't relate atherosclerotic risk factors to recurrent stenosis (17).

There is not a correlation between postoperative symptoms and recurrent stenosis in carotid TEA. This confirm the clinical significance of postendarterectomy lesion and primary atherosclerotic plaque (17).

The duplex scanner permits to evaluate directly the carotid artery and also to identify the postoperative morphology of the vessel wall.

Now is well established the importance in the morphology of the primary atherosclerotic plaque, which may be undestimated in angiographic examination of abdominal aorta (14).

In our opinion the B-mode examination is useful in postoperative aortic TEA to study evolution of the aortic wall.

REFERENCES

1. Pearce W.H.; Blackburn D., Ricco J.B. et al. (1983). Direct and indirect tests for carotid artery lesions. In: Bergan J.J., Yao J.S. Eds. "Cerebrovascular Insufficiency" p. 179 (New York: Gune & Stratton).
2. O'Donnel T.F.; Callow A.D. (1986). B-mode ultrasound in evalua-

tion of carotid endarterectomy: an anatomic study. In "Reoperative arterial surgery". - Gune & Stratton Eds., New York, 81.

3. Taylor K.J.W.; Burns P.N., Woodcock J.P. et al. (1985): ultrasonic pulsed Doppler analysis of blood flow in deep abdominal and pelvic vessels. Radiology, 154: 487.

4. Jager K., Bollinger A., Valli C. et al. (1986): Measurement of mesenteric blood flow by duplex scanner. J. Vasc. Surg.: 3; 464.

5. Reilly L.M.; Lusby R.J.; Hughes L. et al. (1983): Carotid plaque histology using real-time ultrasonography: clinical and therapeutic implications. Ann. J. Surg. 146; 188.

6. Curti T.; Zacà F.; Trianni M.; Cifiello B.I.; et al. (1986): Comprobacion anatomo-patologica del diagnostico non invasivo: estudio con duplex scanner del ateroma carotideo. Angiologia 38 (5): 275.

7. Imparato A.M.; Riles T.S.; Mintzer R.; Baumann F.G. (1983): The importance of hemorrage in the relationship between gross morphologic characteristics and cerebral symptoms in 376 carotid artery plaques. Ann. Surg. 197: 195.

8. Lusby R.J.; Ferrel L.D.; Ehrenfeld W.K.; Stoney R.J.; Wylie E.J. (1982): Carotid plaque hemorrhage. Its role in production of cerebral ischemia. Arch. Surg. 117: 1479.

9. Callow A.D. (1980): Recurrent stenosis after carotid endarterectomy. A limited survey. In: Bernard V.M. Towne J.B. (eds.) "Complications in vascular surgery" p. 259 (New York - Gune & Stratton).

10. Stoney R.J.; String S.T. (1976): Recurrent carotid stenosis. Surgery 80: 705.

11. Cannon J.A.; Kawakami I.G. (1961): The present status of aorto iliac endarterectomy for obliterative atherosclerosis. Arch. Surg. 82, 813.

12. Szylagy D.E., Smith R.F.; Whitney D.G. (1964): The durability of aorto iliac endarterectomy. A roentgenologic and pathologic study of late recurrence. Arch. Surg. 89, 827.

13. Karmody A.M., Powers S.R., Monaco V.J., Leather R.P. (1976): "Blue toe" syndrome. Arch. Surg. 111: 1263-1268.

14. Machleder H.I.; Takiff H.; Lois J.F. et al. (1986): Aortic mural thrombus: an occult source of arterial thromboembolism. J. Vasc. Surg. 4 (5): 473.

15. Stella A.; Gessaroli M.; Cifiello B.I.; Mirelli M.; Bacchini P. (1987): Ateroembolie periferiche: evoluzione dell'ateroma aorto-iliaco. Arch. Chir. Torac. Cardiov. (in press.).

16. Nichols B.T., Rittgers G.E.; Norris C.S.; et al. (1984): Noninvasive detection of renal artery stenosis. Bruit, 8: 26.

17. Clagett G.P.; Robinowitz M.; Youkey J.R. et al. (1986): Morphogenesis and clinicopathologic characteristics of recurrent carotid disease. J. Vasc. Surg. 3 (1): 10.

Index